June 16, 2007

Dear Marica,

I hope this book helps you through all the challenging times to come.

Enjoy motherhood

Children are truely a gift from God.

Much Love from

Kupna Angie

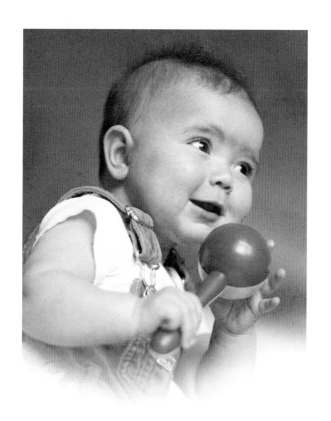

CANADIAN MEDICAL ASSOCIATION

BABY & CHILD
HEALTH

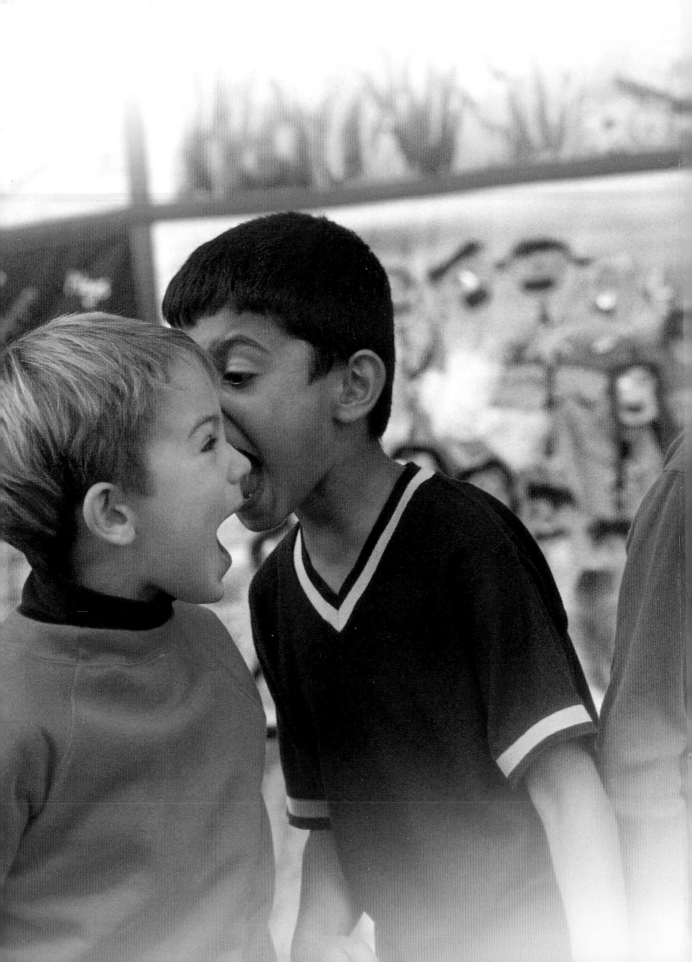

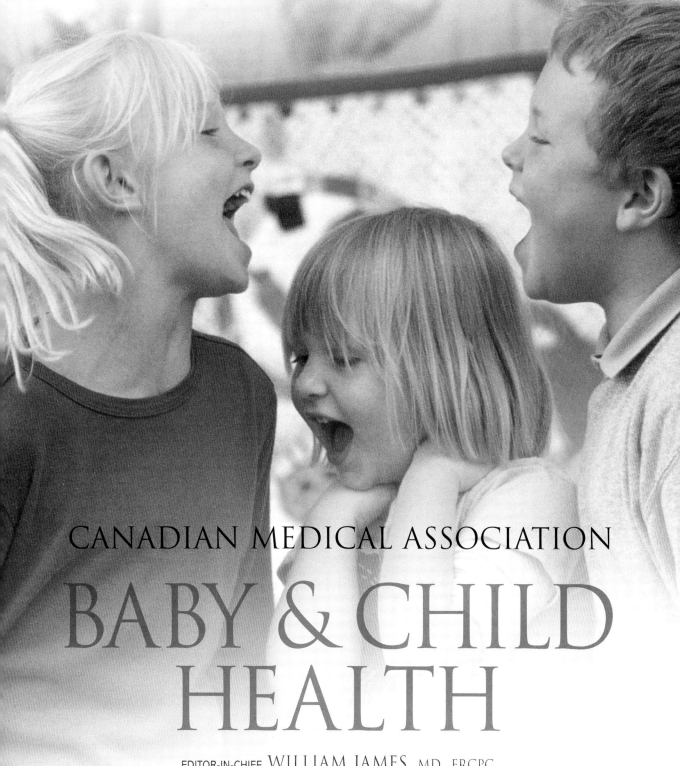

CANADIAN MEDICAL ASSOCIATION

BABY & CHILD HEALTH

EDITOR-IN-CHIEF WILLIAM JAMES, MD, FRCPC

MEDICAL EDITOR CATHERINE YOUNGER-LEWIS, MD, MJ

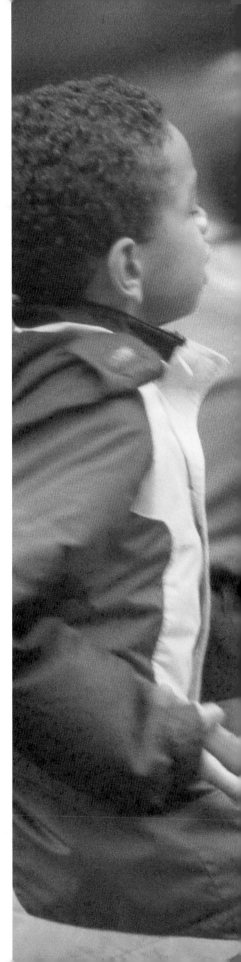

Editor, Canada Julia Roles
Project editor, Canada Ian Whitelaw
Senior editors Julia North, Salima Hirani, Jill Hamilton
Art editor Nicola Rodway
Project editors Jinny Johnson, Kathy Fahey, Pip Morgan, Madeline Farbman
Designers Ted Kinsey, Briony Chappell
DTP designer Karen Constanti
Production controller Shwe Zin Win
Managing editors Anna Davidson, Liz Coghill
Managing art editors Emma Forge, Glenda Fisher
Photography art direction Sally Smallwood
Photography Ruth Jenkinson
Jacket designer Katy Wall
Jacket editor Claire Tennant-Scull
Art director Carole Ash
Publishing director Corinne Roberts

The *Canadian Medical Association BABY AND CHILD HEALTH* provides general information about baby and child health care. The information in this book is intended to complement, not substitute for, the advice of your child's doctor. Before starting any medical treatment or medical program, you should consult with your child's doctor, who can discuss your child's individual needs and counsel you about symptoms and treatment. If you have questions regarding how the information in this book applies to your child, speak to your child's doctor.

The naming of any organization, product, or alternative therapy in this book does not imply endorsement by the CMA or by the publisher; the omission of any such name does not imply disapproval by the CMA or by the publisher. Neither the publisher nor the CMA assumes any responsibility for liability arising from any error or omission from the book, or from the use of any information contained in it.

The information and advice in this book apply equally to children of both sexes, except where noted. To indicate this, we have chosen to alternate between masculine and feminine pronouns when referring to children, as well as to doctors, throughout the book.

First Canadian Edition, 2005

Dorling Kindersley is represented in Canada by
Tourmaline Editions Inc.
662 King Street West, Suite 304
Toronto, Ontario M5V 1M7

National Library of Canada Cataloguing in Publication

Canadian Medical Association baby & child health / William James, editor-in-chief ; Catherine Younger-Lewis, medical editor. -- Canadian ed.

Includes index.
ISBN 1-55363-040-8

1. Pediatrics--Popular works. 2. Infants--Health and hygiene--Popular works.
3. Children--Health and hygiene--Popular works. 4. Child development--Popular works.
I. James, William II. Younger-Lewis, Catherine III. Canadian Medical Association
IV. Title: Baby & child health. V. Title: Baby and child health.

RJ61.C348 2005   618.92   C2004-902266-0

Reproduced in Singapore by Colourscan
Printed and bound in Singapore by Star Standard

04 05 06 07 08 10 9 8 7 6 5 4 3 2 1

Discover more at
www.dk.com

FOREWORD

One of the great privileges of medical practice is the opportunity to share with parents in the health care of their children. The Canadian Medical Association and its members are proud to have this responsibility because it allows us to play a role in the development of Canada's most important resource – our children.

We are very fortunate to have access to a health care system that provides high-quality medical care to all children, regardless of family economics. As parents, you also have access to a wealth of medical information on all aspects of your children's health.

Canadian Medical Association BABY AND CHILD HEALTH integrates much of the quality information available. It discusses, in a reliable and straightforward manner, topics such as vaccination, child care, and nutrition. It also answers many of the questions that will arise as your baby grows. When should I call the doctor? Is my baby crying too much? Is my toddler developing normally? Is my child's behavior normal? Issues such as emotional and social development are discussed in detail. Clear diagnostic charts are also provided to help parents confront the problems that develop in childhood, from teething and fevers to rashes and breathing problems.

This how-to manual will be useful to both new and established parents for many years as their children grow.

Albert J. Schumacher, MD
President, Canadian Medical Association

CONTENTS

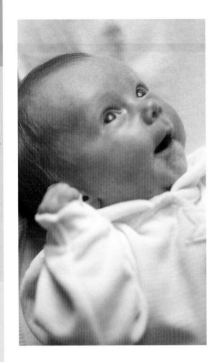

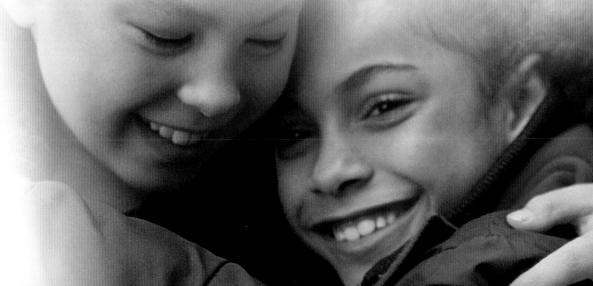

INTRODUCTION

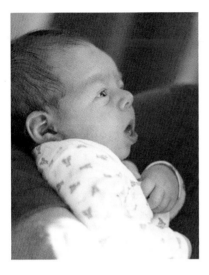

Child rearing can be quite a challenge, but *Canadian Medical Association* BABY AND CHILD HEALTH – along with a large dose of common sense – can help ease any strains and difficulties that may accompany this vital role, and can give our children a better opportunity to develop into happy, healthy, and successful adults.

My 35 years as a pediatrician have been fascinating and rewarding. Each day is different from the day before, and kids really do "say the darndest things," asking questions on everything from health to their favorite hockey team. Children's knowledge of right from wrong becomes evident early in life, and reflects the influence of parents, teachers, grandparents and, hopefully, their doctors. I have never yet met a child in whom I couldn't see great potential to grow and develop into a fine adult.

Prevention is the key to a healthy life and lifestyle. Prevention begins before your baby is born, with appropriate prenatal care, and abstinence from smoking, alcohol, and non-prescription drugs. Do your homework. Get to know what community support groups are available. Think about what you will do if you and your partner both work. Who will provide day-to-day care? Use family support as much as possible. Along with friends, family members can be essential caregivers, allowing you to get away for a few hours a day. Remember to make your baby's first trip home a safe one; get a properly installed car seat.

> "I have never yet met a child in whom I couldn't see great potential to grow and develop into a fine adult."

Making the journey from infancy to adolescence as smooth as possible is one of the principal goals of *Canadian Medical*

Association BABY AND CHILD HEALTH. Through each stage of your child's development you'll find new questions arising – about physical, emotional, and social issues. This book, with its many tip boxes, information panels, and examples, guides you and helps you find your own answers.

The health benefits of breastfeeding are well established, and breastfeeding is an excellent start to mother–infant bonding. If you are unable to breastfeed, consult your doctor for an

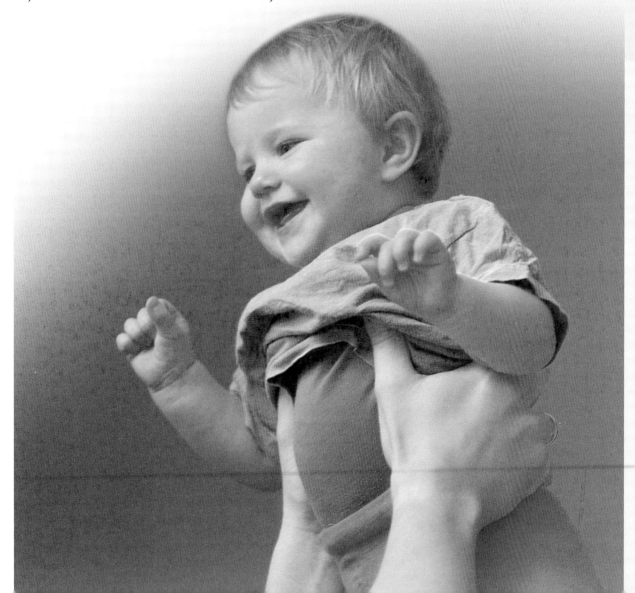

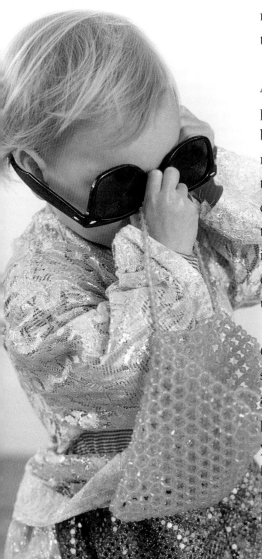

alternative formula. This book provides guidelines for the introduction of solids, but remember that every baby has different needs and your physician's guidance is important.

Get to know your child. Learn what your baby's cry means. Does it mean hunger, pain, or illness? Does your baby need a diaper change or just want a cuddle? As your child gets older, continue to communicate, whether by reading, singing, or, later, by asking about his or her day. In other words, be there for your child. As far as I'm concerned, this is one of the most effective means of developing and maintaining your relationship with your child, right through to adulthood.

All children suffer minor illness, accidents, and behavioral problems. Starting from the newborn, this comprehensive book delves into health-related issues and the questions most frequently asked by concerned parents. It then follows the growing child through the various stages of his or her development, with a compilation of illnesses and conditions that may affect children up to their teen years. Finally, there is a guide to first aid, showing how to deal with childhood emergencies and minor common problems, followed by a useful addresses and resources section.

Canadian Medical Association BABY AND CHILD HEALTH should complement your own instincts and the care and advice of your child's physician. I urge you to form a strong partnership with him or her, for the best possible health for your child. We hope parents will apply the information found in this book to make informed choices that will maintain good health, prevent illness, and establish a healthy lifestyle for their child.

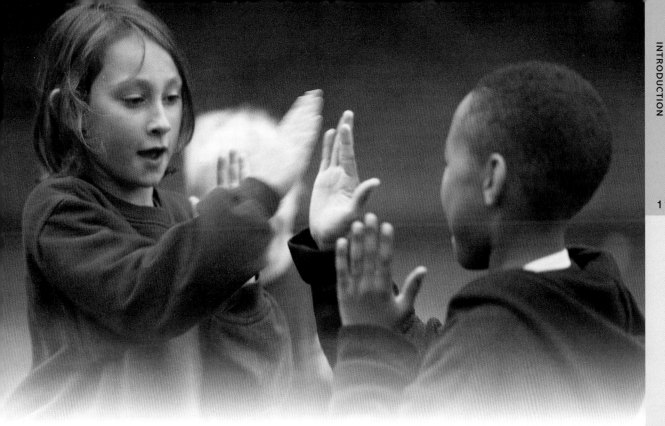

"I urge you to form a strong partnership with your child's physician, for the best possible health of your child."

I wish to thank the wonderful staff at the Canadian Medical Association for their patience with me and their support in publishing this book on child care. Without the numerous reviewers and their expertise, advice, and sound judgement, along with their attention to detail, this book would not have reached the high quality we have all worked to achieve. Finally, I wish to dedicate this book to my patients, who taught me how to be tolerant, to be a better doctor, and to understand their needs; and I would like to thank my three daughters, who have taught me how to parent and how to be a better listener. I appreciate that more than they will ever realize. They have all played a major role in my development as a person, and hopefully this will be reflected in this book.

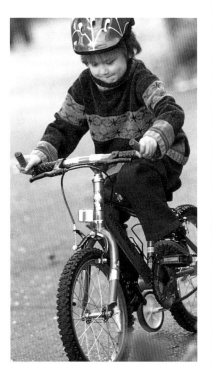

William James, MD, FRCPC

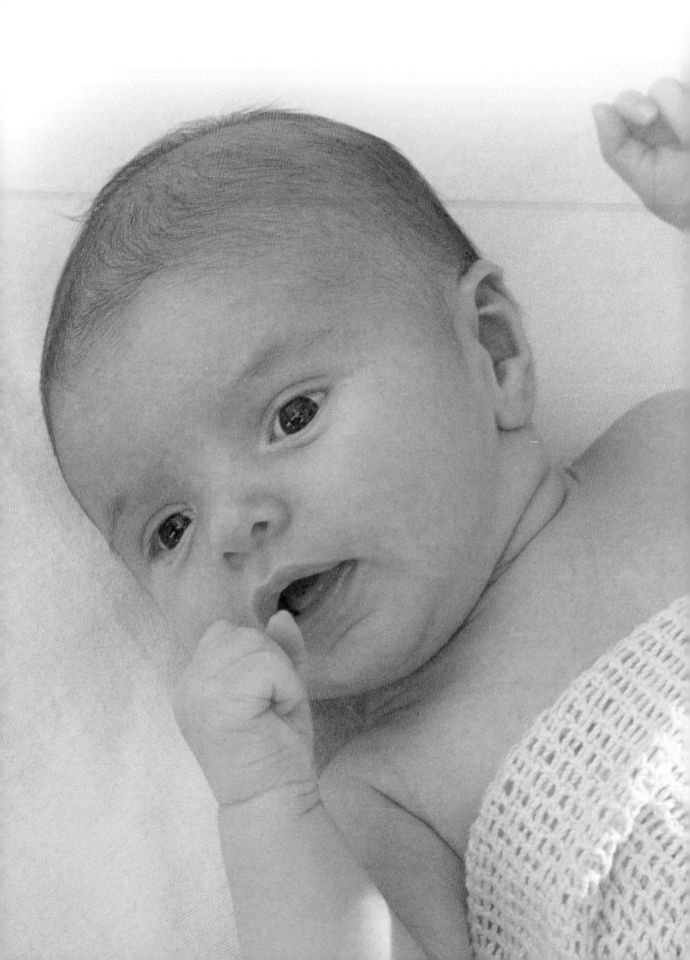

YOUR NEW BABY

CHAPTER ONE

Caring for your newborn baby may seem daunting at first, and you may be unsure about health matters that concern him. This chapter has been written to help guide you through the first weeks and months with your new baby. It provides practical advice and information on subjects such as feeding, sleep, and general development.

FIRST DAYS

Most babies are born perfectly healthy and adapt immediately to the outside world. But any minor setbacks in your baby's health can be upsetting, especially in the first few days after the birth when you are still adjusting to becoming parents. Be reassured that most of these clear up by themselves, or with minimal medical help, within a very short space of time.

Characteristics

Listed below are traits that are often characteristic of newborns but which disappear in the first few weeks.

Misshapen head. Caused by the descent through the birth canal.

Puffy face and puffy, sticky eyes, sometimes with a crossed eye.

Milia. Small white spots caused by blocked sebaceous glands, usually around the nose, cheeks, and forehead.

Swollen genitals and breasts. In girls as well as boys, due to maternal hormones. The breasts may briefly secrete a small amount of fluid.

Skin issues. Babies often have red, blotchy rashes. Extremities may look bluish due to poor circulation. Many babies have jaundice (yellow skin and eyes) in the first week.

Vernix. A thick white coating, and/or lanugo (fine downy hair), may be present on babies born prematurely.

Babies born late may have dry, flaky skin and long finger- and toenails.

HOW YOUR NEWBORN LOOKS

Newborn babies often look wrinkly and rather scrunched up, and do not get that appealing pink chubby look for a few weeks. Some characteristics at birth may worry parents, but they are normal and soon disappear. The most common traits are listed at left.

Some babies are born with minor physical abnormalities that can be corrected with minor surgery or need no treatment. These include extra digits, webbing between two toes, skin tags, and tongue tie, when the tissue under the tongue is tight.

After a hospital birth, your baby will be examined by a doctor. He may receive a hearing screening, a hepatitis B immunization, a vitamin K injection, and antibiotic eye ointment to prevent infection. Between 24 hours and 7 days of age, he will be tested for phenylketonuria (PKU), congenital hypothyroidism, and other rare but serious medical conditions. If the PKU test was done before 24 hours, the test will be repeated by the third week of life.

BIRTHMARKS

A baby may also be born with a variety of common birthmarks. "Stork bites" are small, pink patches that usually disappear in the first year. Strawberry hemangiomas start as red spots and grow into small raised red areas with white marks. They may increase in size over the first year, then shrink and disappear by age 10. Port-wine stains are dark red, irregular patches that do not fade with time. Mongolian spots are blue-black pigmented areas common in dark-skinned babies. They are often found on the buttocks and usually fade in the first year.

FIRST STOOLS

For the first 24–48 hours after birth, babies pass meconium, a sticky green-black mixture of bile and mucus. Your baby's stools will start to change once he starts to feed. Breastfed babies have loose, mustard-colored stools with little odor. Bottlefed babies have firmer, brown stools that may have an odor. Most babies produce stools after every feeding. Discuss any changes in stools with your doctor.

WHAT YOUR NEW BABY CAN DO

Babies have certain reflexes at birth, which slowly disappear within the first three months.
• Your baby sucks on anything placed in his mouth (the sucking reflex).
• He turns in the direction of something brushed against his cheek (the rooting reflex).
• Your baby grasps a finger placed in his hand (the grasp reflex).

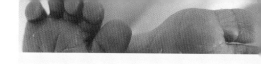

- When your baby is held upright with his feet on a flat surface, he makes walking movements with his legs (walking reflex).
- When startled, your baby throws his arms and legs out wide, then slowly curls them up toward his body (the startle, or Moro, reflex).

He blinks in bright light and can focus on objects up to 20–25 cm (8–10 in) away. He quickly learns your voice and smell.

BONDING

The newborn period is an important time for mother and baby to begin bonding. Fathers need to bond too, and should concentrate on developing their own relationship with their baby.

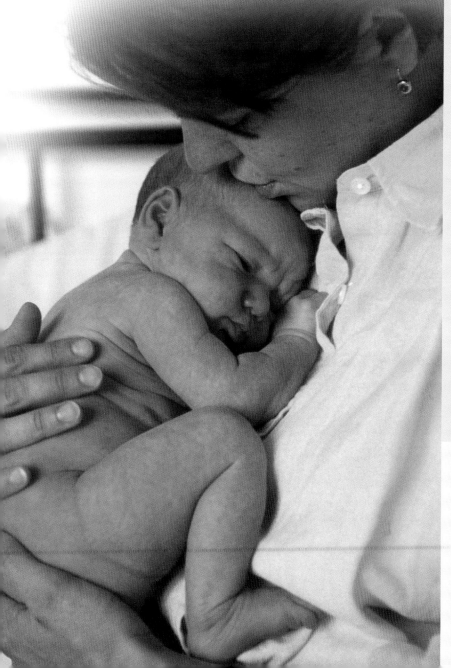

THE APGAR SCORE

Your baby is carefully checked at birth and soon after by a doctor. The Apgar score (named after Dr. Virginia Apgar, who first devised it) is assessed in the delivery room 1 minute and again 5 minutes after your baby's birth. It assesses five key elements of a newborn baby's health.

FEATURE	SCORE
Heartbeat	
Over 100 beats per minute	2
Under 100 beats per minute	1
Absent	0
Breathing	
Regular	2
Irregular, weak	1
Absent	0
Muscle tone	
Active movement	2
Some	1
Limp	0
Reflexes (response to stimuli)	
Crying or sneezing	2
Grimacing	1
Absent	0
Skin color	
Pink	2
Blue extremities	1
Blue	0

Although the Apgar score cannot predict how healthy a child will be when he grows up, it can alert personnel that a new baby may need extra observation or assistance.

FEEDING CHOICES

THERE ARE MANY FEEDING OPTIONS FOR BABIES. Breastfeeding is considered the healthiest for mother and baby because of the nutritional advantages, disease-fighting qualities, and hormones of breastmilk. However, infant formulas are an acceptable alternative. Each mother must have complete, accurate information in order to make the best feeding decision for herself and her family.

Choices

In modern life, there are more choices than ever, as listed below:

Exclusive breastfeeding The infant feeds directly at the breast, and does not receive any other foods or liquids until solid foods are gradually added to the diet.

- Considered the most natural choice, with all possible advantages
- Viewed as convenient by most women, once breastfeeding is established in the first month or so
- Difficult if mother must attend school or work outside the home. If the baby cannot stay with the mother, then expressed breastmilk or formula in a bottle is typically used during their separation (*see below*)

Exclusive bottlefeeding The infant receives the mother's pumped or hand-expressed breastmilk and/or formula from a bottle.

Mixed feeding The infant receives both breastmilk and formula, and may breastfeed directly or take either type of milk from a bottle.

BREASTFEEDING

Feeding your baby provides more than good nutrition and health benefits. It also gives you a chance to hold your newborn close, cuddle him, and make eye contact. These are relaxing and enjoyable moments for both of you and they bring you closer together emotionally.

Before your baby arrives you should seriously consider breastfeeding your newborn. The Canadian Pediatric Society believes that breastfeeding is the optimal source of nutrition through the first year of life. Exclusive breastfeeding is recommended for at least 4 months, with the introduction of complementary foods between 4 and 6 months. Solid foods are gradually added while continuing breastfeeding until at least the baby's first year. (*For more information on starting solids, see p.38.*) Thereafter, breastfeeding can be continued for as long as both mother and baby desire it.

Because of its nutritional composition, human milk is the ideal food for human infants. Babies who are breastfed are found to be less likely to suffer from ear infections or severe diarrhea. They are also less likely to develop allergies. Formula-fed babies are more likely to need treatment for one of these problems. Recent information indicates that breastfeeding plays a small but significant role in the prevention of overweight and diabetes, both in childhood and in later years. In addition, there is some evidence that for mothers, breastfeeding reduces the risk of certain types of cancer and may prevent hip fractures later in life.

Despite the many advantages of breastfeeding for both infant and mother, there may be personal or medical reasons that breastfeeding will not work for you. Discuss your specific concerns, doubts, or fears with someone knowledgeable such as your doctor or lactation specialist. Starting with bottlefeeding and then trying to switch to breastfeeding is more difficult and complicated than switching from breastfeeding to bottlefeeding. Most breastfed babies can easily learn to take bottlefeedings between 1–3 months of age, if necessary.

BOTTLEFEEDING – INFANT FORMULA

If you decide not to breastfeed your baby, commercial infant formula is an acceptable alternative to human milk because it provides the necessary nutrients for your baby. Iron-fortified formula is usually recommended. Your doctor will help you select a cow's-milk-based or soy-based formula that is best for your baby.

Cow's-milk-based formula contains cow's milk protein in a form that is safe for infants. You should not give your baby any regular cow's milk until after twelve months of age. You should not give her reduced-fat (2 percent, 1 percent, or skim) milk before her second birthday.

When you bottlefeed you can keep track of the amount of formula that you feed your baby to be sure that she has received an adequate amount of milk. Formulas are available in powders, concentrates, and ready-to-feed liquid forms. Read the labels carefully to be sure you are preparing the formula correctly. Bottlefed newborns generally drink 30-90 millilitres (ml) per feeding, while older infants may take up to about 250 ml. You will be giving about six to eight feedings per day (depending on the age of your baby) for the first 6 months.

BURPING

If your baby swallows air during a feeding, it can cause discomfort later, but burping her may help avoid this problem. Breastfed babies often take in less air than bottlefed babies while feeding because their mouths form an airtight seal around the nipple; you may notice that they burp less. If your baby is nursing, you can burp her after she feeds on each breast; if she is bottlefeeding, you can try burping her after every 60–90 ml of formula, or more frequently if necessary.

You can burp your baby by sitting her on your lap and supporting her head under her chin so that the windpipe stays straight; or you can lay her against your shoulder. Pat her back gently and rhythmically. Place a cloth under your baby's chin to protect your clothing from any milk coming back up. Since not all babies burp with every feeding, you can try burping her for a few minutes and then stop if there's no response.

MORE CHOICES: TIMING OF FEEDINGS

Deciding how to feed your baby is a personal choice. However, you need to communicate your approach to others involved in the baby's care, such as grandparents or babysitters.

Feeding on demand means responding to your baby's needs by feeding her whenever she seems to be hungry. This may mean feeding 8–12 times a day or more. Many child care experts recommend this method because babies learn to eat according to appetite. Children whose needs are met promptly will tend to be more secure and confident as they grow up.

Feeding on a schedule usually involves feedings at specific intervals, often every three or four hours. New parents may find this method easier to handle, since they know when the next feeding is due. However, a schedule should be flexible enough to respond to obvious hunger cues.

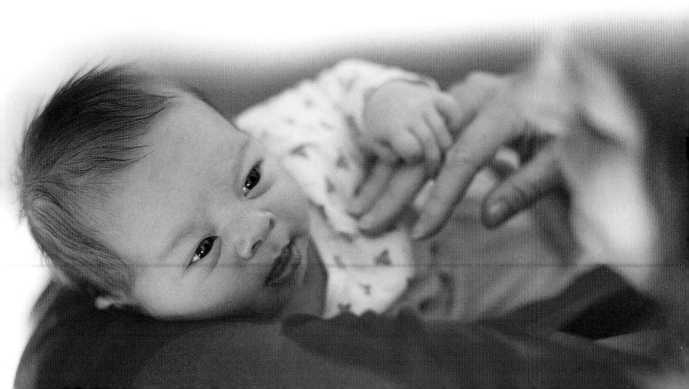

BREASTFEEDING

B Y BREASTFEEDING YOU CAN BE SURE THAT YOU ARE giving your baby the best possible start in life. For some mothers and babies, the process goes smoothly from the start; for others it takes extra effort. Rest assured, breastfeeding takes some practice and this is perfectly normal. Once it has been mastered, breastfeeding can be extremely rewarding.

Positioning

Whether you choose to breastfeed sitting, standing, or lying down, make sure your baby is correctly latched on.

Place a pillow behind your back and under your baby to support your back and prevent shoulder and neck aches during seated feedings.

Avoid slouching and bring the baby up to you, rather than bending over.

Your baby's entire body should be lying facing you, not just his head.

His head should be slightly higher than his body.

Until you are accustomed to breastfeeding, it may be easier to see what you are doing if you wear a top that buttons down the front.

To nurse your baby when you are lying down, turn slightly onto one side and place your baby on his side, facing your breast directly.

BEFORE YOUR BABY IS BORN

Learn as much as you can about breastfeeding before your baby is born. Read, watch videos, and talk with other women who have breastfed. Take a breastfeeding class from a hospital or health organization.Talk to your physicians about cultural practices and beliefs that are important to you. It may also be helpful to have support from family and friends.

Your body naturally prepares for breastfeeding when you become pregnant. After the fourth or fifth month of pregnancy, your body is capable of producing milk. The first milk that is produced is colostrum, a thick, yellowish or orangish fluid filled with nutrients that your newborn needs. It also contains substances to protect against infections. While some cultures traditionally do not give babies colostrum, this early milk is very important for your baby's health.

HOW BREASTFEEDING WORKS

Milk production involves the breasts and hormones produced in other parts of the body. It helps to understand the main processes of milk production: "coming in"; "let-down" (milk ejection); and "demand and supply."

"Milk coming in"

Milk "comes in" usually 2–5 days after birth, when colostrum becomes milky white in color and increases rapidly in volume. Signs of milk "coming in" are tenderness and fullness of the breasts and leaking milk. You may see milk around your baby's mouth and hear your baby swallow during feedings.

"Let-down"

The let-down reflex creates the flow of milk from the back of the breast toward the nipple and allows the baby to get the milk from the breast. Let-down is caused by the hormone oxytocin, which is released about every 90 minutes for several days after delivery. Let-down also occurs when the baby suckles properly and the mother is relaxed, or sometimes when the mother hears a baby cry. The let-down reflex may take a few minutes at first. Later, it will occur in seconds, and may occur many times during each feeding.

The signs of let-down are different for everyone but may include strong cramping in your uterus (for a few days after delivery) or a prickle, tingle, or slight pain in your breast. If let-down has occurred, you may notice that your baby swallows more or gulps while feeding, or that milk drips from the breast that is not being used. Some women do not notice any sensations.

"Demand and supply"

The more milk your baby drinks, the more you produce. Called "demand and supply," this allows women to produce enough milk. Expressing milk creates demand also. In general, there is no relationship between breast size and the amount of milk produced.

FIRST FEEDINGS

Put your baby to your breast as soon as you can after birth. Even a brief attempt at suckling will help stimulate milk production and give your baby a chance to learn how to

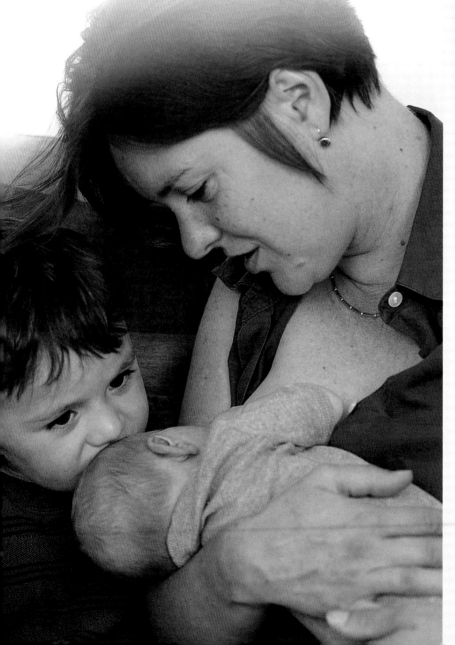

You will notice certain cues or signs that your baby is hungry, such as the following:

- Making small movements as she awakens
- Whimpering or lip-smacking
- Pulling arms or legs up toward her middle
- Stretching or yawning
- Waking and looking alert
- Putting hands toward her mouth
- Making sucking motions
- Moving fists to her mouth
- Becoming more active
- Nuzzling against your breast (she can smell its location even through your clothing).

The following signs will let you know that your baby is getting enough milk:

- Baby feeds frequently, 8–12 times in 24 hours
- Baby is satisfied or content after feedings
- Baby has frequent wet and dirty diapers
- Milk is visible during feedings (leaking, dripping, or around baby's mouth)
- Baby is gaining weight when seen for checkups

INVOLVING FAMILY MEMBERS AND OTHER CAREGIVERS

Fathers, siblings, grandparents, and other caregivers can actively share in all aspects of caring for the baby even if they do not directly feed milk to her. These individuals have an important role that can include playing with, cuddling, or comforting baby and mother. They can hold, burp, diaper, bathe, and carry the baby, as well as assist with household tasks.

suck correctly ("latch on"). Many babies lose a little weight during the first couple days. Your baby needs only about one to two teaspoons per feeding on the first and second days, but his appetite and need for fluids will increase in the next days.

HOW TO NURSE

The keys to successful breastfeeding are relaxation and proper latch-on. A good latch-on means that the baby has opened wide for the breast, and has taken the whole areola – not just the nipple – far back into his mouth.

Help your baby latch on by holding the breast with your free hand. Place your fingers under the breast and rest your thumb lightly on top. Position your baby slightly below the level of the nipple, with his whole body facing you. Be sure your fingers are well back from the areola so they do not get in the way. Touch your breast to the center of your baby's lips so that he opens his mouth wide. This is the "rooting reflex." Then pull your baby in close to the breast. His lips should be curled outward and his lower jaw

and chin well under the breast. The ears and jaw will move rhythmically as he sucks and swallows. If he does not latch on correctly, slide your finger into his mouth and press down on your breast to break the suction and try again.

To take your baby off the breast, gently insert a finger between his mouth and your nipple. This will break the strong suction and avoid your baby pulling on your nipple, which can cause irritation and pain. Alternate the breast you offer first each feeding so that milk supply is stimulated for both breasts and as much milk as possible is removed from each. Until you are able to nurse easily, try feeding in a quiet environment to avoid distractions.

NURSING TWINS

Twins (and other multiple births) obviously present many challenges for new parents. Plan to arrange extra help for the first few months, regardless of your feeding choice. Many women who breastfeed twins find that it is more practical to feed the two babies at the same time, so that the babies can eat and sleep on the same timetable.

EXPRESSING MILK

Expressing milk can be an effective way to continue to give breastmilk if you are away from your baby or uncomfortable feeding in public.

Your nurse, lactation specialist, or doctor can teach you to express by hand, but it takes practice to do it well. You can buy a small pump or rent or buy the electric breast pumps used in hospitals. Talk to your doctor or lactation specialist about the best type for your needs.

Many women prefer to express milk in the morning, when their breasts are often fullest. If you are

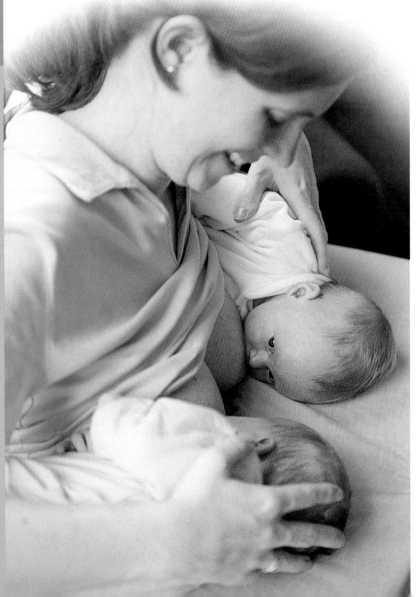

away from your baby for long periods of time, you will need to pump for each feeding that you would normally give your baby.

STORING EXPRESSED MILK

Expressed breastmilk may be stored for later use. It is safe for 4 hours at room temperature, 48 hours in the refrigerator, and 3–6 months in your zero-degree freezer. These guidelines may vary in different locations, so check with your doctor. Store expressed milk in clean small glass or hard plastic containers with tight-fitting lids. Special freezer bags and storage bottles are available for this purpose.

GIVING EXPRESSED MILK

Breastmilk may be given at room temperature shortly after expressing. Warm chilled or frozen breastmilk by swirling the container in a bowl of warm water. You may thaw frozen breastmilk in the refrigerator first. You should never use a microwave to thaw or heat breastmilk – it may heat the breastmilk unevenly and scald your baby. Excessive heat may destroy important nutrients in the breastmilk. Fathers and other caregivers can handle the feeding when a bottle is desirable or necessary.

Bottles

Most experts recommend that you avoid giving your baby bottles until breastfeeding has become well established, which is usually by about 3–6 weeks. If you decide to use a bottle occasionally, it should be possible for the baby to switch from one method to another. You should plan ahead so that you can have some expressed breastmilk on hand for times when the baby will be getting a bottle.

BREASTFEEDING QUESTIONS & ANSWERS

How can I prevent breastfeeding problems?

The keys to successful breastfeeding are relaxation and proper latch-on, as discussed on page 20. These two things, combined with frequent (8–12) feedings per 24 hours will help prevent most problems, including:

- Engorgement – full, swollen breasts caused by tissue swelling and extra milk
- Sore or cracked nipples – usually caused by poor latch-on
- Low milk supply – often caused by a combination of poor latch and infrequent feedings
- Jaundice – a common condition in newborns, seen as yellow-looking skin and eyes. Jaundice may become dangerous if the baby is feeding poorly or has other medical conditions.

How do I handle engorgement?

When your milk comes in, it can do so very quickly. If your baby is not yet nursing very regularly this may lead to painful, swollen (engorged) breasts. Keep draining the breast, either by nursing your baby and/or by expressing milk. Try expressing a little milk before the start of each feeding if your breasts are too swollen to enable your baby to latch on. You do not have to drain the breast each time – nursing small, frequent amounts may be just as effective to help resolve the problem.

How do I treat sore or cracked nipples?

Your doctor, nurse, or lactation specialist can check for proper latch-on. You can treat the nipples with warm moist compresses. Smearing a little breastmilk or purified hypoallergenic lanolin on the nipple can also help. You should not wear plastic-lined nursing pads or use other breast creams.

How do I manage blocked ducts?

A blocked milk duct causes a portion of the breast to feel full and tender. Apply warm moist compresses before every feeding, massage the area, and start each feeding on the affected breast. Drain the breast as well as possible with each feeding. If the blockage has not cleared in 48 hours of treatment, or if you develop a fever, call your doctor.

What is mastitis?

Mastitis is an infection of the breast tissue. Symptoms include breast pain, swelling, redness, fever, chills, muscle aches, headache, or vomiting. The breastmilk is safe for your baby. Continue breastfeeding, and call your doctor as soon as possible.

Do I have enough milk?

During a growth spurt, babies may cry soon after a feeding and appear to be constantly hungry. The mother's breasts often feel "empty" because of the frequent feeding. Remember "demand and supply" – keep feeding as often as the baby needs, and in 3–5 days, the baby usually settles back into his old routines. Supplementing with formula will temporarily satisfy your baby, but will decrease your milk supply in the long run. Call your doctor if your baby always seems hungry in the first two weeks or if he seems to be sick.

My baby is sick or premature. Can I still breastfeed?

If you are separated from your baby after birth, you will be encouraged to express milk frequently, since your baby will gain enormous health benefits from consuming breastmilk. Once you are home, if your baby has to stay in the hospital, you can buy or rent a powerful electric breast pump (see opposite) to maximize the amount of milk you can produce. You can then bring the milk in to the hospital to be fed to your baby.

BOTTLEFEEDING

THE MAJORITY OF BABIES WILL BE BOTTLEFED WITH expressed milk or formula milk at some stage in their development. The key to successful bottlefeeding is organization and hygiene, so that it is both a practical and safe method of feeding. Bottlefeeding has the advantage of enabling other adults to feed a baby, so dads, grandparents, and other caregivers can help out with feedings.

Equipment

If you're bottlefeeding, you'll need to get the following basic equipment.

Bottles: ideally, at least six are required to avoid constantly having to prepare feedings.

Nipples: your doctor can help you determine what's best for your baby. It may take several tries before you find the one your baby prefers. Be certain to check the size of the hole – if the nipple flows too fast for her, she could choke. A hole that is too small may cause her to swallow too much air.

Bottle and nipple brushes: using separate, specially designed brushes can help ensure a thorough cleaning and avoid the risk of cross-contamination.

Formula: different brands of formula are fairly similar in content and are specially formulated to provide all the nutrients your baby needs. Ask your doctor which brand she recommends.

HYGIENE

Hygiene is crucially important during the first few months after birth. Poor hygiene can lead to your baby developing an infection that may require that he be hospitalized. Before you mix formula or give your baby a bottle, wash your hands. You should wash any bottles, nipples, and utensils used to make up the feedings by one of the following methods: in hot, soapy water; in the dishwasher; or for 5–10 minutes in boiling water.

You can keep a freshly made bottle for up to 24 hours in the refrigerator, but you should never reheat any leftover used milk, because it may contain bacteria from your baby's mouth.

MAKING UP BOTTLES

You will soon get used to making up your baby's bottles. You can make up 24 hours' worth of bottles in one batch, then store them in the refrigerator to be used throughout the day. Follow the manufacturer's instructions precisely for mixing the formula with drinking water. You should never dilute or condense the formula, since this will lead to under- or overfeeding your baby. If you use well water or are concerned about the safety of your tap water, you should boil the water for approximately one minute before it

is added to the formula and/or consult your doctor.

Formula or breastmilk that has been refrigerated does not need to be warmed, although most babies prefer that it be at least at room temperature. You should never use a microwave oven to heat bottles since they are not heated evenly. Formula or breastmilk that has been unevenly heated can scald your baby's mouth. A safer way to heat a bottle is to place it in a container of warm water. Test the temperature of the milk on the inside of your wrist to make sure it's not too hot before giving it to your baby.

SWITCHING FROM BREAST TO BOTTLE

If you switch at some stage from breast to bottle, you should aim to do this over a period of at least a couple of weeks, especially if you are changing to formula instead of expressed milk (*see also* Feeding Choices, *p.16, and* Starting Solid Foods, *p. 38*). During this transition period, your baby can get used to the feel of a bottle nipple and the taste of formula. Breastfed babies may initially be very resistant to bottles. It may help to have another adult help with the feeding. Start by giving one bottle a day when your baby seems alert and not extremely hungry. In a few days, introduce another bottle at another time of day. Eventually, you can alternate bottle and breast, and then gradually reduce breastfeeding until both you and your baby agree on the endpoint for nursing.

FEEDING YOUR BABY WITH A BOTTLE

Make sure your back is properly supported when feeding your baby with a bottle. Cradle your baby securely in a semi-upright position with her head supported. Angle the bottle so that the milk fills the top part of the bottle and the nipple. Feed at the rhythm that your baby demands, removing the bottle when she needs a break.

If your baby stops, try stroking her cheek to start her feeding again. If she finishes the bottle and keeps smacking her lips, she may be hungry and you may want to offer her a little more milk. When finished feeding, slide your finger between the nipple and the corner of her mouth to release the bottle.

SAFE FEEDING

Hygiene and organization are of the greatest importance when bottlefeeding.

Wash your hands before mixing formula and giving the bottles.

Clean all bottles, nipples, and utensils used to prepare formulas or express milk. Wash them in hot, soapy water and then rinse them in hot water; run them in the dishwasher; or place them in boiling water for 5–10 minutes.

Formula keeps for a maximum of 24 hours in the refrigerator, which means that you can make up bottles in advance but leftovers must never be reheated. Bacteria in leftover formula can multiply rapidly and make your baby sick.

Never dilute or condense formula. Doing so could make your baby sick.

Shake the warmed bottle to disperse the heat and test the temperature on the inside of your wrist. It should feel slightly warm on your skin, and neither hot nor cold. Do not use a microwave to heat bottles.

Do not switch from your baby's usual formula to other formula types without first seeking medical advice. Occasionally, babies are allergic to cow's milk, so an alternative, such as a soy-based or specialized formula, may need to be used. However, you should not switch unless your doctor advises it (*see p.17*).

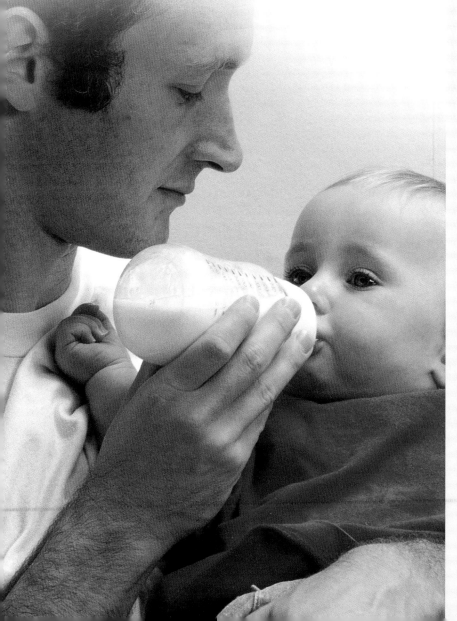

CRYING & COMFORTING

BABIES CRY BECAUSE THEY NEED TO COMMUNICATE THAT something is not right and most parents find it distressing to see or hear an unhappy baby. Although in time you may learn to recognize the various causes of your baby's cries, it may be harder to determine why your baby is crying at first. Be sure to contact your doctor if you are concerned about your baby's crying.

Interpreting cries

Your baby will inevitably cry, and you may find this less upsetting once you understand what his cries mean.

There are many reasons why babies cry and there is little doubt that some babies seem more content and cry less than others.

It may also take you time to learn to recognize the different sorts of cries your baby makes and what they may mean.

Eventually, you may discover that your baby usually cries for one or more of a variety of common reasons. For example, he may be hungry or tired and need food or comfort. His diaper may need changing. He may be uncomfortable because he has gas, or he may have colic (*see opposite*). He may be too hot or too cold, or he may be sick.

There may be times when you cannot console your baby or figure out why he is crying. Contact your doctor if the crying persists or if you are concerned.

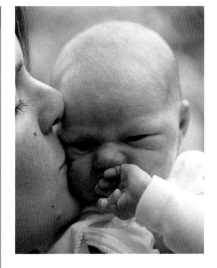

HOW TO CALM YOUR BABY

Most parents will instinctively pick up and cuddle their crying baby and often that is all that is required. Babies like attention. They also like familiar voices, particularly those of their parents, and feel secure when they are in their parents' arms.

However, if cuddling fails to settle your baby, it may be that he is hungry or thirsty, in which case giving him a bit of milk will help. Giving your baby something to suck on, such as your finger or a pacifier, can also be very soothing. When he gets older, he may start to suck his thumb and this too can help your baby stop crying.

Newborns, in particular, cannot yet regulate their temperature very well, so feel the nape of your baby's neck to assess whether he feels hot or cold. As a rule of thumb, he should wear one more layer than you do, although on hot days this may not be suitable.

It may be that your baby is suffering from gas, in which case you can try laying him over your lap or forearm and rubbing his back or gently massaging his tummy. If he has recently been fed, you can also try burping him.

Crying with no apparent reason
If your baby is regularly crying inconsolably during the early evening and is between 3 and 14 weeks, he may be suffering from colic (*see opposite*). During a bout of colic it will probably be difficult to calm your baby. Although there are various remedies that are said to help, some traditional, some alternative, none is a proven cure.

Your baby may cry when he is tired, so you can try swaddling him in a sheet or crib blanket, which may make him feel very secure and, as a result, may help him stop crying and fall asleep as well. Shushing him in a calm, rhythmical way or rocking him, cradled in your arms or lying on his stomach over your forearm (*see opposite*), can also help calm a crying baby. Playing quiet music or white noise may be effective.

As a last resort, many parents find that a drive around the block with the baby in his car safety seat can work wonders for a screaming baby. Less drastically, putting your baby in his stroller for a quick trip in the fresh air often has a similarly calming effect.

If your baby is crying persistently and seems particularly inconsolable, nothing you do seems to have any effect, and you do not think he is suffering from colic, he may be in pain or sick. Trust your instincts and contact your doctor if you are concerned. It may be that there is nothing wrong, but it is better to err on the side of caution.

CRYING IN THE EARLY DAYS

Just as some adults are naturally more cheerful than others, some babies are more content than others. During the first few weeks of your baby's life, you will get to know his personality, whether he is easygoing or more demanding, and you will learn how best to calm him. You should always remember that babies cry for a reason, whether serious or not, and that, until they are older, their only effective method of communicating their needs and emotions is through tears.

CAN I SPOIL MY BABY?

When your baby is very young, you will not be spoiling him by picking him up as soon as he cries. As your baby gets older, however, you may not feel the need to do this quite so quickly, particularly if you know that there is nothing fundamentally wrong with him – he is not hungry or thirsty, his diaper is clean, and he is not sick. Others may offer you well-meaning advice about how to deal with your baby's crying, but remember that crying is your baby's

EVENING CRYING

Between 3 and 14 weeks, some babies develop habitual evening crying that is known as colic. If your baby has colic, he may cry loudly and continuously for up to several hours and will often curl up, as if his tummy is in pain.

Colic is hard to define and diagnose. Some theories say that it is caused either by trapped gas or by spasms in the intestinal tract as it adjusts to digestion in the weeks following birth.

Sometimes hunger, rather than colic, may be a cause of continual evening crying, so try giving an extra feeding.

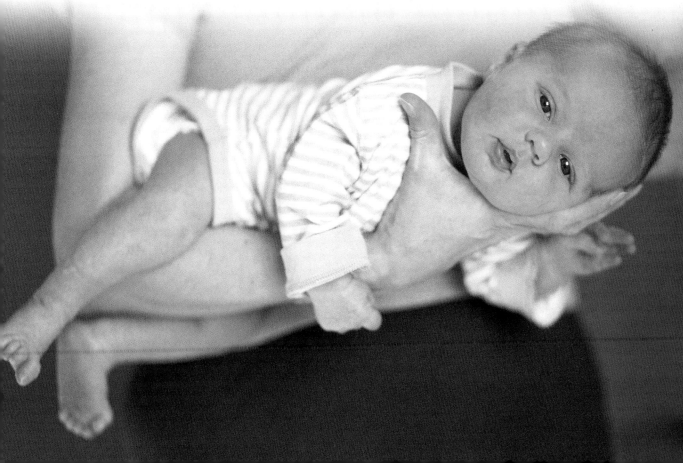

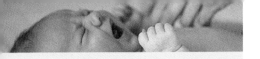

SHAKEN BABY SYNDROME

A frustrated parent or other caregiver may lose control and forcefully shake a baby to try to stop the crying. Since babies cannot fully support their heavy heads, this violent shaking injures a baby's brain. This can lead to death or shaken baby syndrome. Never shake your baby.

Shaken baby syndrome may cause:

- Brain damage and mental retardation
- Vision and/or hearing loss
- Speech problems
- Seizures
- Cerebral palsy

way of communicating. Responding to his needs will help him feel secure and will help him learn how to soothe himself as he grows older.

FATIGUE AND CRYING

After about three months, babies' body clocks start to distinguish between night and day, so they often get tired in the early evening and this can lead to crying (a different type of sound from colicky crying). If this is the case with your baby, he may be ready to go to bed. Keep in mind that babies have to learn how to fall asleep on their own and crying is part of that learning process (*see p.31*).

CRYING AND OLDER BABIES

Older babies (over the age of 6 months or so) are often creatures of habit and if their routine is disrupted, they can become unhappy and unsettled. They may also be very determined, so if, for example, their feeding is late, they might cry until it finally arrives. Equally, they might cry during mealtimes because of a clash with you about a particular food or drink. In short, even though they cannot yet talk, babies are remarkably communicative through their crying.

SHOULD I LET MY OLDER BABY CRY?

Simply because your older baby is crying does not mean that you have to give in to his every wish and, again, only you can decide what your approach will be to any particular circumstance. Despite parents' desire not to upset their children, sometimes it may prove necessary to do so.

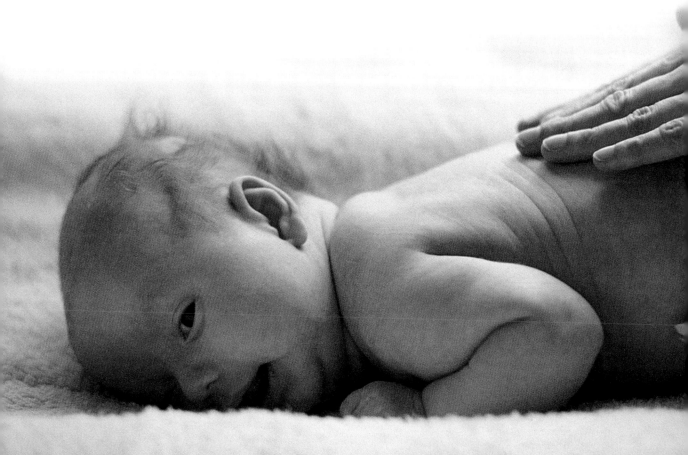

Clearly there are times when it is inappropriate not to soothe your child, but there will also be occasions when you will have to stand firm and let your older baby cry. For example, he may want something that is dangerous. If you always accommodate your baby, he may become inflexible and used to having his own way in everything. Remember that you will not be a bad parent if you follow either path; you will simply be following your own instincts about how you wish to raise your child.

PACIFIERS & THUMB-SUCKING

Opinions on pacifiers and thumb-sucking vary and it will be up to you to decide what your attitude is toward them. If one of these methods works, many parents are simply relieved, since hearing their baby cry can be distressing and their only wish is for the tears to stop.

Thumb-sucking has the advantage that your baby can remove his thumb from his mouth himself if he wants to babble, put something else in his mouth, or simply start crying again. The disadvantage is that a thumb is always readily available and can become a difficult habit for your child to break. Prolonged thumb-sucking may also lead to dental problems in some children.

With a pacifier, the parent can decide when to use it and when to dispense with it, although this may be easier said than done.

Pacifiers are generally not harmful to dental development but, as with thumbsucking, prolonged use may affect the upper teeth or jaw. It is important to think about when and why a pacifier may be used. One suggestion is to use a pacifier only after one year of age, and then only when the baby is in the crib.

WHEN YOUR BABY CRIES

Some ideas to try if your baby does not stop crying:
- Change your baby's diaper.
- Swaddle your baby.
- Feed your baby.
- Offer your baby a pacifier or a finger.
- Rock your baby using slow, rhythmic movements.
- Sing to your baby or play soft, soothing music.
- Take your baby for a walk in a stroller.
- Go for a ride with your baby in the car. Always use a car safety seat.

Some babies seem to cry all the time. If your baby cries a lot and for no obvious reason, speak to your doctor. There may be a medical reason why your baby is crying.

If you are getting angry and feel that you might lose control, try the following:
- Take a deep breath and count to 10.
- Place your baby in a safe place, leave the room, and let your baby cry alone.
- Call someone close to you for emotional support.

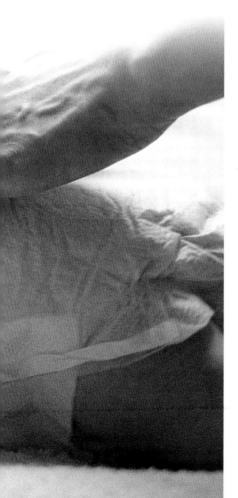

"Remember that crying is your baby's way of communicating. Responding to his needs will help him feel secure and will help him learn how to soothe himself as he grows older."

SLEEP

WHEN SHE IS FIRST BORN, your baby has no notion of night and day and you should be prepared for it to take several weeks, if not months, before she sleeps through the night. Although this does not affect your baby's health, you may find that your own rest is affected because your sleep will inevitably be disrupted during this time.

Beds and bedding

There is a wide range of beds and bedding for babies.

Cradle or bassinet Suitable from birth to about 3 months.

Crib Suitable from birth to about 2–3 years old. Babies may sleep better in a crib than in a cradle.

Pillows, comforters, quilts Not suitable for babies under 12 months. Babies can become overheated or smothered.

Blankets Cotton receiving blankets are best because they are warm yet breathable. Wool can irritate a baby's delicate skin.

Sheets Cotton sheets are best. Avoid synthetic fabrics, which can trap heat. Be sure not to put anything fluffy under your baby.

Crib bumpers Not necessary. If they are used, they should be removed by the time your baby begins to pull to a standing position.

WHO SLEEPS WHERE?

It is up to you where your baby sleeps, and there are issues to consider for all the possible scenarios. You may decide to have your baby sleep in her bedroom or in yours, in her bed or in yours. She may start off in one place, then move on to another when she is a little older.

Some parents like having their baby in the same bedroom with them for the first few weeks, especially if the mother is breastfeeding, because the baby can then be fed in bed during the night with minimal disruption to all concerned. Once a baby is having longer intervals between feedings, she can be put in her own bedroom. If the baby takes a bottle, some parents decide to take turns sleeping in another room so that at least one parent gets a night of uninterrupted sleep, while the other parent is available to feed the baby if she wakes and is hungry.

For comfort or convenience, some parents may take their newborn into bed with them for some or all of the night during the first few weeks. However, sharing a bed can be hazardous under certain conditions, especially if a parent is under the influence of drugs or alcohol. Parents who are concerned about having the baby in the same

bed with them may choose to keep their baby nearby by placing the bassinet or crib in the same room. The disadvantage of having your baby in the same room with you is that newborns can be very noisy sleepers, shuffling and grunting so much that they keep you awake. And even if she is in her own crib, your baby may be distracted by the fact that you are in the same room. If you decide to have your baby in bed, be sure never to place her in a facedown position. Your baby should

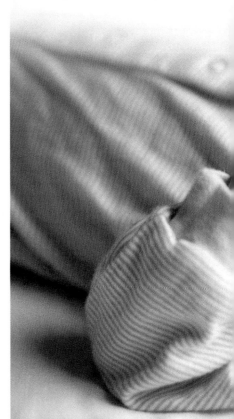

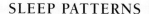

not sleep with you if either parent has been smoking because of the danger of secondhand smoke. You should remove any pillows, loose covers, and soft surfaces from the bed. Move the bed away from the wall or other furniture to prevent possible entrapment.

Once your baby has learned to recognize the parental bed as the place where she sleeps – and this will probably happen within the first three months – it may be very difficult to persuade her to sleep anywhere else. The longer you allow her to sleep with you in your bed, the harder it may be to get your baby accustomed to her own bed. It can put stress on your relationship with your partner if you are not both in agreement on the idea of allowing your baby to share your bed. One of you may end up sleeping poorly or be worried that you might roll over and smother your baby. These and all of the other points discussed in this chapter need to be considered when determining your child's sleeping arrangements.

HOW TO GET YOUR BABY TO GO TO SLEEP

Parents tend to fall into two categories: either they fit their baby into their own lives, or they fit their own lives around their baby's. The parents' attitude toward their baby's sleep habits is very much influenced by which of these two categories they fall into. However, if parents resign themselves in advance to having broken nights of sleep for months on end, if not years, then this can sometimes become a self-fulfilling prophecy.

There are two basic questions to think about when considering babies' sleep. The first is how to get a baby to fall asleep on her own, and the second is how long she is able to sleep at night. While there is much that can be done to teach a baby

SLEEP PATTERNS

The following is a common pattern of sleep for a baby in the first year of life.

First 6 weeks
Until an infant is approximately 6 weeks old, she will be awake for only 6–8 hours per day. She will sleep randomly during the day and the night, because her brain does not yet have the maturity to have developed a cycle of day and night.

6 weeks–3 months
Your baby will sleep less during the day and may start to sleep for longer stretches at night. Her body clock is slowly establishing itself.

3–6 months
Day and night are now established in most babies. Stretches of four hours between feedings are achievable for most babies.

6 months onward
Your baby may be able to sleep for 6-hour stretches, if not more. From 6 months old, many babies no longer need nighttime feeding. If your baby tends to fall back to sleep after only a few sips of breastmilk or formula, she is probably not hungry; quietly encourage her to go back to sleep.

You'll find that establishing a good bedtime routine for your baby (*see p.30*) during her first year can help her establish good sleep habits that may last into childhood. A routine can also make bedtimes easier, because your baby learns the cues that mean it's time for her to go to sleep.

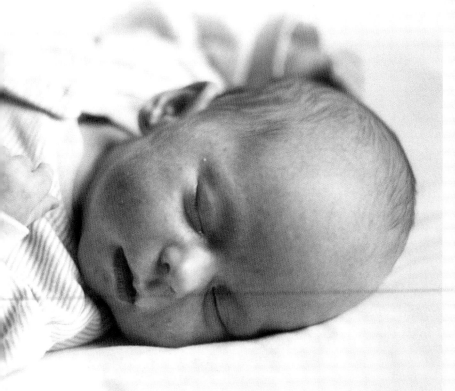

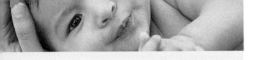

SIDS

Sudden Infant Death Syndrome (SIDS) is the unexpected and unexplainable death of an infant under 1 year old, usually while sleeping. It is very rare, and most often affects babies aged between 2 and 4 months. Recent research has shown that parents can take certain measures to minimize the risk of it happening.

Always put your baby to sleep on her back. Sleeping on the side may be an alternative. Infants with certain medical conditions can sleep prone (on the stomach); consult your doctor. If you place your baby to sleep on her side, alternate one side with the other. Both back and side sleeping have a lower risk of SIDS than sleeping on the stomach.

Do not overdress your baby. She should be lightly clothed for sleep.

Do not overheat your baby's room. The temperature should be comfortable for a lightly clothed adult.

Use cotton bedding, which is warm and breathable. Do not use stuffed toys, comforters, quilts, sheepskins, or pillows in the sleeping environment.

Never smoke in your baby's room or when you are with her. Better still, quit entirely (research shows that if mothers smoke during pregnancy, their baby is 15 times more likely to die of SIDS).

If you smoke, drink, or use drugs, do not sleep in the same bed as your baby.

Place your baby's feet at the bottom of the crib ("feet to foot") to prevent her from wriggling down under the covers.

to fall asleep – since it is a skill that has to be learned – there is less that can be done to help a baby sleep through the night. In addition, during the first three months, a baby's sleep pattern will depend to some extent on whether she is breast- or bottlefed (*see pp.16–17*), because a breastfed baby may wake more often to be fed. The box on page 29 is a rough guide to what sort of sleep patterns you can expect from your baby during her first year.

Learning how to fall asleep on their own is something that comes more easily to some babies than to others. Babies get into habits – both good and bad – extremely fast, but these habits can be changed. The main thing is that you should be consistent and persistent about your baby's sleeping and remember that the longer you leave things, the harder it will be to change them. Your older baby may need to cry a lot at first before falling asleep on her own, but that is part of the learning process.

The importance of bedtime routines

Most sleep experts agree that, for a baby to learn to fall asleep, it helps to establish a bedtime routine. This

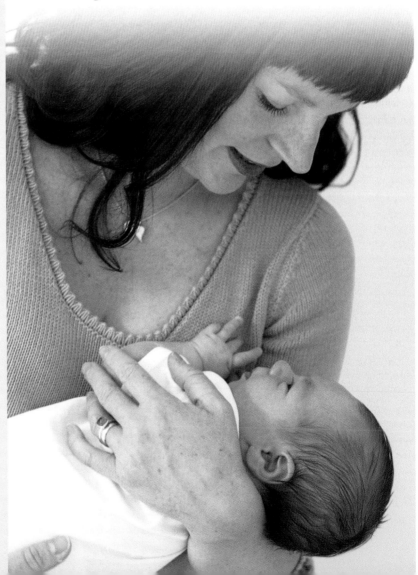

enables your baby to recognize the cues that will tell her it is time to sleep, whether for a daytime nap or at nighttime. It is never too early to introduce a bedtime routine, even if the results of your efforts are not seen until much later.

The aim of an evening routine, aside from giving your baby cues for going to sleep, is to calm her and help her wind down. Try giving your baby a bath, and dress her in different clothes from the ones she was wearing during the day. Feed her in the room in which she sleeps (which should be dimly lit), cuddle her, then put her to bed. Do not linger. The whole process should take you no longer than about 45 minutes from bath to bed.

Bedtime comforts

After a bath, some parents like to read books to their baby, cuddle for a little while, sing, or play soft music. Many find that their baby is comforted by the familiar smell of a soft cloth – perhaps a cotton cloth used during feedings – or by a particular toy. Others find that pacifiers are useful in helping their baby learn to fall asleep on her own. What you need to avoid is stimulating your baby through play at the end of the day.

The final part of the bedtime routine is that your baby should be awake when she is put in her bed so that she can learn to recognize this essential cue for falling asleep. A baby who has already fallen asleep elsewhere before she is put to bed may feel anxious if she wakes because she will not immediately know where she is. So, while it is fine to let your baby fall asleep outside her bed in the first few weeks, you should avoid letting this become a habit as she grows older.

SLEEP QUESTIONS & ANSWERS

When can I expect my baby to sleep through the night?

Some bottlefed babies start sleeping six-hour stretches – what could be called sleeping through the night – from as early as 2 weeks old, but most babies, both breast- and bottlefed ones, will not be doing such long stretches regularly until they are around 3 or 4 months old. Establishing a bedtime routine in the early weeks will eventually help your baby recognize cues for going to sleep.

Why does my 6-month-old baby still feed during the night?

Make sure she is eating enough during the day and that her last meal and bottle are not too early and no more than two hours apart. The bottle should not be taking the place of dinner, but should rather be a way of filling up and settling your baby.

If your baby is waking for a feeding, it may be more out of habit than genuine hunger. Comfort her or offer her a pacifier or her fingers. If she is truly hungry, feeding her may help her fall asleep again.

Why can't I settle my 6-month-old baby when she wakes at night?

If your baby needs increasingly long cuddling or to be taken into your bed in order to settle, try just talking to her and stroking her to reassure her. Avoid picking her up and make sure you stimulate her as little as possible (keep the light off, or very dim, in her room).

You may have to let your baby do some controlled crying (see below); otherwise she will soon realize that if she cries when she wakes, she gets a lot of cuddling with her mother or father and perhaps even a chance to lie in their bed. This can quickly become a habit. The older your baby is, the longer it can take to get her out of the habit of waking and crying.

What is "controlled crying"?

This is a technique that is used to settle babies when they are in their cribs and should only be attempted with babies over 6 months old.

With controlled crying, you leave your baby to cry, initially for five minutes, then go in to reassure her by talking to her and stroking her briefly, but never picking her up. You repeat the process but gradually space out the intervals to 10, 15, 20 minutes and so on, until your baby falls asleep on her own. If your baby is crying hysterically, calm her down first before trying this method.

Controlled crying can be a distressing method, and the older the baby is, the longer it can take to be effective. However, if you are determined and always consistent, controlled crying may work in the end and your baby will have learned to fall asleep on her own.

Why does my baby sleep badly during the day?

Babies like routines and, if you set a pattern to your day, your baby can develop cues for falling asleep. She may also have to do some controlled crying (see above) before naps.

Try to ensure that at least one of your baby's daytime naps is always in the same bed and at about the same time every day. If your baby only falls asleep at random times while you are out and about and only in her stroller or in the car, she will not develop the cues to learn how to sleep in her bed during the day.

In addition, if your baby does not sleep enough during the day, it can make it harder for her to sleep at night, although this may sound contradictory. If your baby becomes fussy and upset in the evening from being overtired during the day, it can make it hard for you to settle her into her crib and get her to sleep.

CARING FOR YOUR BABY

As a new parent, your baby's well-being is your first concern. However, many new parents have no previous experience in caring for a baby: they have never dressed or fed a baby before, changed a diaper, or given a baby a bath. Learning to do these things correctly can be achieved and ensures that your baby stays as healthy as possible.

Keeping healthy

Wash your hands before and after every diaper change.

Use a soft cloth and lukewarm water or mild hypoallergenic wipes to clean the diaper area and allow your baby's skin to air as much as possible.

For the first week or two only give your baby sponge baths.

When bathing your newborn, hold him at all times. Use a mild baby soap or plain water to clean your baby.

Wipe his gums after every feeding. Clean teeth twice a day as soon as the first one appears.

A young baby should wear about one more layer than you do. Cotton is best for clothes and bedding – avoid wool or synthetic fabrics.

CHANGING A DIAPER

If you do not know how, your nurse can show you how to change your baby's diaper. You and your partner can decide what sort of diaper you choose to use; some families prefer disposable diapers while others prefer cloth ones. Whether you decide on disposable or cloth diapers, hygiene is very important for both you and your baby. You should always wash your hands before and after each diaper change.

Cleaning the diaper area

Use cotton balls or a washcloth and lukewarm water, or mild hypoallergenic wipes, to clean your baby's diaper area. (If you are using cloth diapers, make sure that they are thoroughly rinsed of all laundry detergent before they are dried, since laundry detergent residue can irritate your baby's delicate skin.)

Some people recommend using an emollient cream after every diaper change, while others use nothing at all and prefer to let their baby's skin breathe as much as possible. Whatever you decide, you should change your baby's diaper after every feeding and before and after every sleep. The less he sits in a soiled or wet diaper, the less your baby risks developing diaper rash, which is caused when the ammonia in the urine irritates the skin. If your baby does develop diaper rash, you should treat it promptly (*see p.56*); otherwise, the diaper rash may become infected.

Boys and girls

When you are bathing a boy, you should not pull back the foreskin. For a girl, you should gently wipe the labia and vaginal area. Always wipe toward the anus, never away from it, since this can spread bacteria toward the baby's penis or vagina. Remember to clean inside any skin creases, and make sure the skin is totally dry before putting on a clean diaper. Ideally, leave your baby's skin to air as much as possible,

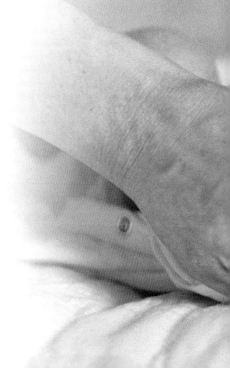

which will let it breathe and help prevent diaper rash. One note of caution, however: if the room is too cold, boys, in particular, will tend to urinate when their diaper is left off.

SPONGE BATHS

Newborn babies are not yet mobile and they do not get dirty quickly, unlike older babies. It is not essential to give your newborn a bath on a daily basis. Instead, you can simply wash your baby's face and bottom, as well as any other part, such as his hands or under his arms, that you would like to clean up a little. This process is called sponge bathing.

How to sponge bathe

You will need a bowl of lukewarm water, some cotton balls or a washcloth, and a soft bath towel. Remember to wash your hands before you begin. Start by carefully wiping your baby's eyes. Dip a cotton ball in the water, squeeze it out, then gently wipe one of your baby's eyes, from the nose outward. Repeat this process with a fresh cotton ball for the other eye to avoid possibly transferring bacteria from one eye to the other. Then wipe the rest of your baby's face and neck using a third cotton ball or soft washcloth, remembering to lift your baby's chin up to clean any folds of skin underneath it. Gently pat the skin dry with the towel. Rinse the washcloth or use additional cotton balls to clean your baby's hands, under his arms, and in the diaper area.

If your baby dislikes washing

If your baby finds it upsetting the first few times you wash him, try talking to him in a soothing voice or singing as you do it. He will soon come to regard being washed as part of his everyday routine.

UMBILICAL STUMP

You should be aware that the stump from your baby's umbilical cord will remain attached to his tummy for around the first two to three weeks after birth. It will gradually dry up and then eventually detach by itself, leaving your baby's belly button.

Sponge bathe your baby until the stump falls off.

Your hospital may apply a special dye to your baby's umbilical cord to help prevent infection.

Redness of the surrounding skin plus discharge or an odor from the stump may be a sign of infection. Consult your doctor.

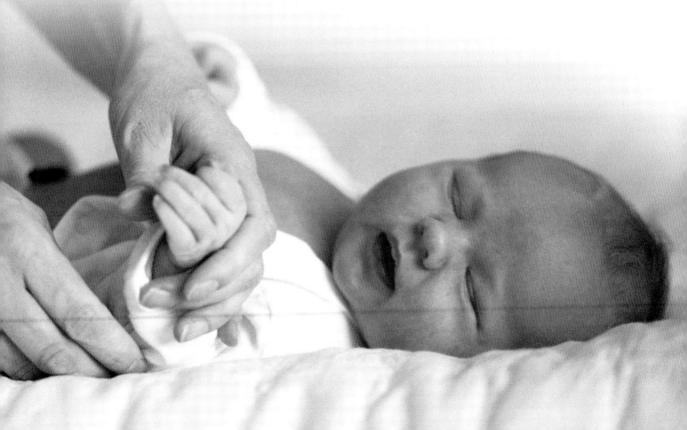

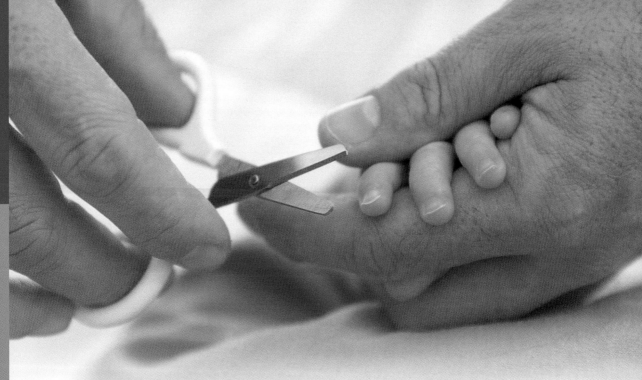

WASHING YOUR BABY'S HAIR

Even if you bathe your baby every day, you do not need to wash his hair more than once a week. To do so, wrap your baby in a towel and hold him along your forearm, so that your hand supports his head. Hold him over the bath and gently wash his hair with a mild baby soap if desired. Rinse well, then pat his head dry with a soft towel.

CARING FOR YOUR BABY'S TEETH & NAILS

Although drooling may begin around 2 months, baby teeth usually do not appear until after 6 months. However, it is not unusual for babies to remain toothless during the whole first year. Wipe your baby's gums after each feeding. As soon as the first tooth appears, clean his teeth using a toothbrush, washcloth, or gauze and plain water. You can begin to use a small amount of fluoride toothpaste as your child gets older. You should keep his finger- and toenails short using nail clippers or small scissors.

CLOTHING & BEDCLOTHES

Babies cannot regulate their body temperature very well for the first few weeks, so it is particularly important that they do not become too hot or too cold. At this stage, your baby should wear one more layer than you are, unless it is very warm weather. An undershirt or onesie, top layer, and pants should be sufficient indoors, although you may want to wrap a cotton receiving blanket around him as well depending on the temperature of the room.

Gradually, as your baby gains greater control of his body temperature, it will no longer be necessary to dress him in one more layer of clothing than you are wearing. When you are outdoors in cold weather, make sure your baby's head, hands, and feet are well covered, since a vast amount of body heat is lost through the head, in particular.

Cotton clothes are best for your baby because they offer warmth and breathability. Do not dress him in wool clothes, such as sweaters and hats, because these may prove too scratchy for infants whose skin is so sensitive. Clothes made from synthetic fabrics, such as polyester fleece, are less breathable, so they may make your baby sweat.

Your baby's bedroom should be kept at a comfortable temperature, and you should never put your baby to sleep near a fire or source of heat. Rather than comforters, use thin sheets and blankets, since these prevent overheating and smothering (*see pp.28–29*).

As with clothes, the best fabric for bedding is cotton because it is breathable yet warm, and you will probably find that a fitted crib sheet, plus two or three receiving blankets, are sufficient for keeping your baby warm at night. If you are not sure whether he is too hot or too cold, feel the nape of his neck, which provides a good indication of his general temperature.

If you think that your baby may be a little cold, it may be best to put another cotton blanket over him, and avoid turning up the heat in the room.

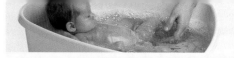

BATHTIME

Your hospital may have explained how to bathe your baby at home, but you will probably be all thumbs the first few times. Parents are sometimes afraid of dropping or injuring their newborn, yet it is crucial that they get used to bathing him from the outset. With an organized routine and a great deal of practice, parents and babies will become very comfortable with bathtime. Sponge baths, rather than full immersion baths, should be given until the umbilical cord has fallen off.

Handling your baby in the bath

Babies like secure handling and are a lot tougher than you think. Hold your baby under his far armpit by reaching around behind his back, thereby allowing his shoulders, neck, and head to rest along your forearm. This position frees up your other hand to wash him or grab anything you need, such as a towel.

It is very important to hold your baby at all times while he is in the bath, at least until he is able to sit up. Even then, you should never leave your baby unattended, even for a split second.

Babies feel quite slippery when they are wet, so baby tubs can be useful because they are compact and there is less room for your baby to move around. Using a baby tub can also place less strain on your back, because you are not reaching down into a large, adult bathtub when you wash your baby.

Bathing your baby

When you are bathing your baby, you should not put any bubblebath or soap in the bathwater, because these can have a drying effect on your baby's already sensitive skin.

Using a very mild hypoallergenic baby bath wash to clean your baby is all that is required.

Bathtime should be a fun time, even if your baby seems anxious or nervous about it at first, so remember to talk and smile a lot throughout. Some babies will be more at ease at first than others, but most will get used to having a bath, however much they protest at the beginning. When he's old enough, give your baby toys to play with in the bath. It also helps if you allow plenty of time for the bath and don't rush.

As your baby gets older, you can get him used to having water on his face or head or having water splashed around him. Don't try this until your baby is confident in the bath, though, or it may frighten him. Many parents like to share a bath with their baby. This can be a wonderful experience, which babies may enjoy and which is safe from birth. Use your baby's bath product instead of your shampoo and soap, and make sure that the temperature of the water is right for your baby, which may be a little cool for you.

Having fun

Bath toys can make bathtimes much more fun and appealing for babies. Look for brightly colored boats and bath books; anything that provides a distraction can help.

When your baby is slightly older and is able to hold things, include plastic cups in the bathtub that he can use to pour water from one to the other or on himself.

Whatever games you are playing, you must remember to always hold your baby securely when he is in the bath. Never leave your baby or young child unattended in the bath, no matter how shallow the water is.

TIPS FOR HAPPY BATHTIMES

Never leave your baby or young child unattended in the bath.

Keep at least one hand on your baby at all times.

When you bathe your baby, keep the bathroom and the room in which you will dress and undress him nice and warm. Newborns get cold very easily and that, together with their frequent dislike of being undressed, often means they cry a lot during bathtime in the early days.

Wear clothes you don't mind getting wet when bathing your baby – you may get wet too.

When sponge bathing, keep other parts of your baby covered. You don't need to wash your baby's hair more than once a week.

Before you put your baby in the bath, gather anything that you will need around you, such as a towel and any toys you may want to include, so that they are within easy reach.

Test the temperature of the water with your elbow, which is more sensitive than your hand. The bathwater should feel warm rather than hot. Never add hot water to a bath while your baby is in it.

If your baby cries whenever you give him a bath, be reassured that most babies outgrow their dislike of baths quite quickly. He will soon come to see bathtime as an enjoyable occasion he shares with his parents.

FIRST WEEKS

THE FIRST WEEKS WITH A NEW BABY CAN BE HECTIC, exhausting, and intensive. You are slowly getting to know your baby and adjusting to the enormous changes that she has brought to your life. For the first few weeks, there is often no pattern to your days or nights, but during that time your baby is developing from being a sleepy newborn into an alert infant.

What to expect

Your baby can respond to the world around her as soon as she is born.

After the first few weeks, some of the reflexes your baby was born with, such as the Moro (startle) and walking reflexes, will have almost or totally disappeared.

She will still be able to focus only a short distance away but can follow you around with her eyes. She will close her eyes in response to bright light or seek out a darker area to look at. It is very rare for babies to be significantly visually impaired, but if by about two months there is little sign of your baby doing the above things, tell the doctor at the 2-month checkup (*see opposite*) or sooner.

Your baby will be startled by loud noises and soothed by the familiar sound of her parents' voices. She may turn her head if she hears them. If your baby seems surprised to see you because she has not heard you approach, or if she is not reacting to loud noises or voices, mention it at the 2-month checkup, even if her hearing was screened at birth.

ADOPTING A ROUTINE

Whatever anyone tells you, it is unusual for a baby to be in any sort of routine before she is 6 weeks old. Bottlefed babies may be feeding more regularly and sleeping for longer stretches than their breastfed peers, but it will still be difficult to predict how long those stretches of sleep will be and when the next bottle is due. So if your baby still feeds or sleeps very erratically by this stage, do not despair. This is very common and things will gradually settle down.

When should I start?

Although 6 weeks is often the time when people start talking about establishing routines, it must be emphasized that this is only an approximate guide.

After the first few weeks, you can start to adopt a daytime and evening routine for your baby, although there is no precise or ideal time to start. The best time is simply when you feel able to. If you are breastfeeding, you are probably feeding on demand, and by now your baby may be feeding efficiently and feedings may take less than about 20 minutes. If you are bottlefeeding, your baby should be having about 6 bottles a day and is probably drinking reasonably quickly at this stage.

Your baby should also not be taking too long to settle after each feeding, so that she can either take a nap afterward or, if she does not seem to be tired, play a little bit. Even young babies like to have company and lying on their own in a bed or sitting in a stroller can get lonely and boring. You can lay your baby out on the floor on a playmat, so that she can enjoy moving her arms and legs around in an unhindered way.

By about 6 weeks, your baby will also be considerably more alert. You can sit her slightly propped up in a reclining baby seat so that she can see and react to what is going on around her. However, you should not let her sit up this way for more than about 15 minutes at a time, a few times a day, and never put the seat on a raised surface – it could fall off.

NAP TIMES

You should be aiming for your baby to have a morning and an afternoon nap, even though this is a pattern that may not establish itself until she is a little older. Don't worry that, by sleeping twice during the day, your baby will not be tired at night. The reverse is often the case: a baby who is deprived of sleep during the day often becomes overtired and finds it hard to settle at night.

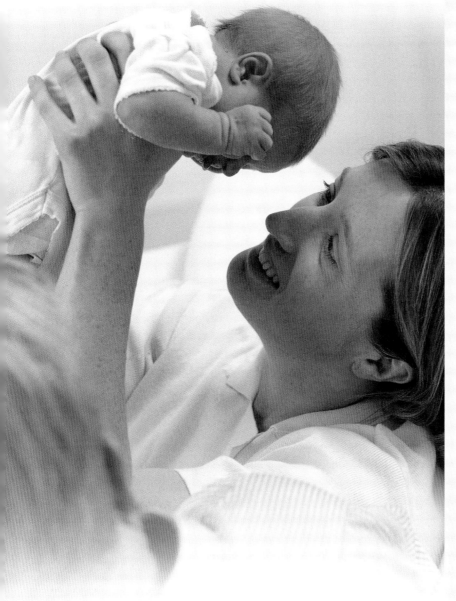

2-MONTH CHECKUP

When a baby is about 2 months old, she will receive her first major checkup since the newborn period.

Your baby will be examined and a number of things relating to her general development will be assessed. These include her size, weight, and head circumference. The doctor will also check her sight and hearing, her reflexes, her heartbeat, and her hip alignment.

Her hip alignment is checked because some babies are born with developmental hip dysplasia, in which the hip joint is unstable and the hips can become dislocated. It is usually treatable if detected in infancy, but if left untreated the child will limp in later life. Girls are more prone to this condition than boys.

If your baby is a boy, the doctor will check to make sure that his testes have both descended completely into the scrotum. If they have not descended by the 2-month check, you may be advised to wait another few months, because undescended testes often descend on their own during this time.

If your baby was born prematurely, this will be taken into account when the doctor assesses her development.

This checkup also gives you the chance to discuss any concerns you might have about your baby's growth or her general progress.

Your baby will receive immunizations at this visit.

BEDTIME

You can also start to introduce an evening routine (*see p.30*), which will eventually help your baby recognize that it is time to go to bed. Evening baths may have the benefit of soothing your baby as well as developing bedtime cues, making her more ready to sleep.

To help you establish a routine, both day and night, you could try keeping a note of feeding and nap times. This will identify any emerging patterns – both good and bad – and will show you clearly when you are progressing in the right direction.

Although you should accept that no routine can always be applied rigidly – parents who fail to realize this may become very tense and frustrated – it is also true that babies like routines. Babies with little pattern to their daytime naps and bedtime often become poor sleepers. If you are content with this, it's fine, but otherwise establishing a routine can benefit all concerned.

STARTING SOLID FOODS

Beginning solid foods and weaning your baby from breastmilk or formula is an important step in his healthy development. Solid foods are usually introduced around age 4–6 months. They provide nutrients for your baby in a variety of flavors, textures and food groups. Feedings can be a messy business, but they are a fun time for babies and parents.

Finger foods

Around 7–9 months of age, infants learn to put objects into their mouths. Once your child can pick up food between his thumb and forefinger, you can try giving him age-appropriate "finger foods." Be sure your child is sitting upright when eating and watch out for choking at all times.

Foods that dissolve easily, such as baby crackers, pieces of bread, plain cookies.

Well-cooked pasta or vegetables, such as peas and cut-up green beans, potatoes, and carrots.

Small pieces of dry food, such as cereal.

Small pieces of soft fruit, such as banana chunks or diced ripe pears. Grapes should be halved lengthwise and then cut again crosswise. Avoid fruits with seeds or pits and large pieces of dried fruit, which may be choking hazards.

Sliced cheese or small pieces of chicken.

WHEN TO START

The Canadian Pediatric Society believes that breastmilk is the optimal source of nutrition through the first year of life, and supports exclusive feeding of breastmilk or formula for at least 4 months.

You can begin to introduce complementary foods into your baby's diet at the age of 4 to 6 months. Consult your doctor for individual advice.

Before 4–6 months, the digestive system is immature and less able to cope with certain foods, so giving solids is more likely to cause food allergies and intolerance. If there is a family history of food allergies, it is advisable to wait until your baby is 6 months old before beginning solid foods. However, if you wait much longer after your child is 6 months old, he may be less willing to accept the new flavors and textures of solid foods.

Developmental cues indicate that your baby is ready to begin eating solids: he is able to sit up by himself for feeding; he is interested in the foods that other people are eating (watching, grabbing, pointing); and he is able to move food from the front to the back of the mouth. At first, your child may push food out of his mouth, but with a little practice will learn to move it back and then swallow.

Continue the same number of daily breastfeedings as you gradually introduce solids. As solid food intake increases, breastmilk supply will gradually decrease. This is a natural, gradual way of "weaning" the baby slowly from the breast. Continue breastfeeding with solid foods for at least 1 year, or longer if desired by mother and baby.

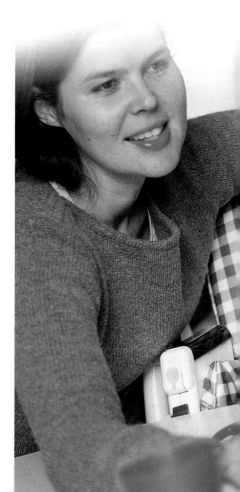

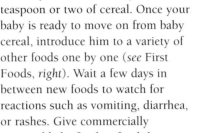

For formula-fed infants, solids should not replace milk. Your baby still needs to drink at least 500 ml (16 ounces) of formula a day until he is about 1 year. Make sure that any food he eats allows him to drink this much formula.

INTRODUCING SOLIDS

Introduce solid foods once a day at a particular meal. Do this for a few days until your baby seems to have mastered eating solids. Once he is eating well at this meal, introduce solids at another meal, until he is having the equivalent of three meals a day, plus his usual intake of milk.

Simple basic food such as infant rice, barley, or oatmeal cereal fortified with iron should be given as the first food. The cereal comes as fine, dry flakes and can be mixed with a little breastmilk or formula. At first you will need only a teaspoon or two of cereal. Once your baby is ready to move on from baby cereal, introduce him to a variety of other foods one by one (*see* First Foods, *right*). Wait a few days in between new foods to watch for reactions such as vomiting, diarrhea, or rashes. Give commercially prepared baby food or food that you have boiled, steamed, or microwaved and then pureed. Do not add butter or salt; your baby doesn't need them. Freeze the food in ice cube trays and put the cubes in labeled freezer bags.

Homemade food has certain advantages. Commercially prepared baby food often has a less distinct taste and feels smoother, so your baby may get used to it and learn to prefer it to "real" food.

FIRST FOODS

The following are types of food that you can safely offer your baby around the age of 6 months. If you are in doubt about any other foods, you should speak to your doctor.

Around 6 months Peas, squash, sweet potatoes, carrots, cauliflower, broccoli, green beans, apples, pears, peaches, plums, and bananas (ripe, uncooked). The breastfed infant can begin chopped meat or poultry at this time, to increase iron intake.

From 6 months Cereal mixed with fruit, wheat-based foods such as bread or pasta.

From around 8 months Ground or finely chopped meat or poultry, mashed cooked egg yolk, dairy products such as full-fat yogurt and cottage cheese (do not give cow's milk as a drink yet), finely chopped citrus fruit or fruit that has pits (removed) such as plums and peaches, and fish (but no shellfish).

From 12 months Whole cooked eggs and whole cow's milk (as a drink). Honey should not be given before the 1st birthday, since it may cause infant botulism, a potentially fatal illness.

Give one new food at a time and wait 2–3 days to see if there is any physical reaction before starting another one. Ask your doctor whether your baby may need vitamin supplements or fluoride.

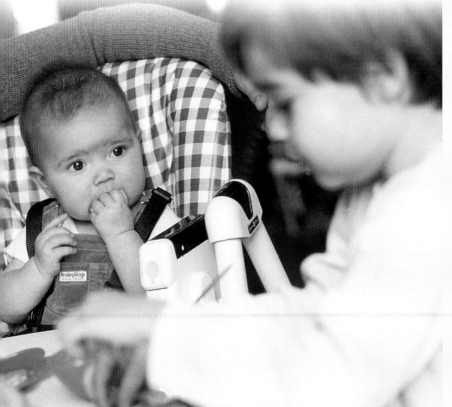

HELPING HIM FEED HIMSELF

From about 8 months, your baby may be able to hold his own bottle and start to drink from a trainer cup, although he may still like a bedtime bottle or breastfeeding for comfort.

At about 7–9 months, babies start putting objects in their mouths, edible or not, and are eager to feed themselves with a spoon or fingers. Both methods are messy but help develop coordination and motor skills. Encourage your baby to feed himself. Eat with him and offer him finger foods (*see p. 38*) or foods he can eat with a spoon.

FOODS TO AVOID

Avoid foods that are nutritionally poor or unhealthy during your baby's first year and beyond. Avoid foods known to cause allergies in susceptible babies, particularly if there is a family history of allergies.

Nutritionally poor or unhealthy foods

Do not give foods with a high salt content. Also avoid low-fat foods. Children need fat in their diets to provide energy essential for the development of the central nervous system. Do not worry about reducing fat as long as your baby has a normal weight gain. Children should drink only whole milk until 2 years of age, when they may switch to reduced-fat dairy products.

Special diets

If you are raising your child on a vegetarian or vegan diet, be vigilant that he is getting the vitamins and minerals required for development of the bones, muscles, nervous system, and brain. People following vegan diets are at a higher risk of vitamin deficiencies. Consult your doctor to ensure that your baby has a balanced diet.

Allergenic foods

At birth, your baby's immune system is not fully developed. If you have a family history of allergic tendencies, your baby may react adversely if certain foods are given too early. An allergic reaction occurs when the immune system produces antibodies to counteract a foreign substance. The most common allergens are wheat, eggs, sesame seeds, shellfish, soy products, nuts, and cow's milk.

Most infants can tolerate eggs at around 8 months. Since egg yolks are thought to be less allergenic than egg whites, start with a mashed, hard-boiled egg yolk, then proceed to a combination of egg yolk and some egg white, and then a complete egg. Do not give scrambled or entire eggs at first. Children at high risk of allergies should avoid eggs during the first two years.

Peanut butter, seeds, and nuts can be a problem for children. Ideally,

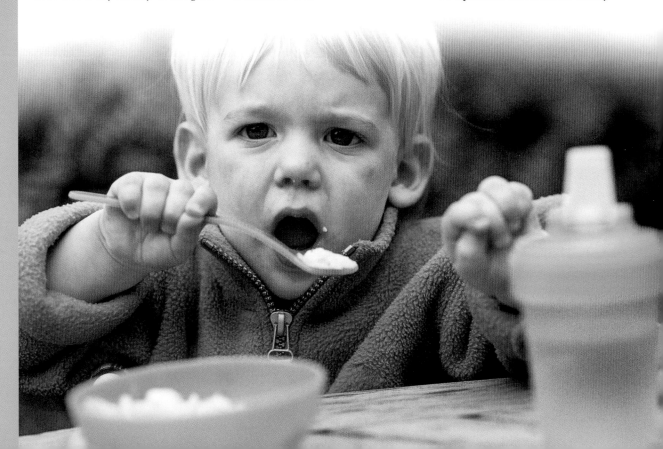

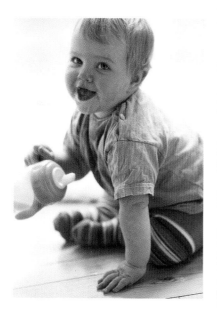

wait until your child is at least 3 years old before introducing nuts or seeds, and do so slowly. Before this, or if your child has a known allergy to nuts, read food labels carefully, since nuts, seeds, and their oils are ingredients in many prepared foods.

Do not give fish until your baby is around 9 months old. When you introduce fish, make very sure that there are no bones. Avoid shellfish until he is at least 3 years old.

When is it safe to give milk?

Regular cow's milk should not be given as a drink before your child is 1 year old, since it is a common cause of food allergy in infancy. However, yogurt, small amounts of cheese, and other dairy products in small quantities are acceptable. Do not switch to soy milk without your doctor's approval, because your child could also be allergic to soy.

If you suspect that your child has an intolerance or allergy (the latter causes an immediate, severe reaction), consult your doctor right away. He or she will evaluate your child and may arrange for tests.

FEEDING QUESTIONS & ANSWERS

How much food should I give my baby?

At first, one tablespoonful of food will be enough. Your baby will soon progress to eating 2–3 tablespoonfuls of food per meal. After that, your baby's appetite will be your best guide. You should try to give him mostly nonsweet foods because he will naturally prefer sweet foods and he may need less encouragement or practice to get used to them.

How do I space out milk and solids during the day?

For breastfed infants, offer the breast as usual. Then, 2–3 times per day offer solids before or after a breastfeeding. Continue to breastfeed on demand, still usually around 8 times per day. For bottlefed babies, many parents find that it works best if they alternate solids with milk. Typically after about 6 months, their baby's meal pattern will be as follows:

Early morning:	milk
Breakfast:	baby rice or cereal
Midmorning:	milk
Lunch:	solids
Midafternoon:	milk
Dinner:	solids
Bedtime:	milk

During the first year, formula-fed babies should continue to drink at least 500 ml (16 fluid ounces) of formula per day.

When should I introduce chunky food?

After 6 months, your baby is able to eat chunkier food, even if he has no teeth. You will be amazed at how efficient his gums are at chewing bits of food.

However, never leave your baby unattended when he is eating chunkier food because he can easily choke on a small piece, especially once he is old enough to feed himself with finger food. To introduce chunks, instead of pureeing the food, mash it up with a fork and, for older babies, chop it up into small pieces. Homemade food will be chunkier than prepared chunky food and will train your baby to chew more effectively.

What should my baby drink?

Aside from breastmilk and formula, water is the best drink, because it is thirst-quenching and not harmful to teeth. Many babies do not take to the taste of water after drinking milk exclusively, which is slightly sweet. So do persist by giving your baby regular little sips. Eventually, most babies get used to the taste of water. Ask your doctor whether it is necessary to boil tap water or use bottled water for your baby.

Is it all right to give my older baby snacks between meals, or should I insist that he eat only "three square meals" a day?

Older babies and small children burn up a lot of energy, but they are usually unable to eat a large amount of food at a single sitting. Snacks can be a useful way to keep a small child's energy levels up and prevent the fussiness that can come from being hungry. Having said this, don't expect your child to eat up his dinner if he's just had a snack an hour or two beforehand. Good snack foods include pieces of soft fruit, bread, and small cubes of cheese.

GOING OUT

ONCE YOU HAVE SETTLED INTO A RHYTHM WITH YOUR BABY, you will begin to want to go out. You don't need to rush into it but you can start, at your own pace, to go for walks, meet with friends, and maybe join clubs and playgroups where you can meet other parents with young babies. This social contact can help you as well as your baby.

Equipment

There are many different ways to take your baby out with you.

Slings and front carriers

These are good for young babies because they have the advantage of leaving your hands free. On the other hand, slings and carriers can be bad for a parent's back as the baby gets heavier. If you use these carriers, be sure to keep your baby's head well supported.

Back carriers

These are good for slightly older babies, once they can hold their heads upright. Back carriers are useful in places where strollers won't go, and leave the parent's hands free. However, back carriers can be bad for a parent's back once children are 2–3 years old.

Strollers

There are many different models of strollers. All-terrain large-wheeled versions and "travel systems" incorporating a car seat are now available. Traditional strollers are often cheaper and offer more flexible seating arrangements.

BENEFITS FOR YOUR BABY

Even young babies like to have variety and can easily become bored. If they never see anything other than the four walls of their home and the same old toys and faces, they can become restless, fussy, and unstimulated.

Simply taking your baby for a daily walk will be of benefit to her. Unless it is really very hot or cold outside, you can take her out in almost any weather. You should make sure she is wrapped up well against the cold and put a rain cover over her stroller if it is raining or snowing. If it is sunny out, you should cover your baby with a sunshade, hat, and clothing and use sunscreen on any exposed areas of the body. The fresh air will stimulate your baby (and then tire her out) and seeing the world around her will interest her as soon as she is a few weeks old.

In addition to taking regular walks, you can take your baby to meet friends and family in places other than your own home. This gets your baby used to mixing with other people and accustomed to different environments, which in turn helps her become more social and adaptable.

You should inquire about what kinds of clubs, activities, and playgroups you might join with your new baby. Your local library may be a source of information for this. Many communities offer parent and baby programs. These playgroups and activities can be a fun and safe opportunity for babies to explore many different ways of playing and interacting with other children of the same age. Babies can develop their social and motor skills while having access to a whole range of different toys and activities that they would not necessarily have at home.

BENEFITS FOR YOU

Many parents who had been working outside the home before having their baby may be surprised at how lonely or isolated they can become when they are at home for weeks with a tiny infant.

In addition, new parents often realize that they know very few people in their area because they had been busy working and had not developed a network of local friends and neighbors.

Although you may not have envisioned yourself participating in parent/child gatherings, you may find that the parents who attend them are a lot like you and that having a baby is a great ice-breaker. These newfound supports can provide you with emotional and practical information and advice.

CAR TRAVEL

The law requires that your baby ride in a car safety seat in a car, and the safest place is in the back seat.

Babies should ride in rear-facing seats as long as possible, at least until 1 year of age. Check the infant seat label for weight and height limits. This style usually has a base that remains in the car and a separate unit with a handle so you can take the seat and baby out of the car without unstrapping her.

Convertible seats may be used rear-facing for smaller babies and forward-facing for larger ones (over 1 year of age), depending on their weight and height

limits. Infants and children are safest in the back seat. Air bags used with seat belts work well to protect older children and adults, but may cause injury to children in car seats or passengers who are not properly positioned. Installing a car seat correctly may be tricky, so you can have a certified child passenger safety technician check it. Only use a second-hand car seat if you know that it has not been recalled or involved in a crash.

YOUR WELL-BEING

Postpartum depression affects at least 10 percent of mothers, and around 50–80 percent suffer from the milder baby blues. To help prevent either of these conditions from developing, it is essential for a new mother to avoid becoming isolated and lonely at a time when she might be feeling vulnerable in her new life.

Try to go for a walk on a regular, if not daily, basis. You can take your baby out with you in a stroller, or strapped into a baby sling or carrier. Fresh air and exercise can make you feel better and can lift your spirits, and will be good for your baby too.

You should also try to have at least some form of adult contact during the day, either by seeing friends or by taking part in some kind of activity at a playgroup, club, or community center.

Whichever parent takes on the role of primary caregiver, making sure that you have sufficient adult company and variety in your day can help your mood enormously. This social contact and change to your routine can have the added benefit that you may rely less heavily on your partner for your emotional and psychological well-being, something that can otherwise be a cause of strain between you.

If sadness or feelings of inadequacy are severe or last longer than the first few months after having a new baby, consult your doctor. Much can be done to treat postpartum depression, and the earlier treatment is started the less likely the condition is to become chronic.

MOVEMENT

Duction the first twelve months of his life, you will see your baby develop from a tiny infant who cannot move by himself and can barely lift his head, to a child who is crawling or even walking. These first twelve months represent the period of most rapid physical and mental development in childhood and they can be a fascinating time for parents.

Childproofing

So that your baby can move around freely and gradually develop his motor skills, childproof your house to minimize the risk of injury (see p.165).

Find a comfortable play mat so that he can enjoy moving around unhindered.

When he is almost able to sit up, do not put him in a bouncing seat, because he may tip it over.

Bouncing chairs must only be put on floors, never on raised surfaces.

Remove unstable pieces of furniture that he may pull down as he tries to haul himself onto his feet.

Put stair gates at the top and bottom of stairs just before he starts to crawl.

Anticipate each new stage in mobility, think how it affects your home and, above all, never leave your baby unattended.

Cover electrical sockets, and keep window treatment strings, electrical cords, and tablecloths out of reach.

PHYSICAL DEVELOPMENT

When your baby is born, his movements consist largely of involuntary or reflex actions. He will curl and uncurl his fingers, for example when he is feeding or sleeping (the grasp reflex); he will throw his arms and legs out when he is startled (the Moro reflex); and he may curl up or kick his legs out if he is crying or in pain.

In order for his motor skills to evolve from involuntary to voluntary, his nervous system needs to develop. This "wiring" takes place from the head downward and from the trunk outward to the fingers and toes. The first parts of the body to develop more deliberate movements are the head and neck. The gross motor skills of the trunk and limbs develop before the fine motor skills of the fingers and toes.

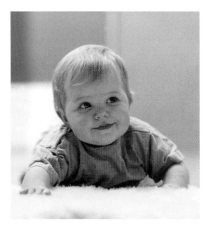

Early development

By the time your baby is 3 months old he can lift his head and, if you place him on his front, he will try to raise his head by supporting himself on his arms. This position also helps your baby exercise his neck and back muscles and is a good way of encouraging him to develop new movements (but remember never to leave him unattended outside his crib or playpen).

The beginnings of movement

Your newborn infant will not be able to roll over, but he will learn to do so at any time between 2 and 5 months old. Since you cannot predict when he will start, never leave him alone on any kind of raised surface, whether it is a bed, changing table, or sofa.

When he is approximately 3 months old, your baby will be able to support his own weight when standing, if he is held. He will flatten his feet out and his legs will be firm. Between 3 and 6 months, he then learns to bounce up and down while standing when held.

His back gradually straightens in the first few months of his life and, when he is 6–9 months old, he learns to sit up unaided. At first, he may tilt sideways or backward, so you may want to surround him with cushions to soften any fall. Soon,

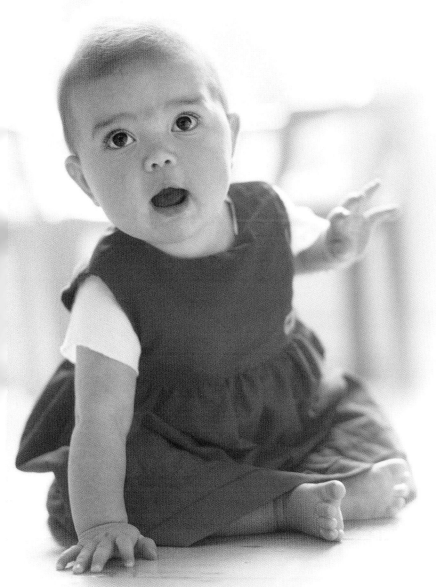

ADDRESSING YOUR CONCERNS

At what stage should I be worried if my baby is still not crawling or walking?

It may be difficult to know whether there is a physical problem with your baby during his first year. It may be that he was late to sit up or that you or your partner were late walkers. If the rest of his physical development and motor skills appear to be progressing normally, there is probably no need for concern but, if his development seems generally slow, seek medical advice.

However, most babies get the urge to pull themselves up on their feet soon after learning to crawl. So, at around 6–10 months old, babies usually start pulling themselves up on any stable – or not-so-stable – object, such as their crib bars or a chair.

"Cruising" and walking

After this, it is a small step between standing and walking, so, at about 9–15 months, most babies start to "cruise" by holding on to furniture or an adult's hands. Your baby will enjoy walking sideways around a low table or walking with you while holding both of your hands. Then, one day, he will let go and take his first few tentative steps alone. This can happen at any time between 8 and 18 months, the average age being around 12 months.

The development of your baby's motor skills is largely dependent on genetics and nervous system development, rather than on practice. If parents were late walkers, it is likely their children will be too. A baby who walks early is no more likely to be a gifted athlete than one who doesn't. Be patient and your baby will develop at his own pace.

however, he will be sitting up confidently and gaining a whole new and exciting perspective on the world.

CRAWLING

The next stage, for most babies, is crawling. Some babies skip this stage entirely, but the vast majority will find a way of getting around that involves either crawling around on their hands and knees or shuffling forward on their bottoms. Crawling of whatever type usually begins between 6 and 10 months. (Remember that, as with all stages of child development, the figures given are simply a guide.) Once your baby can move around independently, there is usually no stopping him. He soon learns to crawl quickly and, if you turn your back for a second, he may be in a totally different place the next time you look. As a result, this stage can be one of the most exhausting because you need to watch your baby constantly.

WALKING

Generally, babies need to go through one stage before moving on to the next, but there are exceptions. Some babies bypass crawling and stay sitting for months on end before getting up, virtually from one day to the next, and starting to walk.

HAND SKILLS

A̲T BIRTH, YOUR BABY WILL NOT BE ABLE TO use her hands in any conscious way but, gradually, she will become aware that they belong to her and that they are very useful for performing a whole range of actions. These hand skills will continue to develop, not only over the first year but over the next few years as she develops her fine motor skills.

Safety

Babies start to put everything into their mouths from about 6 months old. This means that they have to be watched very closely because they can choke on small objects, such as loose change.

Buy special safety plugs for electrical sockets. A curious baby may poke something into one.

Special covers and pads can be bought to protect your baby from sharp table edges and prevent her from pushing things into appliances.

Make sure floor-level cabinets do not contain sharp or dangerous objects. If they do, transfer the contents of the cabinets to a safer place that is locked and out of your child's reach. You could allow her access to one floor-level cabinet that contains objects she can play with. This allows you to accomplish household tasks in the kitchen while your baby enjoys herself in safety.

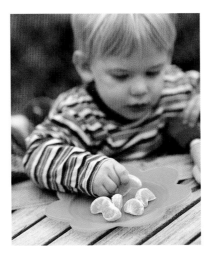

HAND RECOGNITION

By the time she is 3 months old, your baby will have realized that she has hands. This requires her cognitive skills to develop at the same time as her motor skills – her understanding enables her to use her motor skills. When she realizes that these hands belong to her, she will start to move them together.

Between the ages of 3 and 6 months, your baby becomes conscious that there is a cause and effect relationship between reaching out her hand and being able to hold an object such as a rattle. You can encourage her to make this connection by putting toys just out of her reach and letting her practice grabbing them. Your baby also knows how to wave her

hands when she wants something, for example her favorite toy. Since she has now recognized her hands and is gaining control over where she puts them, she is also able to suck her thumb at will.

DROPPING THINGS

The next stage, which occurs at about 6–9 months, is when your baby learns to pass objects from one hand to another. This leads to her noticing that when she is holding something and she opens her hand, it drops. By the end of this stage, dropping things becomes a game that your baby enjoys playing repeatedly: drop the object and watch it being picked up by a cooperative adult. As a result, objects such as bottles or spoons are often used to play the dropping game, particularly if your baby is not especially hungry.

THE PINCER GRIP

Up until now, your baby has been developing the ability to hold larger objects. The gross motor skills that this requires need to be in place before the fine motor skills can progress. Between 7 and 10 months, however, you will notice your baby's increasing ability to use her thumb and index finger to pick up small, detailed objects. The development of this "pincer grip" means that everything from raisins and other finger foods to pieces of dirt, coins, and beads can start to go into your baby's mouth.

The development of fine motor skills coincides with the stage in your baby's cognitive development when she puts unknown things in her mouth in an effort to identify them and explore the world around her. Some babies put things in their mouths more than others, but all will go through this essential phase in their development to some degree. It should not be discouraged, unless your baby is trying to put something that is dangerous into her mouth.

If your baby uses a pacifier, this can sometimes discourage her from putting things into her mouth, since she often will already have the pacifier in her mouth. Although this might seem like a desirable state of

affairs, "mouthing" is an important stage in your baby's development since she uses her hands and mouth to explore her world and should not be hindered. You might try making sure she has her pacifier only when she really needs comfort to give her the opportunity to put clean, safe objects in her mouth instead.

CLAPPING & THROWING

At 9 months, your baby can clap, and by 12 months she can throw things, which comes in handy when, out of anger or frustration, she feels like throwing her toys, spoons, plates, and other objects. This can be a messy period, as she develops both greater physical autonomy and her own independent personality.

ADDRESSING YOUR CONCERNS

If my baby is late in reaching a milestone, should I be worried?
Parents often worry if their baby has not reached a particular developmental milestone by a certain age. Babies develop each skill at their own pace, perhaps reaching one milestone early and another one late. Usually, failure to develop across a range of skills would be a clearer sign of a possible problem than slowness to acquire a single skill. For this reason, it can be difficult to diagnose a physical problem or learning difficulty in the first year. Parents usually have a good instinct about whether or not something is truly wrong. If you have questions, consult your doctor.

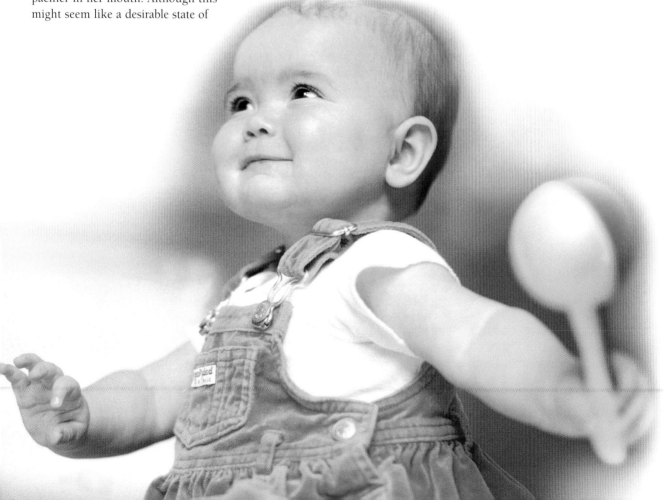

TALKING

A BABY'S ACQUISITION OF LANGUAGE IS, for many parents, the most exciting and fascinating development of all. It seems completely extraordinary that, without any formal teaching, he learns to understand what his parents and other people are saying, figure out the complexities of a sentence, and, usually by the end of his first year, utter his first few words.

Communicating

Tiny babies like adults to talk close-up to them, since their eyes cannot focus very far. Older babies benefit from seeing their parents talk to them and watching their mouths move.

Babies like the speaker's face to show expression, and the smilier it is, the better.

Babies seem to prefer higher-pitched, deliberate talking; this "baby talk," as it is often known, is something that many people seem to do instinctively when they talk directly to a little baby.

Once your baby starts to utter sounds, you can copy them and see if he will do them back to you. This enables your baby to practice making sounds and shows him how conversations work.

Talking out loud to your baby about what you are doing is also an excellent way of teaching him about language. Start reading books to your baby from as early as the newborn period and encourage him to look at pictures.

EARLY COMPREHENSION
In many ways, the most remarkable period of your baby's language acquisition is during his first six months, when research has shown that he is able to distinguish between all the different sounds not only of his native language, but also of other languages with which he has no connection. He may lose this ability from the age of 6 months, as his native language establishes itself as the system of sounds with which he is most familiar. He will then listen for the sounds that are specific to that language and gradually start to make sense of what is being said. This is why babies who are introduced to two languages from birth do not confuse them but simply sort them into separate-sounding codes.

EARLY COMMUNICATION
Your baby learns very soon after birth to recognize the familiar voices of his parents and will be calmed by the sound of them; he may be familiar with them from the time before he was born. By the age of 3 months, he will be squealing and gurgling, usually with pleasure, as an early means of communication. Many babies also love to blow endless raspberries at this age, which helps exercise their facial muscles for speaking.

PREPARING TO TALK
By 4–6 months of age, your baby will start to babble, which involves making a repetitive consonant-vowel sound, often "goo" and "ga" (regardless of which language he will then go on to speak). It was once thought that babbling was simply a meaningless succession of random sounds, but it is now believed that babbling represents a baby's first attempts to practice his speech.

By 6 months, your baby may show the first signs that he is understanding what you are saying to him. However, it is important to remember that there is considerable variation from one child to another.

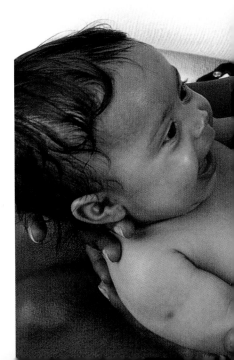

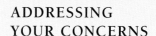

Firstborn children may develop language skills slightly faster than younger siblings, simply because they generally have greater undivided attention from their parents. Older siblings also may ask for things that their younger siblings want or say things that they mean, saving them the trouble of having to say it for themselves. In any case, between the ages of 6 and 9 months your baby will start to understand when you name a familiar person, such as daddy, or an object, such as "ball." He may also start to understand his own name. Around this time, your baby may start to make some single-syllable sounds, although these will not yet be recognizable words.

FIRST WORDS

By the time your baby is between 9 and 12 months, he may understand certain simple commands and questions, such as "No," "Give me," and "Where is…?". He increasingly responds to words, music, and the world around him.

At this stage, your baby may often say "dada" and "mama" as part of his more expressive babbling, which can sound quite melodious, as if he is talking to himself. Babbling can also convey, with surprising effectiveness, whether your baby is happy or angry.

The first few recognizable words your baby utters can occur from about 9 months to when he is over a year old. Sometimes your baby creates his own first word by combining portions of two words or mispronouncing a word (a person's name, for example). The word may not be recognizable to other people, but if he consistently uses it and you understand it, then it counts as a word as far as you and your baby are concerned.

ADDRESSING YOUR CONCERNS

My 12-month-old baby has still not shown signs of saying his first words.

If he appears to understand what you are saying and is successfully communicating by other means such as pointing and babbling, then there is probably no cause for concern. It is simply taking him a little longer to figure out his language (this may be the case with bilingual children and second or subsequent children). Some children bypass the first words stage entirely and, some months later, launch straight into uttering two-word mini-sentences.

He may need to have his hearing checked thoroughly. Children who are slow to speak may have an underlying hearing problem.

If your baby seems to be slow in other areas of his physical or mental development or is not successfully babbling, you should seek medical advice at this stage. You will probably have a gut feeling about whether seeking professional advice is necessary or not, although keep in mind that it may be too early to diagnose any major learning difficulties when your baby is under the age of 1 year.

My 2-year-old's pronunciation of certain sounds is much less clear than her older sister's was at the same age. Does this mean there's a problem?

Again, it may be worth getting her hearing tested just to rule out any possible hearing problems. However, speech development varies from child to child, even within the same family. Most children at the age of 2 mispronounce many sounds, especially "r"s and "l"s. At such an early age there is unlikely to be a problem, but consult your doctor if you are concerned.

SOCIAL SKILLS

Y OUR BABY WILL GAIN INCREASING AWARENESS of the world around her during her first year. She will discover her own separate identity and will learn to interact with people with whom she comes into contact. Learning how to interact with others is an important part of normal development and you can have a great influence on the way that her social skills evolve.

Milestones

6 weeks Your baby may give you his first smile. Many parents believe that their baby smiles earlier than this, and recent research indicates that babies may in fact produce real smiles earlier than 6 weeks.

3–6 months Your baby will be increasingly responsive to you and will watch you with interest.

6–12 months Your baby may begin to show separation anxiety (crying and clinging) when you leave her (*see opposite*).

9–12 months Your baby becomes increasingly responsive to people other than her parents.

12–18 months Your baby will play alongside other babies, sometimes imitating their actions.

15 months Your baby's separation anxiety may begin to lessen, although in some babies it persists into early childhood (*see p.129*).

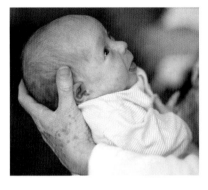

SOCIAL DEVELOPMENT
As early as 6 weeks, if not earlier, your baby will be producing her first smiles – one of the first signs that she is reacting to the world outside. By the time she is 3 months old, she will be looking at her parents with particular interest, following them with her eyes and turning her head toward them as she hears them entering the room.

Between 3 and 6 months old, she is able to play more because she is holding toys and waving her arms around. She now responds more to her parents than to other people, even those she sees regularly.

From 6 months onward, your baby's sense of humor begins to emerge and she will start to laugh and delight in games such as tickling and peekaboo. However, between 6 and 12 months, she may also start to show what is called separation anxiety (*see opposite*), where she starts to cry and

even cling to you if you leave her. This is normal and arises because she now has a sense of people's separate identities and of things existing outside her field of vision (that is, beyond the confines of the room).

RESPONSE TO OTHERS
By the time your baby is 9 months old, she will react warmly to people she knows and may be a little wary of those she does not. She responds to simple questions and can point and babble, so she is increasingly able to interact with other people.

Babies are usually very social, and the more time they can spend with other children of roughly the same age, the more they will develop their social skills. This means that, in addition to learning to play with another child, rather than simply alongside, they learn the notion of sharing and exchanging toys. This is a concept that can be introduced some time during their second year.

Possessiveness
It is important for children to learn that not everything belongs to them, but don't try to introduce the idea of sharing to your child before she is ready. Also, be prepared for your child to take some time to get used to sharing. Like many other things, sharing comes more easily to some children than others.

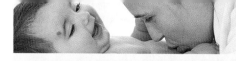

SETTING BOUNDARIES

Babies adore cuddling, kisses, and positive words of encouragement and praise. But at some stage before the end of the first year, you will also have to start saying no to her and set boundaries on her behavior. Children are born with no preset notions of boundaries, but by testing parents and caregivers they learn where the limits of acceptable behavior lie. Only you can decide what the boundaries are for your child, but by being firm and consistent in your approach whatever they are, you will give your child greater confidence and security when she ventures out beyond the immediate family.

Loving your child means providing her with enough social awareness that she will be able to fit in with the world at large, as well as giving her the more usual signs of affection, such as cuddling and kisses, and telling her you love her.

SEPARATION ANXIETY

Separation anxiety, when your child cries and clings if you leave her, is normal but still distressing for most parents. When leaving a crying baby in the care of a trusted person, don't make too much of the situation. Stay calm, provide a distraction such as a toy, then say goodbye quickly, without lingering – lengthy hugs give out alarming signals to your baby. She will usually cease crying within minutes of you leaving.

Knowing you always come back, your baby will realize that she is not being abandoned. This will make her more confident and independent and more comfortable being in the care of others.

ADDRESSING YOUR CONCERNS

My 12-month-old baby isn't interested in playing with other babies – is something wrong?
Babies don't learn to play with their peers until they are much older, usually between the ages of 18 months and 2 years. Up until then, babies tend to play alongside one another, often looking to see what others are doing and sometimes copying them. When the time comes, encourage your baby to interact with other children.

My 6-month-old baby doesn't always respond to noises around her. Is this normal?
Many babies do not always react when they hear even very loud noises around them – it may depend on their mood. If in doubt, get her hearing checked, even if she was screened as a newborn – it may be that she can hear certain sounds but not others. Profound deafness is rare, but hearing difficulties, many of which are treatable, are relatively common. It's important to detect these early so that speech development isn't delayed.

Why doesn't my 6-month-old make eye contact with me?
By this age, she should be eager to look at the world around her and to watch her parents in particular. Failure either to follow you around the room or to notice when you enter her field of vision could indicate a visual impairment. Lack of interest in making actual eye contact when you are near her and talking to her could indicate some form of learning difficulty (see p.147) or possible signs of autism (see p.299 for other symptoms). Talk to your doctor if you are worried.

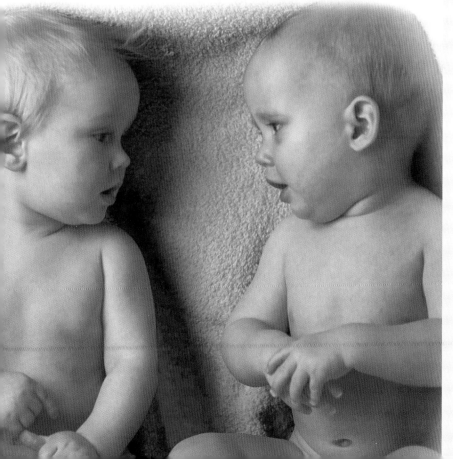

PLAY

CHILDREN ARE NATURALLY CURIOUS AND WILL EXPLORE the world they live in through play, particularly during their early years. One of the most rewarding aspects of having a baby is being able to play with him. This gives you the opportunity to see how his games and imagination develop over months and years and to share unforgettable memories and experiences with him.

Toys and activities

Toys are important for a baby's development, because they stimulate him both mentally and physically. Below are some toys and activities that are appropriate at different stages:

0–3 months
- Mobiles
- Baby gyms
- Musical or squeaky toys

Bold, contrasting colors and shapes are best for all of the above.

3–6 months
- Rattles and toys he can hold easily
- Squeezy, squeaky toys
- Pop-up toys
- Activity mats

6–9 months
- Bells, shakers
- Activity toys that rattle, spin, reflect
- Soft toys
- Easy-stacking toys
- Activity centers

9–12 months
- Push-along toys
- Stacking and sorting toys
- Books (picture/pop-up/activity)
- Songs (especially with actions)

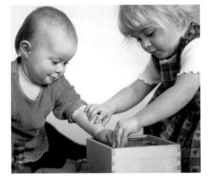

LEARNING THROUGH PLAY

Play will entertain your baby, and, by broadening his knowledge of the world, will have a crucial role in his development. There are many ways to have fun with your baby: some are verbal, musical, or physical games, and some involve toys or everyday household objects. Children, especially very young ones, quickly and easily absorb new experiences and learn from them.

Periodically put your baby on the floor to play tummy-down on the floor so he can see the world from a new angle and learn to push up on his arms. Once your baby is 6 weeks old, try an infant or bouncing seat so that he is propped up to play on the floor. Check the weight and age guidelines provided by the manufacturer. An active baby can tip the seat over so place it on a carpeted floor near you and away from sharp-edged furniture.

Children get tired of constantly playing with the same toys, so consider putting some toys away for a week or so while your baby plays with others, then swap these with the ones that were put away.

Resist the temptation to give your baby toys that are too advanced for his age. These will not make your baby more "intelligent," and he may get frustrated that he cannot play with them properly.

Refrain from too quickly finishing a game for your baby that he finds difficult. Show him how after a period of unsuccessful attempts. Remember to praise his efforts.

WHICH TOYS ARE BEST?

From 0–3 months, your baby can't discriminate well among colors but can distinguish between red and yellow more than blue and green. He prefers things that move (such as mobiles), have a high degree of contrast, and have interesting or complex contours (such as black and white patterns). He also prefers symmetrical designs and circular outlines rather than square ones.

Between 4 and 6 months, your baby will enjoy rattles and other easy-to-hold toys. He will especially like those he can wave around, hit, or squeeze to create a sound. Place toys just out of reach to encourage him to reach out and pick them up.

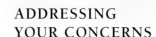

Once your baby is 6–9 months old, he will probably be sitting up and crawling, and this opens up vast possibilities for play. This is the sensory motor stage and he loves toys that rattle, spin, and pop up, as well as jingly bells and shakers. Babies enjoy mirrors at this age, because they are fascinated by their own reflection. Help your baby explore by providing safe, clean toys for him to play with. Many objects will probably go into his mouth, because it has more nerve endings than any other part of his body and is the best way of exploring things.

When he is 9–12 months old, his added mobility and understanding of the world will mean that baby toys that he can push, particularly those in which he can store other toys or objects, become very popular. Stacking and sorting toys and easy-to-hold building blocks are also good. Walkers with moving wheels are dangerous and can cause injury or even death. Do not use them. A safer option for your baby is a stationary activity center with toys and a rotating or bouncing seat.

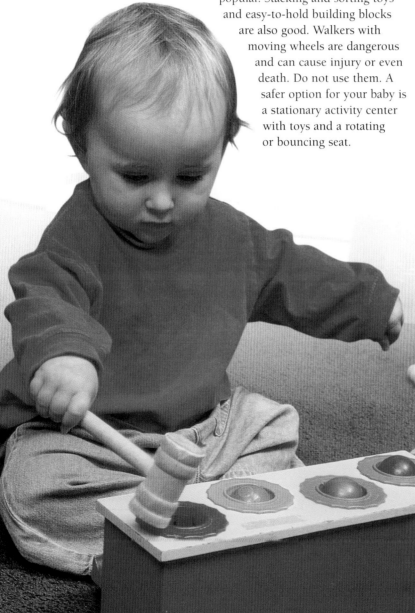

ADDRESSING YOUR CONCERNS

I don't really know how to play with my baby. What is the best way to begin?

Playing with your baby can be fun for you both, and play is essential for developing his mental and physical development. You don't need to buy your baby expensive toys to have a happy playtime.

- Play repetitive games with him and, eventually, he will mimic you.
- Play peekaboo and hiding games.
- Use ordinary objects as toys (boxes, big wooden spoons, saucepans, and lids are favorites, though, as always, you should supervise).
- Accept that messiness is necessary once you have a baby. Enjoy knocking down that pile of blocks.
- Going to a park can be fun and your child will meet other children too. Swings, slides, and climbing gyms will help develop his coordination and self-confidence.

My baby does not seem interested in people or playing.

You should have his hearing checked, because he may have impaired hearing that prevents him from connecting with the outside world.

Although rare, your child may have a learning problem or a disorder of development. Consult your doctor if your child does not seem to enjoy physical contact with you, makes poor eye contact, and has slow language development.

It may be difficult to form any firm judgment during the first year but, if in doubt, consult your doctor for further assessments to be arranged, although it may not be possible to provide a conclusive diagnosis at this early age. Make sure your concerns are taken seriously. If there is a problem, the earlier it is identified, the more help can be given to your child.

GOING BACK TO WORK

I F YOU ARE PLANNING TO GO BACK TO WORK, it is important to do advance preparation before deciding which working and child care arrangements suits your child, you, and your family best. The search for quality child care will involve many factors, including the type of caregiver arrangement, location, and cost.

Child care

Decide what type of child care suits your situation, whether it involves an in-home caregiver, a child care center, or a relative who can help out. Start looking for a caregiver well in advance and check her background, training, and references.

Choose the highest quality child care available – low ratio of children to caregivers, low caregiver turnover rate, and a healthy and safe environment.

Plan practice days where you and your caregiver are both with your baby to ease into the arrangement. Have an in-home caregiver visit you at home, or visit the child care center or family home that you have chosen, before starting care.

Make a backup plan for unexpected circumstances. Determine in advance what you will do if your child is too sick to attend child care or if your caregiver is sick or on vacation.

PREPARING FOR THE TRANSITION

If you are organized for returning to work, you may feel a lot calmer, and the transition between being at home and returning to work will be easier.

If this is your first baby, do your research early concerning the various child care options. For babysitters, nannies, and child care centers, it is never too early to start making inquiries. Have a list of interview questions for potential care providers and select the one that best meets your needs.

If this is not your first baby, plan how your existing caregiver will manage the new baby along with your other children. Routines may have to be adapted.

You can still breastfeed if you are working outside the home.

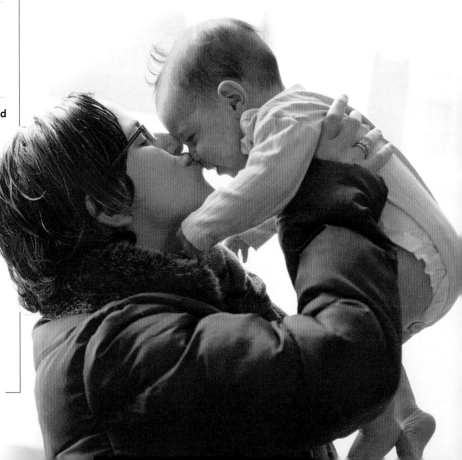

Some options include nursing your baby during your workday breaks if your baby is in a child-care center at your workplace or nearby, or expressing breastmilk while you are at work for your baby to drink later. Plan to breastfeed before going to work and upon returning home. In advance of your return to work, discuss feeding plans with your caregiver and determine if there is a place at work for pumping breastmilk or breastfeeding.

YOUR CAREGIVER

Start writing down your baby's routine a few weeks before going back to work, so that the caregiver can have a written diary of your baby's typical day. You should also allow at least one week's transition time. This allows your caregiver to get to know you, your baby, and your home. You can also show her around any local parks or playgroups and introduce her to other local families and neighbors.

PREPARING MENTALLY

Depending on several factors, you may feel apprehensive about your ability to perform your job.

If possible, go into work for a couple of hours before actually starting back. This will give you a chance to reconnect with your workplace and may make the first true day back much less stressful.

It also helps if you accept that the person who will care for your baby will not do things exactly as you do. This does not mean that things are worse, simply that they are different. Ongoing dialogue with your caregiver is important, but be prepared to explore other child-care options if you are not able to resolve major differences.

PARENTAL BENEFITS QUESTIONS & ANSWERS

Who qualifies for benefits?

If you are an employee, Employment Insurance will probably allow you to receive benefits while you take time off work to care for your new child. Birth mothers receive maternity benefits, and usually also qualify for parental benefits. Both parents, including adoptive parents, can receive parental benefits.

To qualify for these benefits, you must show that your regular weekly earnings have been decreased by more than 40%, and that you have accumulated 600 insured hours in the last 52 weeks or since your last claim.

How much will I receive?

You are entitled to 55% of your salary up to a maximum amount of $413 per week. Your EI payment is a taxable income, and most other income you receive while you are receiving maternity or parental benefits will be deducted dollar for dollar from your benefits. However, certain additional benefits from your employer may not affect your maternity or parental benefits. Your Employment Insurance officer can advise you.

If you are in a low-income family (an income of less than $25,921) with children and are receiving the Canada Child Tax Benefit (CCTB), you are also entitled to Family Supplement.

How do I apply?

To receive maternity or parental benefit you must submit an EI application on-line or in person to your local office. You should apply as soon as you stop working, even if you receive or will receive money when you become unemployed.

Who receives maternity benefits and for how long?

Maternity benefits are payable to the birth mother (or surrogate mother) for a maximum of 15 weeks. You need to prove your pregnancy by signing a statement declaring the expected due or actual date of birth.

You can start collecting maternity benefits as early as 8 weeks before the expected birth date and up to 17 weeks after the actual or expected week, whichever is later.

If your baby is hospitalized, the period during which you can claim maternity benefits can be extended.

Who receives parental benefits?

In addition to maternity benefits, parents can also receive parental benefits, which are payable to either the biological or adoptive parents while they are caring for a new-born or an adopted child, up to a maximum of 35 weeks. You must sign a statement declaring the newborn's date of birth, or, when there is an adoption, the child's date of placement for the purpose of the adoption, and the name and address of the adoption authority.

Parental benefits can be claimed by one parent or shared between the two partners for up to a combined maximum of 35 weeks.

When can I collect this benefit?

Parental benefits for biological parents and their partners are payable from the child's birth date, and for adoptive parents and their partners from the date the child is placed with you. Parental benefits are only available within the 52 weeks following the child's birth or, for adoptive parents, within the 52 weeks from the date the child is placed with you.

If your child is hospitalized, you can choose to claim parental benefits immediately following the child's birth/ placement or when he comes home from the hospital. Each week your child is hospitalized extends the period in which you can claim parental benefits, up to a maximum of 104 weeks.

EVERYDAY CONCERNS

A T SOME STAGE DURING HIS FIRST YEAR, your baby's health will almost certainly cause you concern. In most instances, the problem will be minor and can be solved by you alone. In others, you may need to consult your doctor. You will soon learn to distinguish between the different situations but, if in doubt, always contact your doctor – it is better to be reassured than to worry about your baby's health.

Other problems

The following conditions are common in babies up to 1 year old and are covered in the Diseases & Disorders chapter:

Bronchiolitis, an infection of the smaller airways of the lungs (*see p.228*)

Common cold, a minor viral infection frequent in babies (*see p.221*)

Conjunctivitis, an infection of the membrane covering the eye (*see p.244*)

Croup, a form of laryngitis that affects babies and children (*see p.224*)

Febrile seizures, convulsions that may occur during a fever (*see p.292*)

Gastroenteritis, an infection of the gastrointestinal tract (*see p.254*)

Gingivostomatitis, blisters in the mouth (*see p.247*)

Hernia, protrusion of an organ through a weakness in the abdominal muscle (*see p.260*)

Impetigo, a bacterial infection of the skin (*see p.235*)

Oral thrush, a yeast infection of the mouth (*see p.248*)

Roseola infantum, a mild infection that causes a fever followed by a rash (*see p.267*)

Seborrheic dermatitis, a flaky, oily skin condition (*see p.230*)

DIAPER RASH

Diaper rash causes the skin on your baby's bottom, and sometimes in his crotch and inner legs, to become red and sore. Occasionally the skin can become blistery and infected, in which case your doctor may prescribe a medicated cream or ointment to reduce the inflammation and treat the infection.

Babies' skin is very sensitive, particularly during the first 6 months. Ammonia, which is naturally present in the urine, as well as illness and diarrhea, can all act as a trigger for diaper rash. Some babies are more prone to it than others, but the majority of babies will have diaper rash at some stage. Fortunately, babies' skin heals very quickly, so, with proper treatment, diaper rash should disappear within a few days or a week at most.

If your baby develops diaper rash, use plain warm water to clean the area. Pat your baby's bottom dry

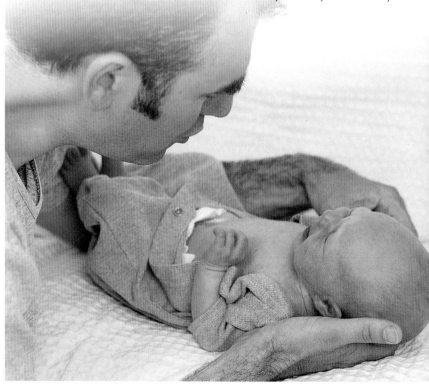

with a soft towel or, better still, let it dry naturally. Leave his bottom uncovered as much as possible. Change his diaper frequently and immediately after every bowel movement or wet diaper. Consult your doctor if there has been no improvement after 3–4 days.

To help prevent or treat diaper rash, you can apply an emollient cream or petroleum jelly during each diaper change, although if you change the diaper frequently, you may not need to do this at all.

GASTROESOPHAGEAL REFLUX DISEASE

Gastroesophageal reflux disease (GERD) is a common problem for babies during the first year of life because the muscle at the entrance to their stomach is weak, which can cause some or all of the stomach contents to be regurgitated. The condition most often develops in the first few weeks after birth but, in most cases, babies outgrow the problem by the time they are 1 year old.

The main symptoms of GERD are persistent vomiting, regurgitation of feedings, crying, irritability, and failure to thrive (if the problem persists). If vomit is bloodstained, see your doctor immediately.

If you think your baby has GERD, consult your doctor. He or she may perform tests for a definitive diagnosis and may also prescribe drugs to help reduce the vomiting.

If your baby has GERD, raise the end of the crib so that his head is slightly higher than his stomach. Burp your baby well and keep him upright for 20–30 minutes after feeding. During the day, put your baby in a reclining chair (or a high chair if he can sit up). Consult your doctor if the problem is persistent and severe. Give food that

is more solid when possible, but do not introduce solids until your baby is old enough (see p.38) and make sure he does not become constipated from lack of fluids.

EARACHES

Earaches are very common in children and inflammation of the middle ear, or otitis media, is the most common cause (see p.240). If your baby has an earache, he may cry and try to pull or rub his ear. He may also have a fever (over 38°C/100.4°F) and may wake at night. Ear infections often occur along with a common cold. Consult your doctor.

TEETHING

Your baby will probably cut his first tooth when he is between 6 months and 1 year old (perhaps slightly older). His final baby, or primary, teeth will emerge when he is around age 3. Although the eruption of the baby teeth at the front of the mouth (the incisors) often causes little or no pain, the eruption of the canines and molars may be more painful.

When teething, your baby may develop red cheeks and sore gums and may drool a lot. He may become irritable, cry more, and sleep poorly. To alleviate pain, try rubbing a teething gel on the gum, letting him chew on something hard and preferably cool (such as a special teething ring) and giving him liquid acetaminophen or ibuprofen. Consult your doctor about the appropriate dose for your child and whether other products may help. While a low-grade temperature may be associated with teething, higher fever and severe diarrhea are rarely symptoms of teething and should prompt you to call your doctor.

CALLING THE DOCTOR

As a general rule of thumb, trust your instinct: if you think there is something wrong with your baby and you are worried, call your doctor.

You should call the doctor when your baby:
- Has a fever higher than 38°C/100.4°F. A baby's temperature can rise and fall very quickly and is a good gauge of whether something, however minor, is wrong.
- Cries more than usual and cannot be calmed.
- Cannot sleep, or sleeps only fitfully.
- Is unusually lethargic or drowsy.
- Has a rash.
- Is not feeding well.
- Vomits more than once during a 24-hour period.
- Is unable to keep down any foods or even water.
- Has diarrhea or any blood in his stools or urine.
- Has sunken or, conversely, swollen fontanelles (soft spots on the head) – see a doctor immediately.
- Is not breathing easily (he may be wheezing or breathing unusually quickly).
- Develops a cough.
- Appears to be in pain or to have developed an infection.

Remember that babies can quickly become dehydrated, so it is important that you see your doctor very soon if your baby is persistently not taking in fluids and/or vomits repeatedly or develops persistent diarrhea. In an emergency situation, seek medical attention immediately.

FEVER IN BABIES

FEVER DEVELOPS WHEN THE BODY'S TEMPERATURE rises significantly above normal. This usually happens when the body is fighting an infection. If your baby is hot or appears listless or irritable, take his temperature (*p.324*): the normal (oral) range is 36–38°C (97–100.4°F); a fever is 38°C (100.4°F) or above.

SYMPTOM	POSSIBLE CAUSE
Is your child under 3 months? Is your child 3–6 months with a temperature greater than 38.3°C (101°F) or over 6 months with a temperature greater than 39.4°C (103°F)?	Fever in babies younger than 3 months is unusual; it may be a sign of a serious illness. Higher fevers in older babies may also be a sign of significant infection.
Does your baby have a bumpy or flat pink rash (Rash with fever, *p.186*)?	Roseola infantum (*p.267*) or another virus.
Does he have a rash made up of tiny red spots that do not disappear (Rash with fever, *p.186*)?	Pinpoint red or purple spots may indicate a serious infection.
Does your baby cry and pull at one ear or wake up screaming?	Inflammation of the middle ear (*p.240*).
If your baby's breathing rate is normal, does he have a cough or a runny nose?	A common cold (*p.221*), or possibly influenza (*p.225*) or another virus.
Is your baby's breathing rate faster than normal?	Pneumonia (*p.227*) or bronchiolitis (*p.228*).
Is your baby vomiting without diarrhea, abnormally drowsy, or unusually irritable?	Meningitis (*p.294*) or other serious infection.
Is your baby vomiting with diarrhea?	Gastroenteritis (*p.254*).
Is your baby wearing a lot of clothing or is the room very warm?	Your baby may have become overheated.
Is your older baby reluctant to eat solid food?	A throat infection, such as tonsillitis (*p.223*) or a mouth infection, such as gingivostomatitis (*p.247*).

DANGER SIGNS

Call your doctor immediately if your baby is
showing one or more of the following symptoms:

- Abnormally rapid breathing
- Noisy breathing
- Difficulty breathing
- Abnormal drowsiness
- Irritability that is unusual for your baby

- Refusing to drink any fluids
- Vomiting that lasts for several hours,
  with or without diarrhea
- A temperature that exceeds 39°C (102°F).

ACTION NEEDED

Urgent! Call your doctor immediately.
Self-help Bringing down a temperature (*right*).

Get medical advice within 24 hours.

Emergency! Call your doctor immediately or seek
medical attention if your baby seems very sick.

Get medical advice within 24 hours.
Self-help Bringing down a temperature (*right*) and
Relieving earache (*p.205*).

If your child makes no improvement within 48 hours,
or if he develops breathing problems or a rash appears,
call your doctor.

Urgent! Call your doctor immediately.
Self-help Bringing down a temperature (*right*).

Urgent! Call your doctor immediately.

Get medical advice within 24 hours, or sooner if you
suspect dehydration.

If you suspect overheating, remove some of your baby's
clothing and reduce the room temperature. If he shows
any of the danger signs (*above*), consult your doctor.

If there is no improvement in 48 hours, call your
doctor. **Self-help** Relieving a sore throat (*p.198*) and
Bringing down a temperature (*right*).

SELF-HELP

Bringing down a temperature

When you bring down your child's high temperature,
he starts to feel less irritable and more comfortable.
If your child is between 3 months and 5 years, you
also reduce the risk of febrile seizures (*p.292*). The
following measures are for a child of any age:

- Remove some of your child's clothing.

- Cool your child with a cloth dipped in lukewarm water
  or in a lukewarm bath. Avoid cold water since this can
  raise the infant's core temperature. Do not use rubbing
  alcohol, which can cause serious problems.

- With your doctor's advice, give the recommended dose
  of acetaminophen. Ibuprofen can be used for a child
  over 6 months, but never give it to a child who is
  dehydrated or vomiting.

- Keep the room at a comfortable temperature.

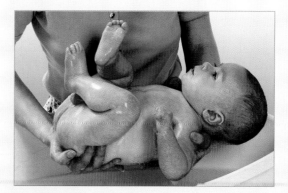

COOLING RELIEF *Give your child a bath in lukewarm water to
help reduce his temperature and give him relief from his fever.*

VOMITING IN BABIES

YOUNG BABIES WHO VOMIT may be suffering from an illness or harmlessly regurgitating small amounts of milk. Contact your doctor immediately if the vomiting continues for several hours or if it is accompanied by small amounts of dark urine, abnormal drowsiness, sunken eyes, or loose skin.

SYMPTOM	POSSIBLE CAUSE	ACTION NEEDED
Does your baby seem well and feed normally but bring up a large amount of milk effortlessly?	Gastroesophageal reflux disease (*p.57*).	Get medical advice within 24 hours.
Does your baby bring up a small amount of milk effortlessly?	Regurgitation is the most likely cause. It may be due to gas and is rarely serious.	**Self-help** Dealing with gas (*p.65*). Check that you are not overfeeding your baby.
If your baby is under 2 months, does she vomit after every feeding?	Pyloric stenosis (*p.260*).	Get medical advice within 24 hours.
Does your baby vomit unpredictably, have a fever, or either appear abnormally drowsy or refuse to eat or drink?	Meningitis (*p.294*) or other serious illness.	**Urgent!** Call your doctor immediately.
Does your baby vomit repeatedly and have diarrhea?	Gastroenteritis (*p.254*).	**Urgent!** Call your doctor immediately. **Self-help** Preventing dehydration (*p.63*).
Does your baby vomit repeatedly and have a cough?	Bronchiolitis (*p.228*) or pertussis (*p.269*).	Get medical advice within 24 hours. **Self-help** Bringing down a temperature (*p.59*) and Relieving a cough (*p.197*).
Does your baby vomit repeatedly and produce a greenish yellow vomit?	Intestinal obstruction (*p.256*).	**Urgent!** Call your doctor immediately. In the meantime, do not give your baby anything to eat or drink.

FEEDING PROBLEMS

PARENTS AND BABIES CAN BOTH SUFFER if difficulties with feeding develop. The first few weeks after birth in particular can be difficult while breastfeeding is established. If your baby is well and gains weight normally, there is probably no cause for concern.

SYMPTOM	POSSIBLE CAUSE	ACTION NEEDED
Is your baby failing to gain weight normally?	Feeding problems or poor nutrition.	Consult your doctor.
Is your baby gaining weight normally yet you are worried you are not producing sufficient milk?	Mothers commonly feel they are not producing sufficient milk if their baby cries a lot and seems difficult to satisfy.	If your baby continues to cry and you are concerned, consult your doctor. See also EXCESSIVE CRYING (pp.64–65).
Is your baby refusing feedings when he is usually eager?	Suddenly refusing to feed may be a sign of a cold (p.221), but it could be more serious.	Get medical advice within 24 hours.
Is your baby usually unwilling to feed but is gaining weight normally?	Some babies need to be coaxed to feed and may even fall asleep while feeding. If the baby seems well, there is no need to worry.	If other symptoms develop or you have any concerns, consult your doctor.
Does your baby feed more often than other babies?	Frequent feeding, as often as once every 2 hours, is normal in breastfed babies, particularly in the first few weeks of life (see Breastfeeding, pp.18–21).	If your are concerned about your baby's feeding, consult your doctor.
Does your baby often cry at the beginning of a feeding?	The breasts may not release milk immediately, or the flow may be too forceful.	**Self-help** If your milk isn't released right away, try to relax. If the flow is too forceful, express some milk before your baby starts to feed.
Does your baby often reject certain solid foods you offer?	Unfamiliar foods and textures may be rejected and even foods that were accepted initially may later be refused.	**Self-help** Keep offering a varied diet to give your baby the best chance of receiving sufficient healthy nutrients (see Starting Solid Foods, pp.38–41).

DIARRHEA IN BABIES

I F YOUR BABY PASSES RUNNY STOOLS twice or more in a row, or intermittently in 24 hours, she probably has diarrhea. Remember, though, that the semifluid stools that breastfed babies often pass is not the same as diarrhea. Babies with diarrhea are prone to dehydration unless you give them plenty of fluids.

SYMPTOM	POSSIBLE CAUSE
Does your baby have a fever – a temperature of 38°C (100.4°F) or above?	Gastroenteritis (*p.254*).
If there is no fever, has the diarrhea lasted for 2 weeks or more, even if it has been intermittent?	A viral infection is the most likely cause. Other possible but much less common causes are allergies to food (*p.252*), giardiasis (*p.262*), celiac disease (*p.256*), and cystic fibrosis (*p.315*).
If your baby has had diarrhea for less than 2 weeks, has she suffered from vomiting, poor feeding, or lethargy in the past few days?	Gastroenteritis (*p.254*).
Have you been giving your baby prescribed medicine for any other disorder?	Your baby's diarrhea could be a side effect of the medicine that she is taking.
Is your baby drinking more juice than usual?	In large quantities, the sugar in fruit juice can lead to diarrhea.
Has your baby's diarrhea appeared within 24 hours of new food being introduced?	New foods may cause diarrhea.
Has your baby not yet been given solid food or have you introduced a new food into your baby's diet more than 24 hours ago?	Reactions to food (*p.252*) or mild gastroenteritis (*p.254*).

Call your doctor immediately if your baby is showing any of the following symptoms:

- Abnormal drowsiness or irritability
- Refusing feedings for several hours
- Vomiting for several hours
- Sunken eyes
- Passing small amounts of urine.

ACTION NEEDED

Get medical advice within 24 hours.
Self-help Preventing dehydration (*right*) and Bringing down a temperature (*p.59*).

Consult your doctor within 24 hours.
Self-help Give small, frequent feedings of your baby's usual milk and solid foods.

Get medical advice within 24 hours.
Self-help Preventing dehydration (*right*) and Bringing down a temperature (*p.59*).

Ask your doctor to find out whether the medicine may be causing your baby's symptoms and whether you should stop giving it.

Limit your child to 120–180 ml (4–6 oz) of 100% juice in children ages 1–6 and 240–360 ml (8–12 oz) in older children. Avoid giving your baby sugary drinks. Choose milk or water whenever possible.

Such episodes are usually short-lived. If it is not, or if it seems to be associated with particular foods, consult your doctor.
Self-help Preventing dehydration (*right*). If you know which food is causing the diarrhea, stop giving it until you see the doctor.

Get medical advice within 24 hours.
Self-help Stop solid food until you see the doctor. Preventing dehydration (*right*).

Preventing dehydration

Water is a vital fluid which must always be replaced after it leaves the body. When a baby loses more water than she is taking in, there is a danger of her becoming dehydrated. Dehydration is extremely serious and may result from conditions such as persistent diarrhea or a fever, or from vomiting for several hours. In each case, it is important to give your child extra fluids. Consult your doctor if you are in any doubt about which rehydrating solution is best to use.

- The best way to give your baby the extra fluids she needs is as a commercially available oral electrolyte rehydrating solution. You can buy these without a prescription.

- Every baby needs to drink between 300 ml (10 fl.oz) and 1,200 ml (40 fl.oz) of fluids each day. Exactly how much fluid depends on the baby's weight – see the table below to find out how much fluid to give your baby every day.

- If your baby's diarrhea is accompanied by vomiting, give her frequent small amounts of rehydrating solution.

This table shows the minimum daily fluid requirement for a normal child. Most children drink more than this. The third column lists the recommended amount of electrolyte solution for a child with mild diarrhea.

ESTIMATED ORAL FLUID AND ELECTROLYTE REQUIREMENTS BY BODY WEIGHT					
Baby's weight		Minimum daily fluid requirements		Electrolyte requirements	
kg	lb	ml	fl.oz	ml	fl.oz
3–3.2	6–7	300	10	470	16
5	11	440	15	680	23
10	22	740	25	1200	40
12	26	830	28	1300	44
15	33	950	32	1500	51
18	40	1100	38	1800	61

EXCESSIVE CRYING

CRYING IS HOW BABIES COMMUNICATE THEIR NEEDS. You may soon be able to distinguish between your baby's different cries. You should never shake a baby. This may lead to blindness, brain damage, or even death. If the crying is inconsolable or sounds unusual, call your doctor immediately.

SYMPTOM	POSSIBLE CAUSE
Does your baby stop crying when you feed him?	Hunger is one of the most common causes of crying in a young baby.
If your baby's crying is unusual, was he reluctant to take the last feeding?	Your baby may be in pain as a result of a disorder, such as inflammation of the middle ear (*p.240*) or gastrointestinal illness (*p.251*).
Does your baby's crying seem to be related to increased tension at home?	Your baby may be unsettled because of a change in routine or increased stress.
Is your baby comforted by drinking or eating?	Thirst or hunger may be causing your baby to cry excessively, especially if the weather is particularly hot, or if he is having a growth spurt.
When you burp your baby, does he stop crying?	Gas (*p.17*).
If your baby is under 3 months, does he cry in late afternoon or early evening?	Colic (*p.25*).
If your baby is 3 months or older, does he stop crying when you pick him up and give him your full attention?	Your baby may need more comforting and parental reassurance than other babies of the same age.

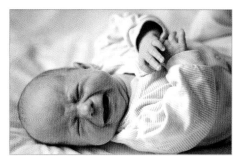

CRY BABY *Crying is the most effective way your baby can attract your attention. You soon learn to recognize whether the cry is urgent or not.*

ACTION NEEDED

Self-help If your baby stops crying after a feeding, you may need to feed more frequently to keep up with the demand.

Urgent! Call your doctor immediately.

Self-help During a period of change, give your baby extra attention. Try to reduce the source of the stress. If you have concerns about your baby's crying, consult your doctor.

Self-help Give your baby age-appropriate liquid or food.

Self-help Dealing with gas (*right*).

Self-help Feed your baby if he is hungry. You can try to calm him by rocking, by patting his back, or by gently massaging his abdomen.

Self-help Cuddle your baby as often as he wants; there is no risk of "spoiling" your child at such a young age.

Dealing with gas

If your baby cries just before a feeding, or if he feeds quickly, he may take in air, which can irritate him when it is trapped in the intestine. The following tips may either prevent gas or help release it:

- If you are bottlefeeding, make sure the hole in the nipple in the bottle is unblocked and the right size.

- Let your baby lie in a semiupright position when he feeds so the milk falls to the bottom of his stomach.

- Burp your baby midway through and after every feeding to release trapped air. Either hold him against your shoulder or sit and put him face down on your lap. Calm him by rubbing him or patting his back.

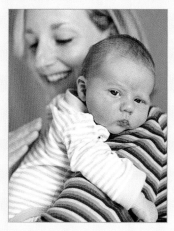

BURPING YOUR BABY *After every feeding, move your baby to a different position, such as upright against your shoulder, so that any gas can be released.*

Calming your baby

See also When Your Baby Cries, *p.27.*

Hands-on techniques
Gently stroke his head or pat his back. Swaddle your baby in a blanket.

Movement
Rock your baby, either in a chair or in your arms as you sway from side to side. Take him for a walk or go for a ride in his car safety seat or stroller.

Sound
A recording of a rhythmic sound, such as your heartbeat (or even the vacuum cleaner) may settle your baby. Singing, talking, or playing soft music may help.

SKIN PROBLEMS

YOUR BABY'S SKIN IS SO SENSITIVE it can easily become inflamed or irritated. If the inflammation or irritation does not fade naturally, or if it is accompanied by any other symptoms, consult your doctor. If your baby seems sick with a fever, see RASH WITH FEVER (*p.186*). If there's no fever, see SPOTS AND RASHES (*p.184*).

SYMPTOM	POSSIBLE CAUSE	ACTION NEEDED
If your baby is under 3 months, does she have an inflamed, scaly rash in two or more of: neck, face, groin, behind the ears, or armpits?	Seborrheic dermatitis (*p.230*).	If the rash does not clear up within a few weeks or if it is extensive or oozing, consult your doctor.
Does your baby have a scaly, itchy rash on the cheeks or around the elbow or knees?	Eczema (*p.234*).	If the rash is extensive, oozing, very itchy, or uncomfortable, consult your doctor.
Does your baby have crusty yellow patches on the scalp?	Cradle cap (*see* Seborrheic dermatitis, *p.230*).	If the crusts are extensive or if other symptoms develop, consult your doctor.
Does your baby have inflamed spots on the genitals or anus?	Diaper rash (*p.56*).	If the rash lasts over a few days or if the skin breaks or blisters, consult your doctor.
Does your baby have spots or blotches anywhere on the body yet is well and feeding normally?	A minor skin irritation.	If the rash lasts over a day or if your baby becomes sick, consult your doctor.

SELF-HELP

Relieving itching

If your child scratches itchy areas, an infection may develop. The following tips may help discourage her:

• When bathing your child, use a nonirritating substance, such as plain water or a mild baby soap. Avoid frequent long baths and the use of bubble-bath products. Make sure that the water is not too hot.

• Dry skin may make itching more severe. Moisturize the skin regularly.

• Avoid rough or irritating fabrics.

• Your doctor may recommend a special bath additive or skin ointment for itching.

SLOW WEIGHT GAIN

I F YOU AND YOUR CHILD SEE THE DOCTOR on a regular basis, you will be able to keep a close eye on how well your baby is putting on weight. Your doctor may have standard growth charts that can help you if you are interested in monitoring your child's weight.

SYMPTOM	POSSIBLE CAUSE	ACTION NEEDED
Does your baby seem sick?	An underlying disorder may be responsible for your baby's failure to gain weight normally.	Consult your doctor.
Are you breastfeeding exclusively?	You may need help with breastfeeding technique or you may not be producing enough milk to provide all the nutrients your baby needs.	If your baby is otherwise healthy, your doctor may recommend a lactation consultant, if available.
Do you mainly breastfeed or bottlefeed your baby according to a routine?	Insufficient milk may be responsible for your baby's failure to gain weight normally.	If there is no normal weight gain within 2 weeks, see your doctor. **Self-help** Offer a feeding when your baby cries, not in a strict routine.
Could you be adding too much water or too little formula to the bottle?	If feedings are too diluted, your baby may not be receiving enough nutrients.	If there is no normal weight gain within 2 weeks, see your doctor. **Self-help** Always follow the instructions for mixing formula.
Does your baby always finish the entire feeding?	Your baby may need more food than the amount you have been offering him.	If there is no normal weight gain within 2 weeks, see your doctor.
Has your baby started on solid foods?	You may not be giving enough solids to meet all your baby's nutritional needs.	See your doctor, who may recommend changes to your baby's diet. (*See also* Starting Solid Foods, *pp.38–41*.)

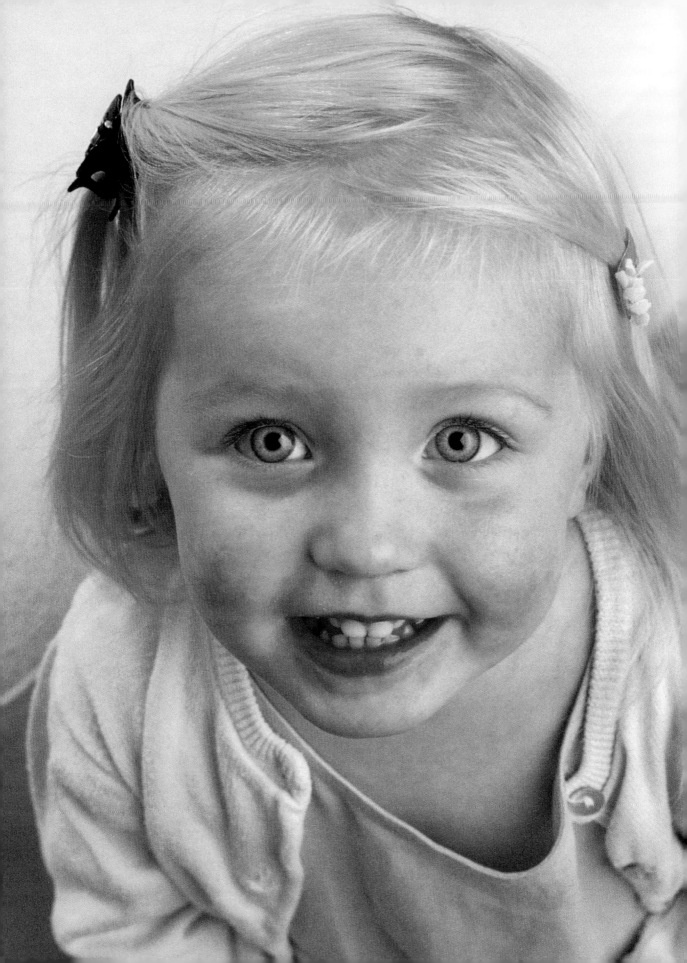

RAISING A HEALTHY CHILD

GROWING UP

Aᴌᴛʜᴏᴜɢʜ ᴀ ᴄʜɪʟᴅ's ʀᴀᴛᴇ ᴏꜰ ɢʀᴏᴡᴛʜ ɪꜱ ᴠᴇʀʏ ʀᴀᴘɪᴅ during the first year of life, it slows down considerably in the second year. Children's rates of development in other areas vary from child to child within a range of what is considered normal. Your child's general development will be checked at each examination to make sure that all is well.

"A child's growth… tends to happen in spurts, and children grow more rapidly in spring and summer than in autumn and winter."

GROWTH

A child's final height tends to reflect her parents' heights, regardless of her size at birth. Tall parents tend to have tall children, and shorter parents, shorter children. As a very rough rule of thumb, at the age of 2 a boy is likely to be about half of his adult height.

But growing taller isn't the only change that occurs after the first year. Your child's head, which at birth was about one-third of the size of an adult's, is almost full size by age 2. Muscles are stronger, bones are less flexible, and the heart is stronger and more proficient at pumping blood, so that the heart rate decreases and blood pressure increases. Digestion of food is more efficient and the immune system is now stronger.

Studies over the years show that children have been getting taller – better nutrition, smaller families, and improved living conditions having played their part. Today, 5-year-olds are, on average, 7–8cm (3–3½in) taller than 100 years ago. A child's growth isn't consistent either – it tends to happen in spurts, and children grow more rapidly in spring and summer than in autumn and winter. A study among 7- to 10-year-olds in Britain showed that between the months of March and July they grew three times more quickly than during their three months of slowest growth.

In between periods of growth, the body seems to rest. Children tend to grow more at night, because higher levels of growth hormone are secreted during sleep. For some children, growth at night can lead to periods of restless sleep. Ensure that your child gets enough sleep throughout childhood.

Rates of growth

Except for the rapid growth during the first year, and a growth spurt around midchildhood, both boys and girls grow at a steady rate of

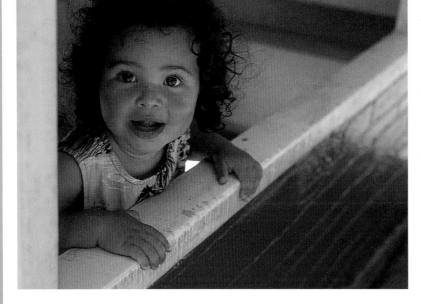

around 5–6cm (2–2½in) a year. Just before puberty, this slows to around 5cm (2in) a year, with boys typically being a little taller than girls. (For girls, puberty usually begins at about 10 years of age and for boys at about 12 years.) During the growth spurt that takes place during puberty, both boys and girls grow about 30–45cm (12–18in), generally reaching mature height by age 16 in girls and age 18 in boys. Not only do girls begin puberty earlier than boys, they tend to grow fastest at the beginning, while boys grow fastest in the last third of puberty. This means that for around two years, girls are often taller than boys of their own age.

Prepuberty growth

In the years leading up to puberty, many girls carry a little extra weight, often referred to as "baby fat." With the rapid growth that occurs at puberty, this extra weight soon disappears. For boys, rapid growth may make them appear underweight for a while, before they fill out. In both cases, this temporary awkwardness may give rise to the typical self-consciousness teenagers feel about their bodies. While most children tend to develop enormous appetites during puberty, some may have a tendency to become weight-conscious and picky about food. For healthy growth, both boys and girls need regular, nutritious meals, without too many snack foods and soft drinks that contain empty calories. In particular, adolescent boys and girls need an adequate intake of calcium from milk, yogurt, and cheese to promote healthy bone growth. This

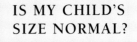

IS MY CHILD'S SIZE NORMAL?

There is a great variation in what is "normal" in terms of a child's height, and although most children follow the normal pattern of growth, there can be individual variations within this. Height is largely an inherited characteristic, and if both parents are tall or short, you can expect their children to be similar heights as adults. However, if you have a tall mother and a short father, for example, initially the baby's birth size will probably reflect the mother's size. During the first two years, the child's true genetic height, inherited from both parents, will emerge.

After the first year, a child's height is of more importance than his weight when it comes to detecting growth problems. A child may lose some weight during illness and growth in height may halt briefly, but after health returns there is usually catch-up growth.

If your child seems consistently small for his age as compared to his peers, or appears shorter than you might expect for your family, it's worth monitoring him for a short period and then consulting your doctor. Measure your child accurately several times over a six-month period, and record it on a growth chart (you can ask for one at your doctor's office). The height of a child with growth delay may not appear low on the chart, but the growth curve won't run parallel to the one on the chart. Monitoring your child's height will give an accurate summary of your concerns when you visit the doctor, and will help with the evaluation.

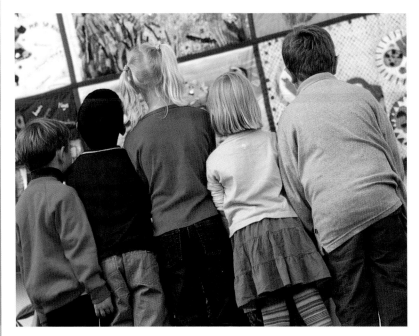

child is physically able to control the muscles of her bottom and bladder, which mature between roughly 18 and 30 months of age. In addition, your child must also be psychologically ready to toilet train. Most children become more independent and eager to please their parents around 18–24 months, so be sure he is physically and emotionally ready before you proceed. It's also worth noting that girls tend to be earlier than boys in their readiness for toilet training.

When should I start?

When your child's bladder is large enough to hold a reasonable quantity of urine and she is aware that she has been urinating or having a bowel movement, then she may be ready for toilet training. It's also important that she is willing to learn. It's a good idea to have a potty around and available in the bathroom for some months before your child is likely to be ready, since this allows your child to get used to sitting on it. She may even occasionally manage to use it successfully, which is a good basis from which to start.

In addition to being able to control her bowel and bladder muscles, there are other skills your child has probably been developing that will come in useful during toilet training. Can she remove her diapers or pants without help? Is she able to sit down on the potty and get up again easily? Is she able to tell you she needs the potty? All these things will make it easier to be successful when the time comes.

Some studies have reported that some children who begin toilet training before the age of 18 months aren't completely trained until after the age of 4, whereas those who

is especially important for girls to help reduce the risk of osteoporosis (brittle bones) later in life. Many teenagers need extra sleep during this period.

Growth delay

Around 3 percent of children are up to two years behind the average for their age in terms of growth, with boys being affected by this ten times more frequently than girls. Children with asthma or eczema also seem more likely to show a pattern of growth delay. This delay in growth may occur in early childhood, but it also may not happen until puberty is expected. Growth delay may be a family trait, with a parent or other family member having had a similar problem at puberty. For the majority of children with delayed growth there is no reason other than being a late developer, and they will catch up in time.

There can be a number of other reasons why a child's growth may be delayed, including a range of

hormonal deficiencies that need treatment. These problems can't be identified without specific tests, such as X-rays of the bones of the hand and wrist to assess the child's bone age and blood tests to check hormone levels.

Some children may have a dietary deficiency, such as anemia, or a problem absorbing food, such as celiac disease. These children will have other symptoms as well, including listlessness and feeling generally unwell. Rarely, psychological distress can affect the production of growth hormone, thereby affecting growth, but levels of distress have to be quite severe for this to happen. In these cases, normal growth resumes once the distress has been alleviated.

TOILET TRAINING

"Toilet training" is a bit of a misnomer, because you can't "train" any child to use a potty or the toilet until she is physically ready. Toilet training is only possible when your

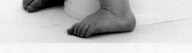

started at around 2 years old were completely trained before their third birthday. Starting to toilet train too early may actually prolong the learning process.

Once your child is ready, consider using a potty chair, which is easier for small children to sit on. Try to make trips to the potty a regular part of your child's daily routine, such as first thing in the morning, after meals, and before naps.

You will also need to give your child regular reminders that she might like to use the potty. Having asked, don't sit her on the potty unless she says yes; otherwise, she won't make the connection for herself. Sometimes she may say no,

and two minutes later realize she actually does feel the urge to go. For the best success in potty training, allow her to recognize and then respond to her own urges to use the toilet.

Some accidents are inevitable, but if your child is ready to manage without a diaper, these should be few. If they do occur, gently remind her what the potty is for, change her, and don't make a fuss. Reacting negatively may make your child resentful and less inclined to try.

Work on the principle of praising your child's efforts and successes and ignoring accidents as much as possible. If, after a week's effort, you find that no progress has been made,

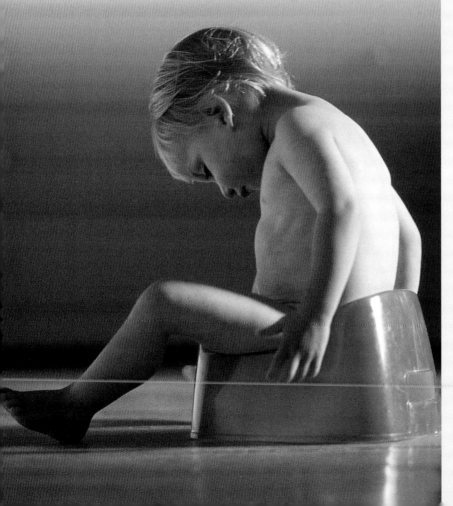

HOW TO START TOILET TRAINING

Start looking for signs that your child is ready to manage without a diaper.

- Has she seen you or other family members use the toilet?
- Is she aware of urinating or having a bowel movement, even when wearing a diaper, and does she tell you?
- Does she sit on and try to use a potty, perhaps before her bath in the evening?

When you feel your child is ready to start learning to use the toilet, the following tips may help.

- Avoid times when your child is coping with changes in her life: a move, a new baby in the family, or some other change to her life. It may be easier for both of you without additional stresses.
- Make sure the potty is easy and comfortable to sit on. For boys, it may be helpful to have one that has a higher splashguard at the front.
- For a boy, you will also have to help him understand that his penis needs to point inside the potty. It's easy for a boy to sit down quickly without checking and find he is going outside the potty.
- Encourage your child to tell you when he or she is about to urinate or have a bowel movement.
- You may have to tolerate several "accidents" before this is clear to your child. If your child does not make progress after a week or so, try going back to diapers for a short time and try again later.
- Carefully decide what words you use to describe body parts, urine, and bowel movements. Remember that other people will also hear those words, so choose proper terms that will not embarrass your child or others.

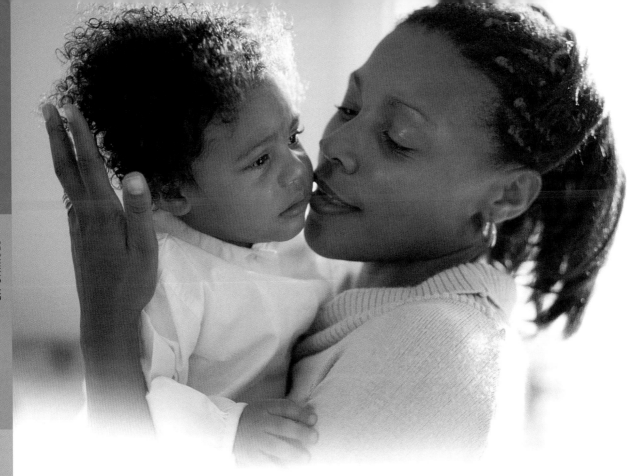

"...being handled and touched is important to babies and children. It gives them a sense of their physical existence"

go back to diapers for a few weeks. It may be that your child is not yet developmentally ready. It's less frustrating for you both if you take a break and try again in a few weeks. Remember that many children are still not trained by age 3, or even by age 4.

Even when your child is happily out of diapers during the day, she may still need a diaper for naps or nighttime, but you can introduce the idea of going without by getting her to use the potty before going to sleep. She may actually have a dry diaper as a consequence, especially when she wakes from her daytime nap, and you can praise her. If she is waking in the morning regularly with a dry diaper, then you can try going without one at night. Make sure you have a protective waterproof cover for the mattress, and that there is enough light at night for her to be able to manage to use the potty or toilet alone.

SENSORY DEVELOPMENT

Although your child was born with all her senses – sight, hearing, taste, touch, and smell – it is only through using them after birth that they continue to develop and mature fully. Sensory development depends on stimulation, which creates the necessary neurological pathways to enable their further development.

Touch

Although your child's sense of touch is by no means fully developed at birth, it is more advanced than her sense of sight, hearing, or even taste. Being handled and touched is very important for babies and children. It gives them a sense of their physical existence and also helps in the development of the nervous system.

A fully developed sense of touch is dependent on nerve endings that can differentiate between, for example, touch and pressure or acceptable temperature and pain. Touch also helps your baby understand the physical world and develop tactile sensitivity and motor skills. As every parent will notice, the mouth is very touch-sensitive in a young child, which is why it is used to explore physical objects. Even at 5 years old, a child's face is still more touch-sensitive than her hands, although using the hands to explore will have become second nature by this age. By her first birthday your child can process information from touch much faster than she could at birth, and by age 6 her ability is almost on a par with the ability of an adult.

Touch is also an extremely important form of nonverbal communication that can comfort a toddler in a tantrum, an 8-year-old with a bruised knee, and a disappointed teenager. The experience of being cuddled and cherished physically helps promote a child's emotional development as well as general health and growth.

Smell

After touch, smell is the most developed sense at birth and is important for a baby who can hardly focus beyond about 16–24cm (8–12in). Smell is useful for early recognition and bonding between parent and offspring. It has also been shown that young children prefer the smell of their siblings to that of other children, which helps create a special sibling bond. Familiar smells add to a child's sense of security, and this can partly explain the attraction of a favorite stuffed animal or blanket.

Taste

Even very young children will show definite and sophisticated tastes for different foods if given

the opportunity to try them. Babies show a natural preference for the sweetness of breastmilk, which is nutritiously advantageous. It also allows the possibility of other flavors to filter through from the family foods eaten by a breastfeeding mother. Taste helps stimulate salivation, swallowing, and tongue movements, which are all important for learning to eat solid food later. Distinguishing between the four different tastes – sweet, sour, salty, and bitter – occurs over time as your child experiences different foods. However, there remains in most of us a natural inclination to sweet and high-fat foods which, like breastmilk for babies, have calming properties.

Hearing

Hearing is quite advanced at birth, because your child has had about 12 weeks' actual listening experience in the womb. The mother's voice is the most familiar and reassuring sound to a baby after birth.

The development of hearing has a number of different aspects. One

of the first to mature is sensitivity to higher and lower frequencies of sound, followed by the ability to locate where a sound is coming from. Younger children may find it difficult to distinguish specific sounds against a noisy background. In fact, this is something for you to keep in mind when your child is learning to talk. Background noise may be distracting for some children. Try to have quiet times when you talk to your child without the television or radio on in the background. Hearing continues to improve until puberty.

Sight

Sight is probably the sense that is least developed at birth, because the eyes need to see things in order to develop and for the brain's ability to interpret images to mature. The eye muscles also need to strengthen.

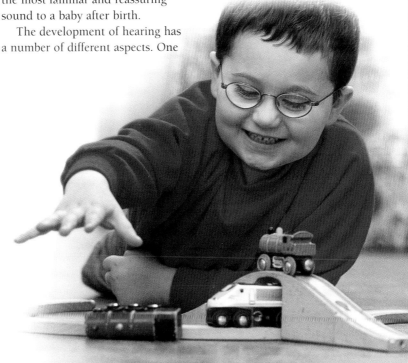

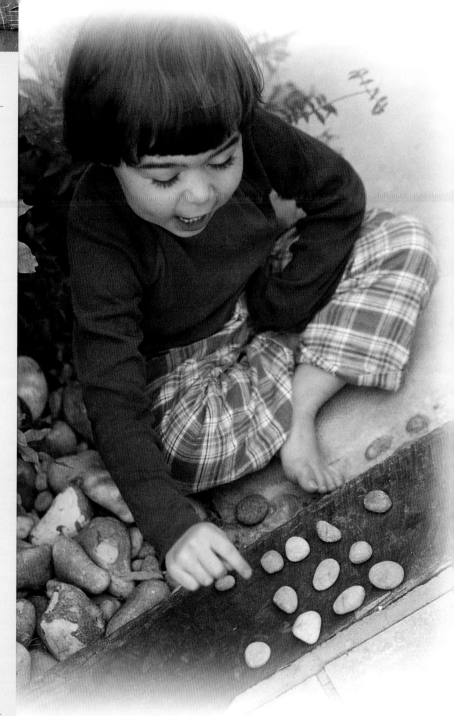

YOUR CHILD'S ATTENTION

Your child's ability to attend to tasks and activities will take some time to mature fully, but there are some things you can do to encourage this process.

- Keep tasks, instructions, and explanations short and simple.
- Provide busy, more fast-paced activities along with quieter ones.
- Choose times when your child seems interested and engaged to focus on one-on-one activities, such as card games or puzzles.
- Consider turning off background noise, such as the television or radio, to reduce distractions.
- Put away all but a few toys at any time so your child isn't distracted.
- Choose an activity appropriate to your child's attention span.
- Engage your child's attention by asking questions and talking about the events of the day.
- Listen to what your child says and respond so that she knows you have heard her.
- Choose activities appropriate for your child's age, which may include reading a book together, doing a jigsaw puzzle, playing board games, building with blocks, or painting.
- Avoid the temptation to over-assist your child, and allow her time to try to figure things out for herself.
- Encourage her to complete an activity, taking frequent breaks if necessary, and praise her efforts.

Some children are more attentive than others. But there are a number of children whose poor concentration or high activity level needs specific help. If you notice a problem, keep in mind your child may be tired or hungry. You may want to keep a record noting specific behaviors or patterns. Be sure to consult your doctor if problem behaviors persist.

One of the first aspects of the eyes to develop is their ability to work together. The ability to see detail takes longer to develop. We refer to someone with normal adult vision as having 20/20 vision, meaning that at 20 feet (the top figure) he or she can see the detail that a normally-sighted person sees at 20 feet (the bottom figure). Babies are born with 20/600 vision. At 20 feet they see what a normal person sees at 600 feet, so they are very nearsighted, with some development needed before the eyes reach maturity. Color vision takes time to develop too. But by the end of the third year, color vision has matured and the development of visual nerves is complete, although many children continue to show a slight degree of nearsightedness until around 10 years of age.

DEVELOPMENT CHECKUPS

Sight and hearing require particular checkups because of their impact on other aspects of physical and intellectual development.

Vision checkups

Your child's eyes will be checked at visits to the doctor with a vision screen starting at about 3 years.

Although babies sometimes seem to have crossed eyes (strabismus), as they develop the ability to use the eyes together it should disappear. However, it's important that crossed eyes don't linger or develop in a baby or an older child. Crossed eyes must be treated; although it won't damage the eye itself, it will affect the development of the brain's visual center and can alter a child's vision permanently if left untreated.

Your child's school may also provide regular vision screening. If any problems are detected or if your child reports vision problems, she may be sent for further evaluation to an ophthalmologist experienced in caring for children. If needed, glasses may be prescribed. Normal vision is necessary for your child's development and for successful performance in school.

Hearing checkups

Some babies will have their hearing checked at birth before they leave hospital. Your baby's hearing will be carefully assessed at visits to the doctor, especially in conjunction with an evaluation of language development. The reason for this is that the ability to hear clearly is essential to the development of speech. Hearing problems in young children should be treated promptly to assure appropriate development of speech expression and comprehension.

Slight deafness may be caused by something as temporary as a blocked ear due to a cold. Repeated ear infections or chronic fluid in the middle ear, in which a persistently blocked ear may impair hearing (*see p.241*), need prompt treatment.

If you have any concerns about your child's hearing, you should discuss them with your doctor as soon as possible. Even if there is nothing wrong, it is better to be reassured.

DEVELOPMENT OF CONCENTRATION

The development of concentration comes more easily to some children than to others, but it's worth encouraging early because it is essential for learning.

The attention span of a young child is naturally short and is easily affected by fatigue, hunger, thirst, or being unsettled in some way. Young children also have a lot of energy and may find it difficult to settle down, but even very young children may be encouraged to focus on a particular activity briefly.

Parents will notice short periods of focused behavior in their baby, encouraged by talking and playing one-on-one. But it's not until toward the end of the first year that the area of the brain responsible for concentration, the frontal lobe, is sufficiently developed to make a difference in a child's attention span. At the same time, her ability to ignore things is developing too.

Some children, when they are school age, may show continued poor concentration and need help to gain the skills they need to concentrate for longer periods. It's important to address any problems early because concentration is essential to learning and schoolwork.

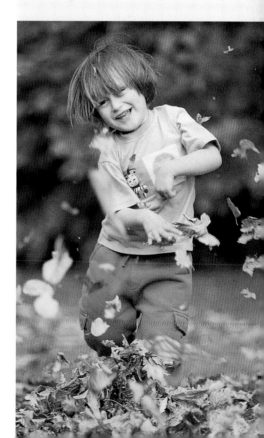

ATTENTION DEFICIT HYPERACTIVITY DISORDER (ADHD)

Below is a list of symptoms that may be associated with ADHD (*see p.299*). Keep in mind that many preschool children who do not have ADHD exhibit these behaviors and later outgrow them as they mature; ADHD is not normally diagnosed until a child is school-age or older.

- Inattention
- Hyperactivity
- Impulsivity
- Academic underachievement
- Behavioral problems

If you think your child may have ADHD, consult your doctor to determine if an evaluation is needed. ADHD is the most researched of all childhood behavioral disorders. Children referred for an ADHD evaluation should have a thorough assessment, with observations of behavior by parents, teachers, and other caregivers.

PHYSICAL SKILLS

Bᴇʏ ᴛʜᴇ ᴇɴᴅ ᴏꜰ ᴛʜᴇ ꜰɪʀsᴛ ʏᴇᴀʀ, ᴍᴏsᴛ ʙᴀʙɪᴇs ʜᴀᴠᴇ the physical strength and motivation to move to the next stage of developing their "gross motor skills," learning to walk and then to run, jump, and hop. As a child grows older, developing a range of physical skills through active play and starting to take care of herself will help her develop self-confidence and independence.

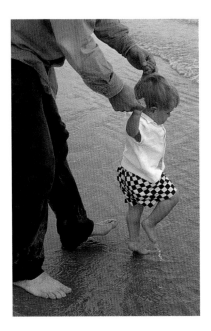

ABOUT MOVEMENT MILESTONES

We use milestones as markers for developmental stages, but all children are individual, so while one child might walk at 10 months, another might not be ready until 14 months or later. Both of these ages are within the normal range. What is true about milestones, however, is that all children follow the same sequence of development even if they reach each of the milestones at slightly different stages. Quite literally, you can't run before you can walk.

It's also worth remembering that some children are, by nature, much more physically active than others. The quieter, more contemplative child may simply have less motivation to explore and so may have less inclination to start walking than another child. So it is important for all children that the parents encourage a balance of activities, alternating more active games with quieter ones.

Try not to be too anxious as your child moves toward greater mobility. She will need to feel your confidence in her ability to be able to manage new activities in order to feel confidence in herself. Encourage her and offer assistance only when it is needed, rather than imposing it on her.

"...progress is individual, but all children show the same sequence of development...you can't run before you can walk"

Walking

Before walking, your child has probably practiced standing upright, holding on to you, or the furniture. Supported by you, she has probably taken practice steps, all of which help strengthen the leg muscles in preparation for independent walking. These practice steps, often taken by side-stepping from one piece of furniture to another (sometimes referred to as "cruising"), are useful preliminaries to independent walking.

The next stage in walking is to balance unsupported. Your child is likely to be a bit wobbly at first while she adjusts to the new sensation of standing upright alone. If standing upright feels too insecure, she will probably sit down suddenly to avoid falling over. Eventually, with feet planted wide apart, toes pointing outward and arms raised to the sides to aid balance, she will take the first few steps unassisted. These are inevitably a bit cautious and the whole attempt may end with your child suddenly sitting down or collapsing into your arms, but progress from here is usually fast.

Running

Early walking has a certain lurching momentum, which isn't quite the same as deliberate running. Initially the "go" mechanism in the brain is more effective than the "stop" mechanism, so toddlers tend to launch themselves into walking at speed, then sit down to stop. With practice, as she finds her center of gravity toward the end of the second year and her legs are less widely spaced, walking becomes easier to control. Prior to running effectively, your child also has to learn to stop, start, and change direction. Once her leg muscles strengthen and her coordination improves, running becomes more natural. You'll probably find that your child will be running by the end of her second year.

Jumping

At 2 years of age, your child may try to jump, but somehow her feet don't quite leave the floor. It may be manageable for your child to try jumping off a low object while holding your hand. By 3 years, with practice and as muscles strengthen, your child can master jumping easily. At first your child will tend to raise her feet high when she jumps, bending her knees to take the impact when she lands.

Hopping

Like jumping, hopping on one leg is an activity that your child may try before she has the required muscle strength. In addition, your child might not yet have the ability to balance for hopping. Even standing on one leg requires adjustment for balancing in a more lopsided way and takes practice. Encourage your child to hop from leg to leg, which isn't too far removed from jumping, and then to try hopping on one leg

FIRST SHOES

While your baby is learning to walk, it is easier for her to have bare feet. Close contact with the surface on which she is walking provides a greater sense of stability, which is lost when feet are in shoes. Allow her a lot of opportunities for safe, barefoot exploration; if you do put her in shoes, choose the softest ones and make sure they have nonslip soles. Wearing shoes too early may interfere with the growth of your baby's feet. This also applies to socks and footed pajamas if they're too small and are worn for long periods.

Shoes only become necessary once your child begins walking outside, and then her feet need to be accurately measured and shoes properly fitted. If your child is walking confidently before shoes are fitted, the adjustment to wearing shoes is easier. Special features designed to shape and support the feet make shoes more expensive and have no proven benefit for the average child.

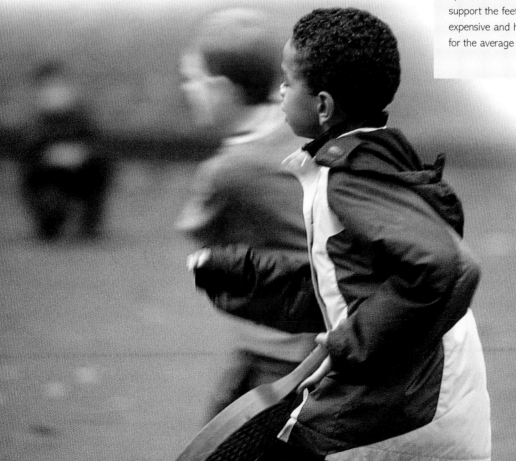

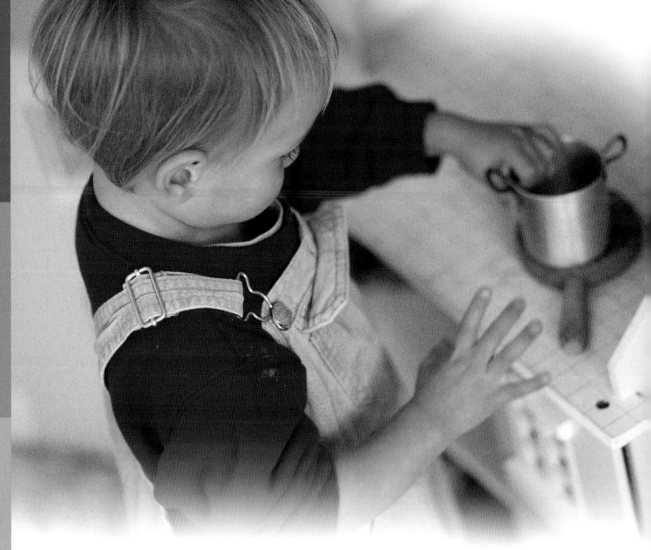

before alternating sides. Your child will probably be able to hop before she can stand still on one leg.

Standing on tiptoe

Standing and walking on tiptoe is another way to challenge and assist the development of balance and coordination. You will probably find that your child naturally stands on tiptoe in order to reach or see something more easily. She may not even realize she is doing it. Toward their third birthday, most children can stand and then walk on tiptoe.

Kicking a ball

At first your child's balance isn't good enough to give a ball a hefty kick, and it's more a case of pushing the ball a distance with the foot. By 3 years of age, most children can kick a ball some distance and will generally favor one foot for kicking over the other. This is normal. Just as we are right- or left-handed, we also tend to be right- or left-footed.

Throwing and catching a ball

Throwing a ball isn't possible until babies have learned to let go of an object deliberately, which usually happens toward the end of the first year. You may not want to encourage your child to throw things until she is old enough to understand that some things may be thrown but others may not. Catching a ball is harder than throwing one because it relies on hand-eye coordination.

You will probably notice that when your child first practices catching a ball, she will hold out both hands but keep her eyes on your face, in anticipation of what will happen rather than watching the ball. Again, these are skills that require practice, and some children are more naturally skilled and coordinated at these activities than others. But by age 3, most children can catch a ball from a short distance, as long as it is a reasonably large size and soft.

Climbing stairs

At 2 years old your toddler can probably manage the stairs, placing two feet on each step and supported by the handrail or wall. The big difference at 3 years is that she can probably walk upstairs using alternate feet, although coming down she may continue using two feet on each step, supported by the wall or handrail. It's worth encouraging your child to climb stairs safely, and you should discourage her from carrying anything on the stairs while she is learning to manage them.

DEVELOPMENT OF FINE MOTOR SKILLS

Fine motor skills refer to those that develop in the hands and fingers. What began with your 2-month-old swatting at a toy has progressed considerably by the end of the first year, but there's a still a great deal more development to come.

For example, whereas your baby used to tightly grasp a toy in her fist until she dropped it accidentally, releasing the toy now becomes deliberate. Around her first birthday, she can use her hand to pick something up, move it from hand to hand, or to another place, and let it go. Simple though this seems, it is an important new skill, giving her more control over her environment. This grasping of objects now begins to refine into the ability to use the fingers and the thumb to pick up an object, and then the ability to use just the thumb and forefinger, known as the pincer grip. You will probably notice your child's development of the pincer grip in the increased efficiency with which she can manage finger foods, although eating with a spoon may still be difficult and messy.

At birth babies have developed very few bones in the wrist, restricting movement. As these bones grow it becomes easier to make a twisting movement with the hand, so at around 15 months your child will have greater dexterity in her hand movements. By 18 months she will also be able to hold objects between the thumb and fingers and let go voluntarily. This means she can place objects such as building blocks one on top of the other and manage large, simple puzzles. Developing hand-eye coordination also contributes to success in activities such as these.

More sophisticated hand movements, such as poking, squeezing, rolling, and twisting, are being practiced as your child plays, especially with something like play dough. At 2 years old, being able to hold a crayon or marker means that scribbling on paper, the forerunner to drawing and writing, is an exciting new activity. It is also at this stage that hand preference (the hand your

child consistently uses for things such as throwing, scribbling, and using a spoon) becomes evident. Handedness is genetically determined, and although small children will continue to swap hands for some activities, their use of the dominant hand soon becomes consistent.

At 3 years old, a child should be able to manage to eat with a spoon and fork, dress herself (with help with buttons and laces), play with construction toys designed for her age group, thread large beads on a string, and copy simple line patterns, such as a circle or a cross, with a crayon on paper. All these activities both demonstrate and encourage manual dexterity on which greater skills, such as fastening buttons, tying shoelaces, and using scissors, will be built.

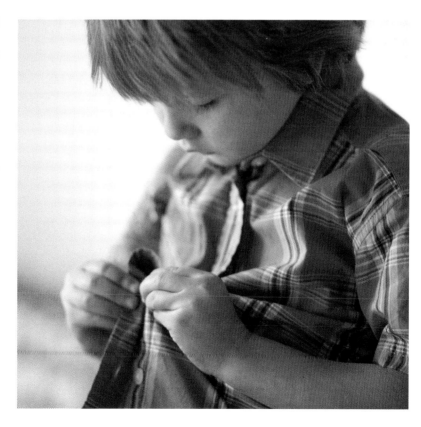

"...your child's increasing mobility coincides with a greater desire for independence...you should work toward instilling a sense of caution in your child"

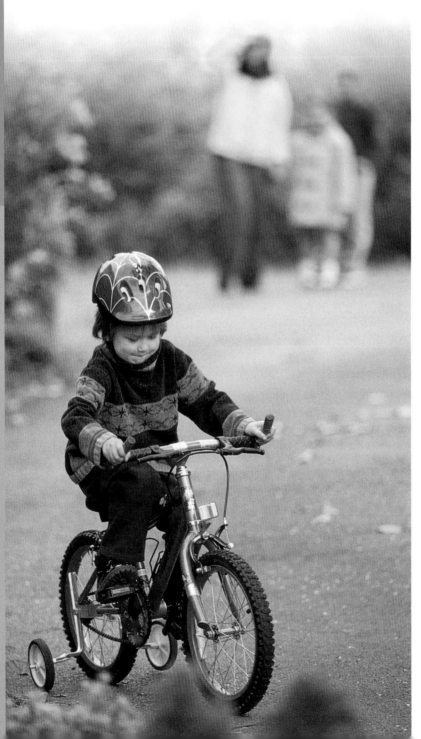

SAFETY

As your child's mobility and instinct to explore the world increase, you will need to consider safety issues. It can be an exhausting time for parents while a child's intellectual ability catches up to her physical ability and she can understand some of the safety measures you need to enforce. Your child's increasing mobility coincides with a growing desire for independence, leading to a battle of wills which, when it comes to safety, you need to win.

While it's essential to take standard precautions to avoid hazards, you should also work toward instilling a sense of caution in your child, on which she can build her own instinct for self-preservation. This includes allowing your child to try things, with your guidance, to help her understand why some things are unsafe.

It's also important to establish those rules that are nonnegotiable. At first it's simplest to say to your child that she must simply follow the rules, for example about car safety, which apply to everyone. As your child grows, you can explain more fully why we take the precautions to keep safe, reinforcing the message at every opportunity.

You may need to repeat information again and again, because, due to young children's short memories and lack of experience, they won't necessarily take it in the first, second, or even the third time.

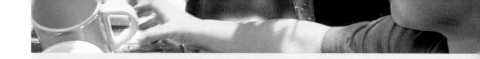

KEEPING YOUR CHILD SAFE

Toys and safety

As your child becomes increasingly coordinated and mobile, she will begin to do things such as riding a tricycle or a bike (with training wheels at first). Older children may learn to ride a scooter or a skateboard. These can be a lot of fun and learning to use them correctly will also increase your child's confidence. However, it is vital that your child is supervised and always wears the appropriate safety equipment, especially a helmet, when participating in these activities.

"Stranger danger"

The unfortunate truth is that children are more at risk from people they know than from strangers. Introducing the idea of a "stranger" can be unnecessarily scary and ineffectual and may also reduce your child's confidence, so it is better to establish some straightforward rules that apply to every situation.

• Teach your child from an early age that she must never go anywhere with anyone, even a friend or neighbor, without first checking that it is all right with her parent or caregiver.

• Tell your child that only good secrets should be kept, like birthday surprises. Anything that feels wrong to her should be shared with you and you will never be upset with her for telling you something.

• As your child grows, discuss what behavior in another person might make her feel uncomfortable so she can learn to trust her instincts.

• As soon as she is old enough (about age 5), teach your child your home phone number and address. Check periodically that she can still remember them.

Road safety

Injuries to child pedestrians tend to occur when they are crossing the street or playing in or near a road. A young child cannot judge distance or speed effectively and often cannot see nor be seen above or around a vehicle, all of which make roads extremely hazardous. At the earliest opportunity, even when your child is still in a stroller, start explaining about road safety. Remember, most children do not have the skills to handle traffic situations safely until at least 10 years of age. Here are important road safety rules.

• Always cross at a marked pedestrian crossing when available.

• Even at a marked pedestrian crossing, wait to be sure the cars stop. Otherwise you can't be certain that the driver has seen you.

• For children too young to cross on their own, always stop when you reach the curb and only cross holding an adult's hand.

• Stop, look, and listen before crossing. When teaching your child about road safety, ask her to tell you if she thinks it's safe to cross, which helps her learn to concentrate.

• Avoid crossing streets between parked cars, which obscure vision.

• Wear light-reflecting strips on your coat, especially at night.

• Avoid playing games in the street.

Safety in the car

If your child is correctly restrained in the car, she is significantly less likely to be killed in a crash, so the use of a child safety seat and seat belts is a must even on the shortest trips. Holding a child on your lap is never a safe option.

• As soon as your child is old enough, encourage her to take responsibility for her own proper restraint in the car. However, you should always check that it's secure, and praise her efforts to be safe.

• Child safety door locks can prevent children from opening the door from the inside. Check to see if your vehicle has this feature.

• Make it clear that buttons and handles in cars are not for play.

Safety in the yard

The yard can be an enjoyable place to play, but make sure it's safe and has appropriate supervision. Any garden tools, including garden chemicals, must be stored securely out of the reach of children.

• Make sure your child knows that she must never eat any flowers, leaves, or berries, since many common plants (such as hydrangeas, chrysanthemums, and certain mushrooms) are poisonous.

• Encourage your child to wash her hands after playing in the yard, and especially before eating.

Safety in the kitchen

A kitchen can be hazardous, but it's also where a child is likely to spend time. So teach safety rules and keep the kitchen as safe as possible (see p.166).

• Show what's hot so your child learns why it's important not to touch. Don't rely on her to remember this, though, and keep all hot dishes, pots, and appliances, well out of her reach. The same applies to sharp utensils.

• No running in the kitchen should always be the rule.

Water safety

Small children should never be left unattended around water, no matter how shallow. You should never leave a child alone in the bath, even for just a few seconds. Fit garden ponds with a mesh grid or fill them in, and always supervise children in wading or swimming pools. Check your area's bylaws for rules about protective fences around swimming pools.

THINKING
& UNDERSTANDING

CHILDREN LEARN THROUGH TRIAL AND ERROR, exploration, interaction, quiet times, and making mistakes. Young children learn primarily through play, and they learn best when they are relaxed and having fun. Older children should be encouraged to do their homework on their own as much as possible, and to take responsibility for getting it done.

> "...keep in mind that a balance between physical activity and quieter activity is important"

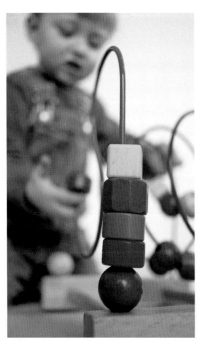

HOW CHILDREN LEARN

Providing learning opportunities for your child doesn't mean that you need a large number of educational toys, or that you must do structured activities. Understanding roughly the stage of development your child has reached, and meeting her need for activities that engage her and enable her to practice new skills, demands a certain amount of commitment and input. In the long run, though, this commitment pays dividends when your child becomes happily absorbed in an activity after you have shown her how. Even better, she may discover new skills and create different activities, adding to the basics you have taught her. Keep in mind, too, that some children need more input than others to stay focused, and that achieving a good balance between physical activity and quieter activities is important.

Your child doesn't need a huge number of toys, but what she does need are play materials. These include materials that allow her opportunities to express herself, develop her fine motor skills, and extend her imagination: crayons and paper to scribble on, old clothes for dressing up, modeling clay and building blocks, all of which will allow her the chance for exploration and discovery.

Children also learn by imitation. Long before they can understand the meaning of what they do, children imitate the behavior of others. They then apply meaning later. Imitation also allows the beginnings of imaginative play, which is an important component of learning because it aids creativity, problem-solving, and role-play and enables a child to imagine how other people feel in different situations. All of these things contribute to a child's emotional development as well as to her learning.

Learning social skills

Playing with other children will help your child learn about social interaction with her own peer group. Children lack the experience to understand different behaviors, so it's an opportunity to learn how to negotiate and compromise, how to be assertive and handle rejection, and how to make friends and have fun. These important social skills can only be learned by spending time with other children. Some children find it more difficult to learn these things than others, and

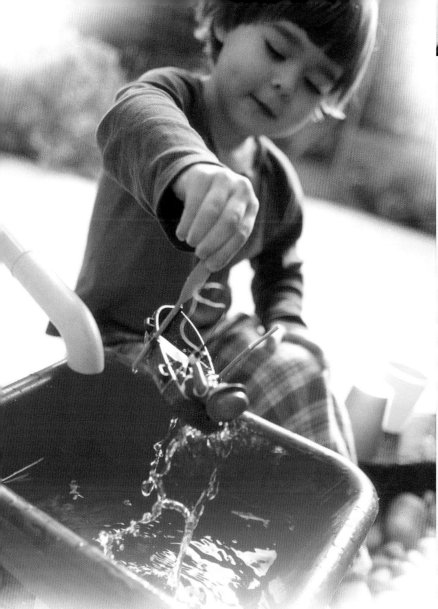

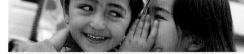

in any case your child will probably need some help from you at first to develop ways to deal with social situations. Showing your belief that she can manage and enjoy friendships will help your child feel confident that she can do this.

Regular one-on-one interaction with you is important, especially for language development in a younger child. Although you may feel as if you are with your child 24 hours a day, there may be a lot of routine activity going on during which you are not particularly "tuned in" to your child. Children need some time

every day when they are given undivided attention. Complete attention all the time would be too intense and intrusive, but for several regular periods every day you should try to make your child the focus of your attention. During this time you and your child could share an activity, read a book together, talk about the day in a relaxed way, or discuss feelings or events, all of which allow your child to feel cherished. Making sure your child gets some one-on-one attention can help build your child's self-esteem.

Learning and language

Language development is essential to a young child's learning. Through language your child can ask questions, name objects, and express ideas and feelings, all of which contribute to her learning. And if you listen to her attentively, taking turns in conversation, then she will learn how to do that too. Try not to correct early language mistakes overtly; just repeat back what has been said, speaking correctly and clearly. Hearing words pronounced correctly will also help her later in identifying written words.

Quiet times are also important to young children. They need periods of reflection to make sense of what they learn; they are not sponges that merely absorb information. Intelligence is the ability to use what you know and to build on it, and that requires the evolution of a thinking process that only time for reflection can supply. It is even important for children to be bored sometimes, because it's through the experience of occasional boredom that they can develop the resourcefulness and imagination to overcome it. Constantly providing activities and structured things for

your child to do can actually deprive her of this opportunity to develop independence and imagination.

The ability to learn through experience also relies on the development of memory. One reason that young children like repetition of enjoyable experiences – of games, stories, or activities, for example – is that it reinforces what has happened before and starts creating memories.

Learning in the classroom
Once your child starts school, she will begin to learn in a more formal way. Much early learning takes place in groups, so it's important for your

child to know how to get along with other children. For this reason, attending a playgroup or preschool may be beneficial. It's also important for your child to know how to listen and take turns.

LEARNING DIFFICULTIES
The term "learning disability" covers the full range of anything that makes learning difficult for a child. A learning disability may be something specific, such as dyslexia, or something more general, such as developmental delay. If there is no obvious problem at birth, parents are often the first to notice that there

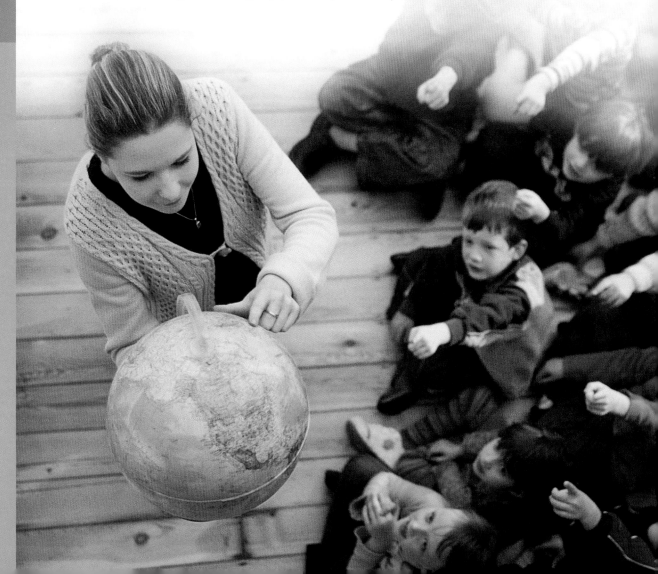

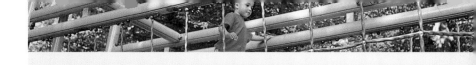

may be a problem with their child's development. A learning disability might also be identified by a doctor during a routine checkup, or in later years by a teacher when a child starts school.

One of the benefits of the routine checkups performed in the first few years of life is that they monitor each milestone and when your child reaches it, which can give an early indication of any emerging problem. The earlier any learning disability is picked up, the better, because early intervention means a child's particular needs can be met more adequately. Vision and hearing tests are also part of these checkups and are similarly important in identifying problems early.

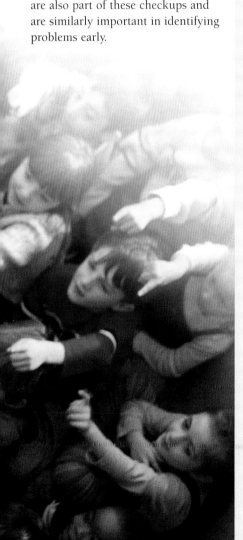

ENCOURAGING CONFIDENCE

Confident children find the world a much easier place to negotiate, and their confidence comes primarily from feeling unconditionally loved and accepted for who they are. Confident children have an expectation that they will be able to manage, or that there will be someone to help them overcome a difficulty. Some children are more naturally confident than others, depending on their personality, but there is much that you can do to encourage confidence in your child from infancy to teens.

Children need to know that they matter, their feelings are respected, their needs will be met, and their opinions listened to, even if you may not agree with them. They need to feel your confidence in them, and to feel that they can meet your realistic expectations – a child needs to feel loved for who she is and not just for her achievements. Your child will want to please you, and will take pleasure in your pleasure, giving her the confidence to keep trying.

- Praise your child's efforts as well as her achievements.
- When she misbehaves, make it clear that it's her behavior you disapprove of, not her.
- Never humiliate a child if she can't manage a task or activity, saying she is clumsy or stupid.
- Don't over-assist when she is trying to do something; she will feel she can't manage alone. Ask if she needs some help rather than imposing it on her.
- When accidents happen, avoid over-reacting or making it personal, and instead show her how to fix it.
- Find an activity your child enjoys, and encourage her – succeeding at something makes her feel confident about trying other things.

- Encourage your child to speak for herself rather than always answering for her.
- Encourage basic skills, such as swimming or riding a bike, which give a child a sense of achievement and means she can participate in activities with other children.
- When giving your child instructions, promote the positive rather than the negative. Instead of saying, "Be careful you don't spill it" try, "Use both hands and you'll be fine."
- Don't make comparisons between your child and her siblings or other children.
- Don't dismiss your child's negative feelings about something, or over-praise something she is dissatisfied with. Instead, offer alternatives, or suggest taking a break before the frustration becomes overwhelming.
- Try to avoid expressing your anxieties about her ability to manage alone, especially when she is facing a new situation, such as starting school or taking an exam.
- Emphasize to your child that making a mistake is an opportunity to learn how to handle a situation and not the end of the world.

What also gives a child confidence is the ability to cope with new situations. For example, being able to put on her own shoes or use a pair of scissors before starting school can help your child feel that she is competent, which will in turn give her greater confidence in trying new activities. For this reason, it is important to encourage children to manage age-appropriate tasks on their own, rather than always doing things for them. You should be careful not to give your child more difficult tasks before she is ready.

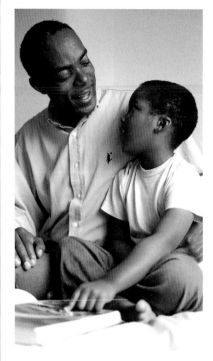

The severity of learning disabilities varies widely; they are usually described as ranging from mild to moderate to severe. When a learning disability is suspected, accurate assessment by a specially trained professional is needed to clarify the type and extent of the disability, so that appropriate learning support can be provided. This support allows a child to reach her own potential, in spite of any limitations. Early support and help for a child with a learning disability can also prevent the frustrations that may arise from it, which often cause additional problems with behavior. Many children in Canada participate in a special education program or require extra help to manage in a mainstream school. Other children, whose needs are greater, may need to attend a special school.

READING

Encouraging your child's interest and pleasure in books from infancy is an essential precursor to reading. From the first time you sit your baby on your knee and look at a board book together, you are beginning the journey that leads to independent reading. At this stage you aren't teaching your baby to read but are simply introducing the idea that books provide a source of entertainment and information. Sharing books also provides relaxed, one-on-one time with your child, talking together, which aids language development.

An important stage before reading is being able to recognize word sounds and to differentiate between letter sounds. These abilities develop from talking with your child and from repeating what she has said correctly. For example, if she points to a picture of a dog in a book and says "woof," you can say "Yes, that's a dog. And dogs go 'woof.'" You could use this as an opportunity to ask her, "What color is the dog?" to develop the conversation. Try to limit background noise when you are talking to your child in this way, so that she can hear your words clearly.

Your child's first books should also include a selection of rhymes, because repetition and rhyming help develop an idea of how language – written and spoken – works. Rhymes help develop memory in young children who don't yet have much language – and they are also fun. Other books include stories or songs. You will probably find that your child enjoys the same book read over and over again, and this is normal.

It's worth taking your child to visit your local library, which will have a children's section and a librarian who can help you choose books appropriate for your child. Many libraries hold special story times for young children.

Learning the alphabet

In due time, learning the alphabet should include learning not only the letter names, but also the letter sounds. And check that the letter sounds are correct – "s" should be for sun, not shoe. Although individual word recognition forms part of the way in which children learn to read, they also need to understand how the building blocks of words – the letters – work together. Repetition is helpful when learning the alphabet. You may be able to help your child by teaching her the "alphabet song," showing her letters in books and on signs, and pointing out the letter names and sounds in your usual conversations.

"...from the first time you look at a book with your child, you are beginning the journey that leads to independent reading"

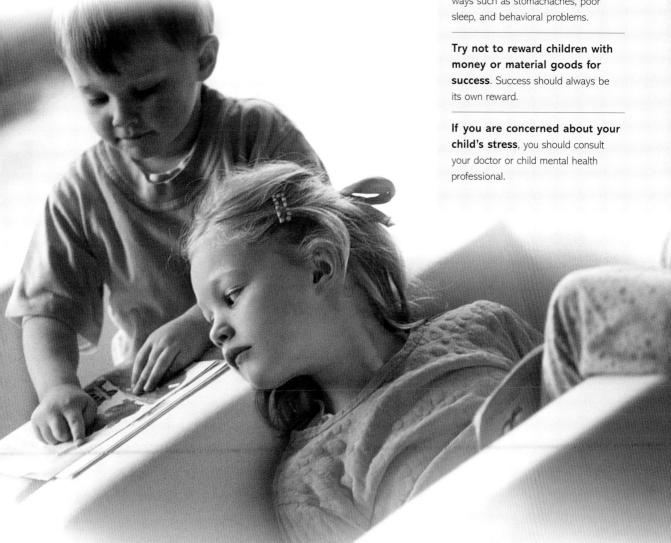

PUSHY PARENTS

While all parents want what's best for their child, it's sometimes hard to get the balance right between doing what you feel is right and following your child's inclinations. With the best intentions in the world, many parents know what their child needs to do to succeed but overlook what she enjoys doing. It can be very tempting to impose your own interests on your child, but if you take it too far you may end up by causing only resentment and resistance. If you always wanted to play the piano, take lessons yourself.

Homework, after-school activities, and private coaching are all becoming more prevalent as children start school. For an 8-year-old to spend six hours at school, followed by additional activities afterward, and an hour of homework every night with perhaps an instrument to practice as well, may be overwhelming. Children need freedom to relax and the personal space to develop their own ideas and interests. Encouraging your child's own interests is important, so try as much as possible to take the lead from your child.

DON'T OVERDO IT

It's worth keeping in mind how pushing a child too far can backfire.

If children's time is over-structured, they may never learn to be self-motivated, which is essential to future successful learning.

A continuous emphasis on the next achievement for achievement's sake reduces the sense children have of taking pleasure in a task. Whatever they do, it isn't good enough when the emphasis is always on the next thing.

Stress isn't good for a child's health, and it can show up in physical ways such as stomachaches, poor sleep, and behavioral problems.

Try not to reward children with money or material goods for success. Success should always be its own reward.

If you are concerned about your child's stress, you should consult your doctor or child mental health professional.

LANGUAGE
& COMMUNICATION

Most of us take our children's speech and language development for granted because it seems to happen so naturally. It is a fascinating process, both because of the speed with which it takes place and because children almost seem to teach themselves. A child's early vocalizations are often the subject of pride and amusement as parents begin to see their young child as a person in his own right.

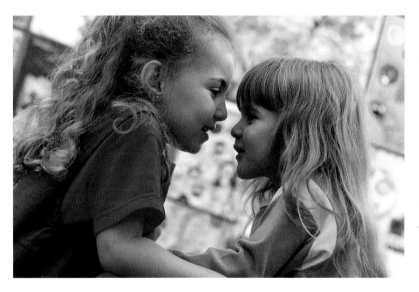

"...language is essential for school 'readiness,' enabling communication in both the classroom and the playground"

LANGUAGE IN THE PRESCHOOL PERIOD

After the acquisition of early speech and a small repertoire of single words, toddlers gradually start using two- or three-word sentences and we soon forget their early faltering steps into language. Instead we start to respond to our children as conversational partners. Of course, children in these early stages are focused on what they see or feel and may not engage in actual conversations. But it is not long before they start to be able to comment on what others are doing,

and by 4 years of age children are able to sense what other people are thinking and respond appropriately. By this age children are also using complex sentences, many of which resemble adult sentences. They continue to make errors, for example in the way they use irregular verbs (saying "go-ed" for "went" or "see-ed" for "saw"), and they often make minor errors with their pronounciation, but these are perfectly normal steps on the road to fluency.

Language and communication are essential for school "readiness." It is often assumed that most speech and language development occurs before children start kindergarten (at about age 5), and indeed for many children this is true.

By the time they enter school, children need to have developed listening and attention skills to allow them to cope in the classroom. They also need the verbal comprehension and expressive language skills to understand what their teacher is saying, to respond when asked questions, and to create stories about their experiences. Children's language skills also allow them to communicate with their peers in the playground and to form the strong social bonds that are essential for a child to be happy in school. Finally, children need to develop the early reading and counting skills that will allow them to go on to tackle new subjects in class, which form the foundation of the broader curriculum on which their later education will be based.

LANGUAGE & OTHER DEVELOPMENT

Sometimes people think that language and communication are separate from other things that a child does. In fact, speech and language development is closely related to your child's sensory abilities – for example, it is much

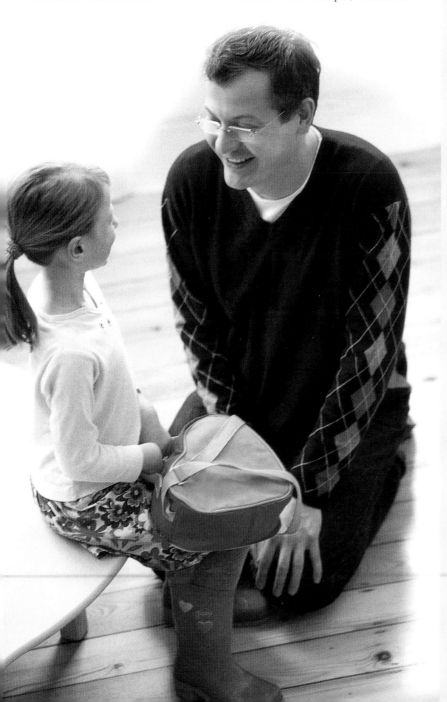

EARLY LANGUAGE SKILLS

There are a few key things parents can do to help the early stages of their child's language development:

Actively engaging in the earliest communication with your baby gives the message that communication is important and makes her want to try to get her meaning across.

Helping your child listen carefully can be invaluable to early language development. High levels of background noise may make it difficult for a child to "tune in" effectively.

Engaging in early verbal interaction with your young child and responding to whatever interests her, rather than talking at her, helps her focus on the meaning of words and pick out consistent patterns of sounds and words.

Once your child has started to speak, interacting with her and repeating back what she has said helps her see that what she has to say is meaningful to those around her. Don't forget that young children love familiar rituals and they often want to go on repeating things that they like saying for a long time.

Reading books to your child can be a useful way to help her concentrate on language. Children love to listen to an adult talking about the pictures in the book.

easier to learn to speak if your child can hear and see effectively. This is not to say that children who cannot see or hear will not learn to speak, just that they may find it more difficult. Language and communication skills are also closely related to the ability to walk, manipulate objects with the fingers, play with toys and other objects, remember things and listen, and pay attention. Language is related to a child's overall development, and while there can be differences in the route that children take through the process, generally children who are managing well in one area of development tend to do well in other areas as well.

WHERE LANGUAGE CAN GO WRONG

There are some children who struggle with the whole process of acquiring speech and language. They may not understand as well as their peers or pick up words as quickly; they may not be able to get their words out fluently and they may start to stammer; they may not produce the sounds at all or may mix them up and be unintelligible to everyone except their closest family members. These problems, and how to separate them from what is "normal" development, are outlined in the box, opposite. Parents may need to talk through their concerns with their doctor or a speech and

language professional before assuming that there is something wrong with their child's language development. Having said that, early speech and language difficulties can lead to problems in school and therefore need to be taken seriously.

HOW CAN I PROMOTE MY CHILD'S LANGUAGE DEVELOPMENT?

Parents may be uncertain as to whether they should "teach" speech and language to their child or whether they should just leave their child to do it themselves, assuming that there is little that can be done to help. We now recognize that children's brains are designed to

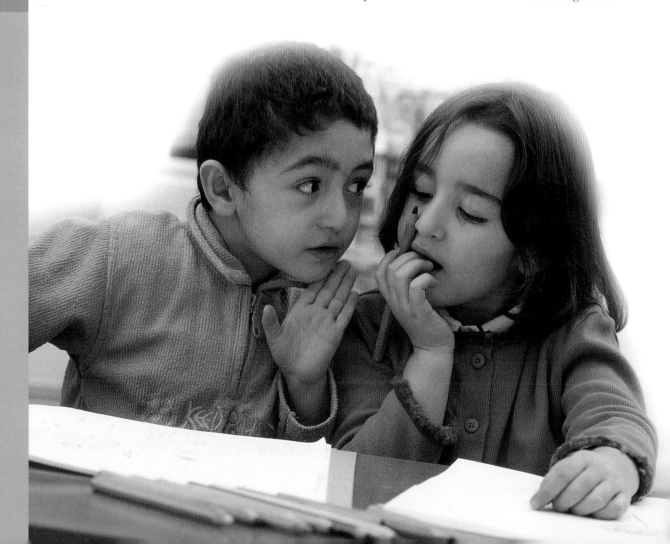

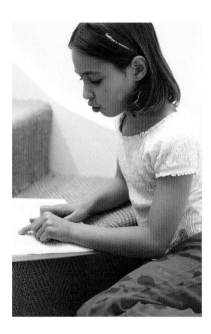

acquire language as much as their bodies are designed to grow, given the necessary nutrition. Generally, children do develop language and communication skills without much deliberate teaching from their parents. Of course, it is a different situation when we are talking about things such as teaching children the meaning of specific words, speaking grammatically, and the use of what we consider polite expressions. Aspects of written language are also deliberately taught, for example, the use of punctuation.

Although there may be relatively little to teach about language, children always benefit from being listened to, so that they come to believe that what they have to say is important. Listening to your child will give her confidence and make her want to contribute to conversations at home and at school. It is this confidence in her own ideas and her ability to communicate them effectively that will carry her forward to being a competent communicator as an adult.

OUTLINE OF NORMAL LANGUAGE DEVELOPMENT IN THE PRESCHOOL YEARS

2–3 YEARS
- Good range of sounds, although may have difficulties making certain sounds.
- Two- and three-word phrases.
- Language used for a variety of purposes – possession/assertion/refusal/attribution and so forth.
- Able to find two or three objects on request.

Seek advice if:
- Poor control of facial muscles.
- People outside the family do not understand much of what is said.
- No word combinations by age 2.
- Very restricted vocabulary.
- Unable to find two objects on request by age 2.

3–4 YEARS
- Most speech sounds correct. May have difficulties with /ch/ or /j/.
- Intelligibility may decline when excited.
- Talks increasingly fluently.
- Able to refer to past and future events. Marks past tense with -ed, but may be some confusion with irregular verbs, e.g. "I go-ed to the park."
- Able to understand concepts such as color, size, etc.
- Will understand most of what a parent is saying.

Seek advice if:
- Very limited repertoire of sounds and much of what is said is unintelligible.
- Nonfluency that is common in younger children persists.
- Little feeling of interaction in conversation, either because the child says very little or because the child continues to echo what is said to her.
- Restricted use of verbs or adjectives.
- Comprehension outside everyday context very limited. May still not be aware of the function of objects.

4–5 YEARS
- Completely intelligible except for occasional errors.
- Grammatical errors may persist but rarely affect the meaning.
- 4–6 word sentences used consistently.
- Question forms, such as "why?", now common.
- Able to construct own stories.
- Can now understand abstract words, e.g. "always."
- Understands and can reconstruct a story sequence from a book.

Seek advice if:
- Much speech is still unintelligible.
- Pattern of stammering may be emerging – especially if beginning "blocking" on certain words or sounds.
- Increasing awareness of problems and frustration with language.
- Child avoiding situations where she must talk, e.g. preschool.
- Continues to respond in single words or uses very simple grammatical structures.
- Little idea of tense.
- Cannot retell a story.
- May be able to understand enough to manage familiar routines but cannot cope if structure changes.
- Child often isolated because cannot deal with the verbal level of peers.

General points to look out for:
- Family history of speech or language difficulties.
- Any history of hearing difficulties.
- Concerns about parent/child interaction.
- Difficulties with behavior or attention.

If you have doubts about your child's speech and language development, see your doctor for an evaluation and possible referral to a speech and language therapist.

LIVING AS A FAMILY

THERE ARE MANY DIFFERENT KINDS OF FAMILIES. Children whose parents are married, children whose parents are cohabiting, single-parent households, foster families, and stepfamilies are only a few of them. Each family has different characteristics and issues, and what works for one family doesn't necessarily work for another. You need to find your own "style" as a family that works for you.

"...the challenge is to arrange a way of living that works for you and your children"

FAMILIES TODAY

Being a parent has never been easy and it isn't any easier today. Combining work with bringing up children can often be a complicated juggling act. Children face many different kinds of pressures, too, including more school homework and tests than ever before.

You probably aren't short on advice, from relatives, friends, health professionals, books, and magazines.

The challenge is to use this information to arrange a way of living as a family that works for you and your children and gives them the healthiest possible start in life.

Various approaches may help you. Accepting that stress is inevitable, and planning how to deal with it, is a good start. For instance, if your toddler always has tantrums in the morning when your older child needs to get to school, try getting

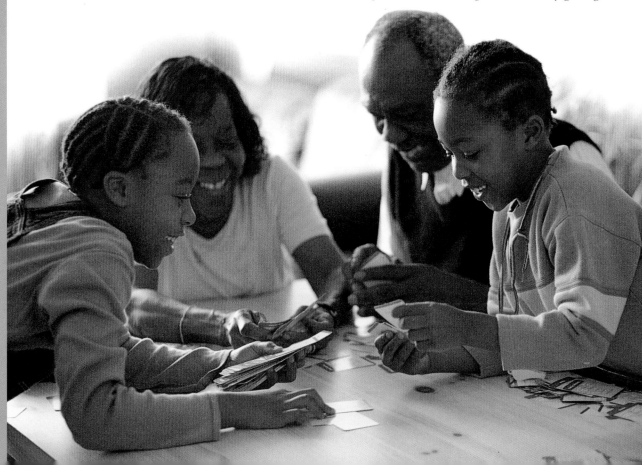

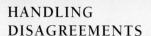

up a little earlier to allow extra time. This way, it is a little easier to get everyone out of the house in time.

GETTING ALONG WITH YOUR PARTNER

It can often be difficult to agree with a partner on child care issues, but your child will benefit if you are consistent, even on small things. For example, your child will be confused if your partner insists she eat all her vegetables and you don't. She may learn to play you against each other. Agree on a line with your partner and stick to it. If you find it difficult to agree, try to avoid arguing in front of your child. If you can't come to an agreement on a matter of your child's health or safety, get another opinion from someone qualified to advise you.

If sharing household chores is an issue for you and your partner, outside help with cleaning or laundry can make a big difference if you can afford it. Or you could organize a babysitting arrangement with your partner, a relative, or friend to give you time to do chores yourself. Make an effort to get to know other families. Many parents say they benefit tremendously from friendships with other parents in terms of discussing problems and supporting each other.

Remember, too, to make time for yourself, even if it's a short, uninterrupted time, to take a bath or read a book. It can be easy to forget your own needs when children are around. Plan time alone with your partner as well.

RELATIONSHIPS BETWEEN SIBLINGS

The arrival of a new baby is the starting point of a relationship that will greatly affect your child's life.

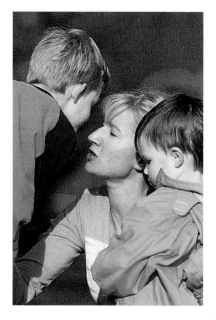

As they grow together, your children may go back and forth from being best friends to rivals. You may see them attacking each other physically and verbally and also ganging up on you to defend each other. Sibling rivalry is a normal, healthy part of growing up together. Children feel a sense of freedom and security with their siblings that they don't with other children. This feeling lets them try out all kinds of emotions that they wouldn't dare show anyone else. Sibling rivalry is usually at its peak in the early years, but be prepared for rivalry to last into your children's teenage years and sometimes even into adulthood.

How you can help

Parents can do a lot to help smooth the relationships between their children. Preparing your older child for a new arrival is a good starting point. Initiate a discussion when your pregnancy becomes fairly obvious. There are a lot of good books that can help. If your child is under age 4, though, he won't

HANDLING DISAGREEMENTS

As children grow up they are bound to fight. It's best to try to let them work out their own disputes as much as you can, because this will help them develop problem-solving and negotiating skills. However, if they are not resolving their own argument or if there is a chance that someone might get hurt, you do need to step in.

Try to act as an arbitrator and avoid blaming one child or the other as much as possible. Ask what's going on – getting a straight answer may not be easy. Ask them to apologize to each other and if they won't, try walking away and saying "I'm not happy about that." The chances are that they will make up later on. You could try talking about the incident with your children later when things have calmed down, suggesting what they could have done instead.

Sly behavior is more difficult to deal with. For example, one child might hide something that's precious to the other. If you confront that child, you'll probably get a denial. If you can be sure that the child did commit the act, tell him you know he did it and that it's hurtful to you and his brother.

Comparison and competition are natural between siblings. Regardless of who wins, always praise your children simply for joining in. It is important to avoid comparing things outside your child's control, for example physical characteristics or academic achievement.

When your children are playing well together, be positive. Simply saying "you played very nicely together this afternoon" will give them the message that you appreciate it when they get along well.

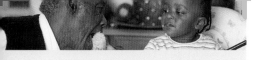

GRANDPARENTS

Many people find that becoming a parent puts their own relationship with their parents into a different perspective. Seeing things from a parent's point of view may give you a new empathy for your parents. You may also think about your own childhood, what you enjoyed and valued, and perhaps about any mistakes that you would like to avoid with your own children.

The role that grandparents play in your child's life depends very much on where they live, what kind of people they are, and how physically able they are. If they live nearby, they can help out in practical ways, for example by babysitting. But even if they live far away, grandparents can still be a source of support and often develop special relationships with their grandchildren, which can be rewarding on both sides.

There are bound to be some differences in the way you and people from an older generation approach child care. For example, your mother may have strong views about early toilet training with which you don't agree. Try to discuss differences in opinion openly with your child's grandparents on both sides of the family. You could explain that your child will benefit from consistency and that you would like them to follow the same basic rules as you do at home.

Many grandparents say that one of the joys of having grandchildren is that they can indulge them for a short time. Be careful not to ask grandparents for more help than they feel they would like, or are able, to give.

really understand pictures of the baby in the uterus. It might be better to read him a story about another child or an animal who becomes a big brother or sister.

Once the baby is born, the way you introduce her is important. It might help if your baby is in a crib, or being held by someone else, when your older child meets his sibling for the first time. Having your arms free to hug your older child, and spending your first few minutes giving him your full attention, is particularly important. Having a present ready for your older child from the baby may be a useful tactic. These things make your older child feel special and also introduces the idea of give and take.

Some studies have demonstrated that the way a mother interacts with the new baby affects the future relationship between the siblings. It is very natural to feel protective, but if you are overly protective of your new baby an older child may be more likely to feel resentful and show aggression as a result.

Try to spend time with your older child alone. You don't have to plan any special activity or expedition;

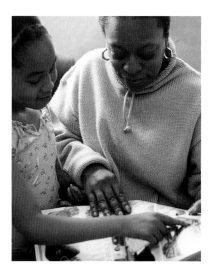

just being together, reading a book, or watching a favorite video, may help your older child to feel better. However, it can be difficult to find the time for this and you will notice that you don't have as much time to rest as you might have had with your first child. Be sure to ask for help from family and friends when you need it. Arranging for someone to spend some time with your older child so you can tend to your new baby, or vice versa, is also a good idea if you can manage it.

RELATIONSHIPS WITH OLDER CHILDREN

Your child's character might seem to change overnight as he approaches puberty. One moment he will be striving for more independence, making him appear difficult, pushing boundaries, and creating arguments. The next, he may seem childish again. This behavior can be tiring and frustrating for parents.

Your child will probably want to start spending less time doing family activities and more time with friends as he enters puberty. This is an important step for him in gaining a sense of his own identity, distinct from his family. These friendships are not just about learning to get along with other people but are also about identifying with a peer group.

Real disagreements can begin to emerge as your child starts to develop views of his own that are not necessarily shared by you. Even if you do seem to have frequent disagreements, your child is still likely to hold you in high regard (although he probably won't let you know this). The rejections and conflicts you may experience often have little to do with your personality but happen simply because you are

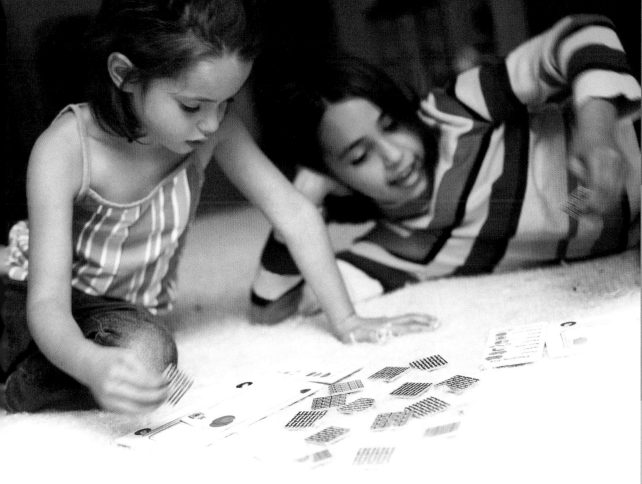

his parent, from whom your child must increasingly separate himself if he is to have his own life.

Rules and negotiation

It will help you if you and your partner discuss discipline in advance of any behavioral incidents. Just as when your child was younger, the key here is for parents to agree between themselves and support each other. Having one parent always allying himself with a child against the other parent can be a recipe for disaster.

Set rules and limits, outlining what you and your partner consider acceptable behavior and what you don't. However quickly your child seems to be growing up, you are still his provider and it is reasonable that you should decide on the ground rules. These should be clear, so that everybody knows where they stand, and they should be applied consistently. However, ground rules should be reasonable and become less restrictive as older children become more responsible.

You will need to figure out what you and your partner consider important and what you don't, so that there aren't too many rules. While some issues will not be negotiable, there should be room for bargaining on others. Sanctions such as grounding, when a child loses the privilege of going out with his friends, or loss of allowance, will work better if they are established in advance. Consequences should never be threatened if they are not going to be carried out if rules are broken. If you do this, warnings soon lose all meaning.

Rules actually help your child feel safe during this transitional phase. Paradoxically, your child also needs

"...as they grow together, your children may go back and forth from being best friends to rivals"

"...your child needs rules to rebel against...rebellion and the questioning of authority is a normal part of growing up"

rules to rebel against, and rebellion and questioning of authority is a normal part of growing up. Rules also help your child think things through and start to develop his own set of values and morals.

Listening to your child
If your child seems upset, ask him what he is thinking. He may confide in you, but don't worry if he doesn't want to talk right away. Talk to him whenever you have an opportunity, such as travel time in the car. Parents are often chauffeuring their children around, and these car trips can be good opportunities to listen to your child's views and to discuss

things. Your child may also appreciate spending time alone with you now and then, perhaps going for a walk, seeing a movie, or going to a hockey game.

The most important thing is to listen to your child. You will only be able to offer advice and comfort to your child if he knows that you are a sympathetic listener and won't immediately react with a judgment or criticism.

WHEN PARENTS SEPARATE OR DIVORCE
Parents are more likely to separate or divorce than ever before. Each year in Canada, 70,000 or more divorces occur. When parents' relationships dissolve, a child's life is turned upside down. However,

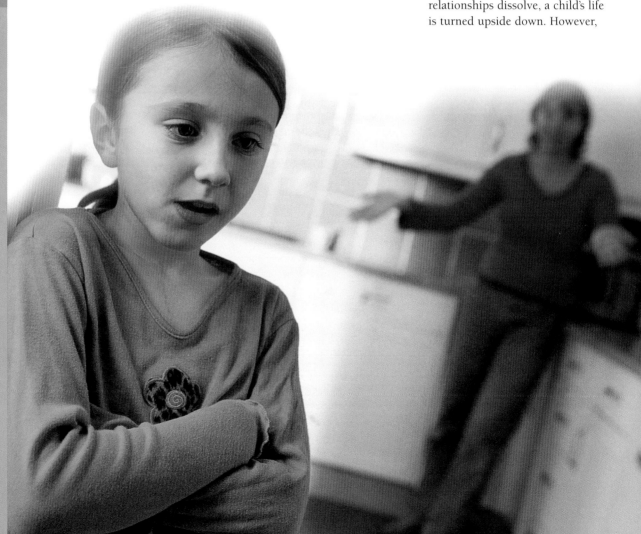

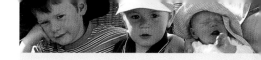

research shows that if the breakup is handled carefully and sensitively, harm can be minimized.

The parent's divorce or separation can be a very confusing time for a child. He might feel a bewildering range of emotions, from anger and rejection to concern that he has done something to cause the split. A child can feel a tremendous sense of loss, which in some ways may feel like a bereavement.

How children are affected

Emotional and behavioral problems are common in children when their parents separate or divorce. If parents have been fighting for some time, these problems can emerge long before the actual separation. The separation may cause a child to feel that his loyalties are pulled in two directions. As a consequence, he may suddenly have trouble concentrating at school when he did not before. Some children may have difficulty expressing their feelings.

When parents split up, the father is often the one to leave the family home and the relationship between fathers and children is more likely to be the one that may later suffer. Research shows the importance of a father's involvement to a child's well-being and performance at school. Children need to know that both parents still love them and will continue to be involved in their lives and that they can still love both their parents.

Preparing for the separation or divorce

A good starting place for helping your child through this difficult time would be for both parents to write a plan together, setting out how they will continue to share responsibility for co-parenting. The plan should be flexible, reflecting the temperaments and changing needs of each child, and specify how each parent will try to meet these needs.

It may be a good idea to give a concrete, practical role to the parent who has left home; for example, picking the children up after sports practice once a week. Keeping a consistent approach between parents to issues such as discipline and treats is still important.

It is also worthwhile for you to discuss maintaining contact with grandparents. Not only are they likely to be important in your child's life and want to remain involved, the grandparents may also be able to give support and help to both parents, as well as to the children.

Making it easier

Although parents may want to protect their child from distress, children will probably sense that something is wrong. Talk with your child early and often about separation, divorce, and custody issues. Speak in open, simple terms and try not to place any blame on your spouse. Also, make sure to let your child know he's not at fault for the divorce or separation.

Children may turn to relatives, neighbors, friends, and teachers for support. In addition, counseling may be worthwhile for children or parents dealing with changes in the family. Parents may also benefit from objective mediation to help settle custody disagreements.

In time, most children learn to cope with the changes brought on by divorce. Parents can help with the adjustment process by maintaining a strong, loving relationship with their child and by putting their child's needs above their own differences.

HOW CHILDREN REACT TO SEPARATION OR DIVORCE

Children respond to a separation or divorce in a variety of ways, depending on factors such as age, temperament, experiences, and family support. The following are normal behaviors parents can anticipate. However, if any of these behaviors become excessive, speak to your doctor.

Children under age 3 may display:

- Sadness
- Fear of others
- Problems eating or sleeping
- Trouble with toilet training
- Tantrums or outbursts

School-age children may display:

- Moodiness
- Problems eating or sleeping
- Trouble at school
- Desire for their parents to reunite
- Anger

Adolescents may display:

- Emotional withdrawal from friends and/or family
- Aggression
- Problems eating or sleeping
- Risk-taking behaviors such as the use of drugs
- Concern with the financial impact of divorce on the family
- Depression

Be patient with any questions your child may have. You may not have all the answers, but listening carefully to your child's questions, feelings, and worries can help your child feel safe and more comfortable.

PLAY

WHEN WE THINK OF CHILDREN, we invariably think of them playing. Playing is what being a child is all about, for both older and younger children. Play keeps your child happy and busy, and is vital for mental, physical, and social development. Although some parents may believe that play has little importance, play is actually children's work. It is how they learn and discover the world.

> "...play is children's own unique and natural way of learning"

WHY PLAY IS IMPORTANT

Adults consider play to be fun. It is a time for recreation, amusement, stress relief, and interacting with others. It is something they might do to take a break from work.

Children are somewhat different. The phrase "play is children's work" has a lot of truth in it. For children, play isn't motivated by the need for relaxation, although it can be relaxing. Instead, play is children's

own unique and natural way of learning. A child needs to learn in order to survive. That may sound dramatic, but from the earliest months, play is the main means by which your child can acquire the skills she needs to learn and grow physically, mentally, and socially.

You don't, for example, teach your child to talk using books and tapes the way you would teach a second language to an adult. Instead

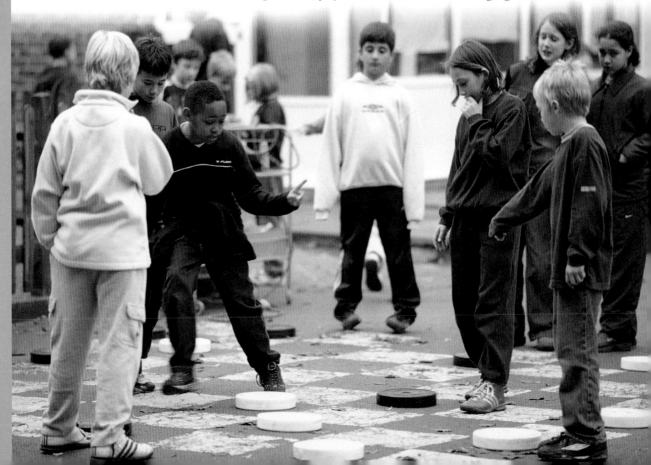

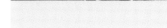

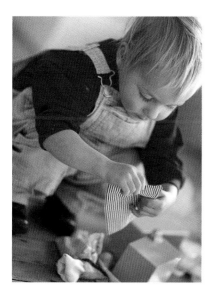

you sing nursery rhymes to her and look at picture books together, and slowly she starts to understand the basis of language. Instead of signing your child up for a crash course in physics, you buy her a rattle – when she shakes it and discovers it makes a sound she realizes that she can make things happen. It's an early lesson in cause and effect.

Different types of play have different roles. Physical play, for example, is essential for developing your child's strength, balance, and coordination. Messy play – exploring water, mud, and sand – helps your child find out about the physical world around her.

Playing with other children teaches your child vital social skills, such as cooperation and empathy. Playing also enables your child to develop problem-solving and communication skills. There's only one ball and both children want it; what's the best solution and how is it best conveyed?

In these ways, play is a constructive activity as well as being essential for the development of a happy, healthy child.

ENCOURAGING PLAY – WHAT YOU CAN DO

Children love to play. And while it helps for parents to appreciate the purpose and meaning of play, it is important to remember that play is also about having fun.

With that in mind, there's a lot you can do to facilitate your child's play. From the earliest age your child will enjoy toys. They don't need to be expensive or numerous, but they should be appropriate for your child's age. You can get great value out of toys that will grow with your child. For example, simple building or construction kits, which you can add to over the years, can be played with again and again.

Children also need opportunities to play. Toys are no good if your child never has the time to play with them. Giving your child uninterrupted time to play at turning her bedroom into a store, for example, can be more valuable than buying the latest game or whisking her off to a new activity. Child care needs and the desire to provide a "head start" can tempt many parents to overfill their children's lives with classes and extracurricular activities.

Stimulation

New environments can provide fresh and exciting stimulation. While your 4-year-old may still enjoy building tents out of blankets and chairs, your 8-year-old will be looking for new challenges. Going for a picnic in the woods, for example, may inspire your older child to attempt to create a whole new kind of shelter using leaves, stones, and sticks.

Stimulating play opportunities can be increasingly hard to provide as your child gets older. Outdoor play is especially important in

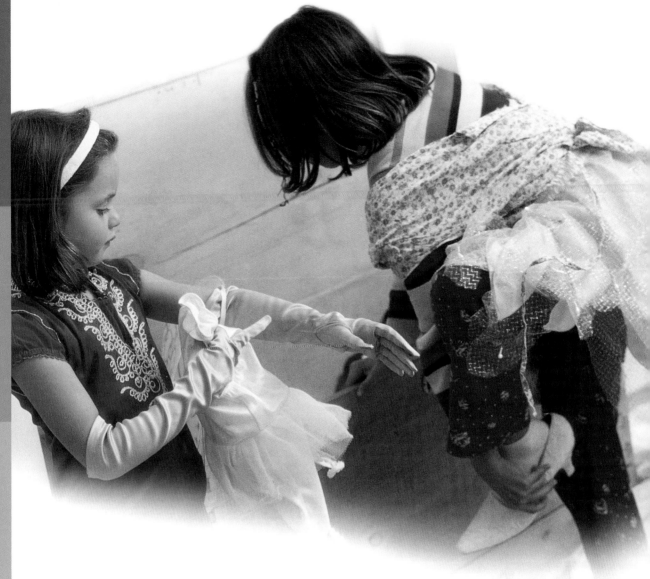

"It's not uncommon for young children
to invent imaginary playmates."

offering children the chance to build
their confidence, make decisions,
and develop skills in terms of risk
assessment. Yet some children may
get bored by parks and playgrounds
if they are taken there too often.
Some parents prefer their children
not to ride bikes or skateboards,
nor climb jungle gyms or trees
because of the risk of injury. Parents
may be wary of offering them the
freedom in their environment that
they experienced as children because

of the increase in street traffic and
the fear of "stranger danger."

How far you are prepared to go
to give your child a sense of freedom
and adventure is an individual
matter. To a certain extent it will
depend on where you live and the
age and maturity of your child. For
many families, supervised activities –
hiking in the mountains or staying
at a campsite close to the beach –
give their children the chance they
need to spread their wings safely.

FANTASY PLAY
Watching your child play make-
believe is one of the real pleasures of
parenthood. Your toddler pretends to
sip from a plastic cup. Your preschool
child turns a broomstick into a horse
and the bunk bed into a castle, and
insists you call him "Sir Knight"
when you call him in for lunch. By
the time he's in kindergarten, your
child is still enjoying fantasy play,
only now he is more likely to be
the director of the story, turning

his action figures into a mountain rescue team and manipulating all the characters to help his story come to life. Some children may prefer to share their fantasy play, so siblings and friends become part of the cast. Others become absorbed in a private imaginary world. It's not uncommon for young children to invent imaginary playmates.

PLAYING WITH YOUR CHILD

From day one you are your child's preferred playmate and, whether you like it or not, your child will spend hours encouraging you to join in with her favorite activities. For some parents, play comes naturally. For others, dressing up as a pirate and sailing in a makeshift ship is not very enticing, especially while chores pile up.

Play, however, is one of the primary ways parents and children bond. And while ignoring the chores can be hard, if you want to nurture a good relationship with your child it may be worth postponing the housework for a while.

Playing together is also a social activity. It is one of the major ways in which a child learns how to relate to other people. Think of the hours you and your baby spent passing a rattle backward and forward. This kind of give and take is your child's first experience of turn-taking, a skill which in later years will be the foundation of good relationships.

Making compromises

At certain periods of your child's development you may feel more in tune with her needs. Some parents, for example, are very baby-oriented and love cuddling and tickling games. You may be bored by playing "pretend" games but happy to sit for

half an hour and color. If this is the case, there's no point feeling guilty or forcing yourself to do an activity you dislike. Your child will sense your disinterest. Try to find activities that you both enjoy. If you are actually having fun instead of just pretending to enjoy yourself, your child will be much more likely to see the activity as worthwhile.

TV, COMPUTERS, VIDEO GAMES – GOOD OR BAD?

Many parents comment that their children spend a good deal of time on the computer or watching TV. But how much is too much? And is it all bad? It's unlikely that snuggling up with your older child on the sofa a couple of evenings a week to watch a favorite program will adversely affect her. Television and computers can be a valuable source of information. Used carefully, they can broaden your child's outlook on the world.

However, if you leave your child to her own devices she may spend many hours mesmerized in front of the screen. The obvious worry is that your child may be viewing inappropriate material. Many computer games, TV shows, and commercials display violence, sexual and other stereotypes, and marketing aimed at children. Watch programs with your child and discuss the content in the context of your own family values.

Of equal concern is that a child who is sitting indoors in front of a screen all day is inactive and solitary.

Limit your child to a reasonable amount of time each day, or a certain number of hours a week, for watching programs or playing on the computer. When enforcing limits, a kitchen timer can prevent arguments when the time's up.

MEDIA EXPOSURE

Recommendations from the Canadian Pediatric Society:

Develop good media habits well before children start school.

Keep television sets and the Internet out of children's bedrooms.

Learn about Canadian and American rating systems.

Monitor the shows children and adolescents watch. Encourage informational, educational, and nonviolent programs.

Talk to your child about stereotypical and violent images in the media.

Look at your own media habits and set a good example.

Encourage alternative activities such as reading, sports, hobbies, or creative play.

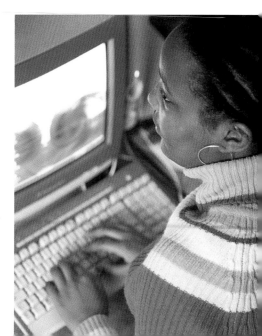

EXERCISE

KEEPING CHILDREN PHYSICALLY FIT IS ESSENTIAL FOR THEIR HEALTH. Whether your child is naturally athletic or not, and whether or not you are interested in sports yourself, there are a lot of fun ways to help keep her active. Encouraging activity from an early age will get your child into good habits that will help her stay healthy into adolescence and adulthood.

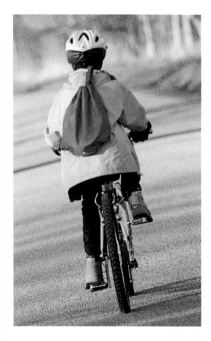

WHY EXERCISE IS IMPORTANT

At a glance, it may appear we are a nation obsessed with health. Pick up a flyer from your local community center and you will see a vast range of activities from which to choose. Magazines and newspapers are crammed with advice on diet and exercise. But sadly, children today are getting fatter, not fitter.

Making sure your child is physically fit and healthy is vital for her health and well-being. Getting off the couch and into action helps build a healthy heart, develop strong muscles and bones, and reduce body fat. It also has a positive impact on your child's well-being. During exercise, for example, chemicals called endorphins are released by the brain, causing the body to feel more relaxed. Doing well at a chosen activity also helps boost a child's self-esteem. Participating in sports and activities also has social benefits. It gives children a chance to mix with others, make friends, and learn about the "give and take" needed to keep play fun and fair.

Encouraging children to exercise also helps them stay fit in later life. Research has shown that physically active children are more likely to remain active in later life. Physically fit adults have less chance of developing serious diseases including heart disease, diabetes, and osteoporosis.

HOW MUCH EXERCISE IS RIGHT FOR MY CHILD?

How do you know whether or not your child is getting all the physical activity she needs? Research has shown that to maintain necessary

"...getting off the couch and into action helps build healthy hearts, muscles, and bones"

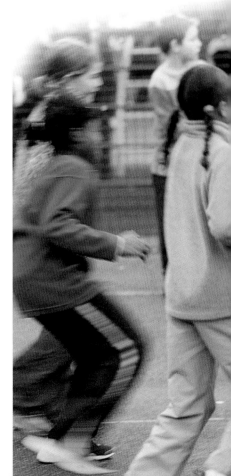

levels of fitness, children of all ages need to have regular physical activity. Examples of moderate-intensity activities include brisk walking, swimming, dancing, active play, bicycling, and most sports.

Health experts recommend that children take part in activities that are beneficial for developing and maintaining muscular strength and flexibility and bone health. Activities such as climbing, skipping, jumping, and gymnastics are good for this.

It is probably most important to choose a type of activity that your child enjoys. For example, a child who walks briskly to and from school, plays outside most days, does a regular activity such as soccer or dancing, and joins in with family activities on weekends is probably averaging the recommended level of exercise over the week.

FAMILY ACTIVITIES

At younger ages, children find almost any activity more attractive if their parents are involved too. Putting the emphasis on fun and family participation rather than physical activity per se can inspire even the most sedentary child. If your child sees the value you attach to being out and about and on the move, they are more likely to see it as worthwhile as well.

Try planning specific physical activities for the whole family on weekends, such as swimming,

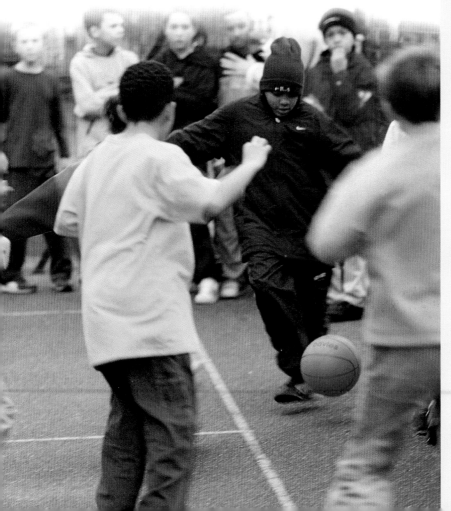

IS YOUR FAMILY ACTIVE ENOUGH?

Use this simple question-and-answer guide to find out whether your family is getting enough exercise.

Do you and your child do such activities as going walking, hiking, or biking together?
Yes/No

Do you and your partner participate in sports or fitness classes, or work out?
Yes/No

Does your child spend less than 2 hours a day watching television, playing video games, or using the computer?
Yes/No

Does your child participate in physical activity programs at school?
Yes/No

Does your child participate in physical activities or sports that are not school based?
Yes/No

Here's how to interpret your answers:

All yes
Congratulations! You are setting a great example for your child and she is learning to make physical activity part of her lifestyle.

All no
Time to get moving – both you and your child!

A mix of yes and no
Look at where you answered no – is it an area that needs improvement?

Adapted from the Family Health – Active Living Quiz
Copyright © Heart & Stroke Foundation of Canada

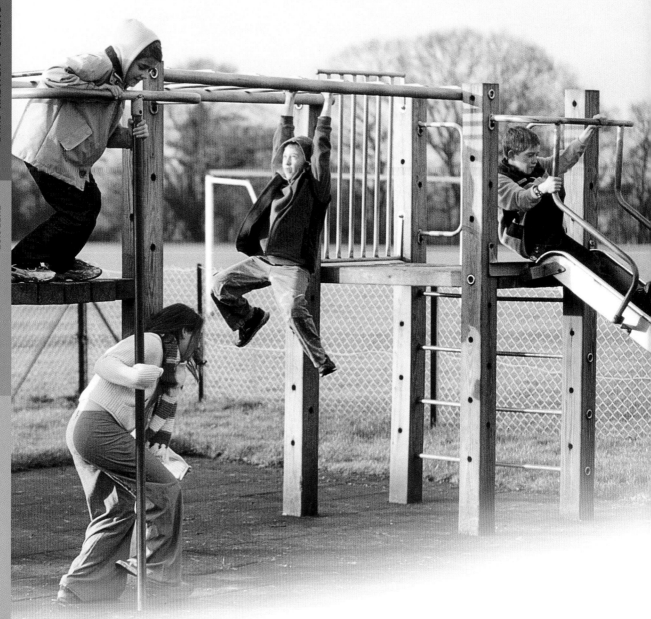

bicycling, ice-skating, and walking. Planning ahead can help keep it fun. A child probably won't enjoy being marched across a hilltop just because it's good for them, but take a picnic and a kite and it will be an afternoon to remember.

Getting a family membership at your local community or recreation center may also be a good idea. In addition to the fun you can have doing activities together, structured activities for preschool and school-age children will probably also be included in the membership.

You don't always need to go out for the day to be active. If you have a yard, make the most of it. When you can't face another game of soccer, get your children to help you with garden chores, such as digging up the weeds or raking the leaves. Make a big pile and then let them jump in the middle.

As summer fades and winter sets in, it's easy to become less active and spend more time indoors, but with the right outdoor clothes there's no excuse. Dress your children in a warm fleece, a ski jacket, and warm waterproof boots and they may have great fun throwing snowballs or splashing in puddles outside.

On rainy days you can have active fun indoors as well, especially with younger children. Putting on a tape or CD and dancing is good for you and your child. Hopping, skipping, and jumping games don't require

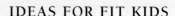

much room either, but for safety's sake, be sure to keep clear of any toys or furniture.

Small children are naturally active and love movement, so it won't take much effort to get them going. If you are active yourself and have healthy habits, your children will follow your example. Walking or bicycling to stores instead of jumping in the car can make a big difference. If being active becomes a natural part of your child's day, she is more likely to keep it up for the rest of her life.

PHYSICAL FUN FOR CHILDREN UNDER AGE 5

Toddlers and preschoolers often don't need much encouragement when it comes to being active. Once they are mobile, most young children seem to be permanently on the go and parents need to find constructive ways to channel this natural energy. Activities where parents participate as well are best for the under-3s, while a preschool child may be happy to join in an activity with you just watching. Music and movement and toddler gymnastics are popular choices. Classes like these help children learn a whole variety of skills, such as climbing and jumping, and encourage coordination, balance, and agility. Your child can build her muscles while having fun too. Swimming within arm's reach of a supervising adult can also be a good choice. Children over 4 years may be ready for formal swimming lessons.

At this age, it's especially important to balance periods when your child is expending physical energy with quieter times when she can recharge her batteries. Children don't know their own limits and can find it difficult to

wind down. Overactive children can become sleep-deprived, which may in turn lead to behavioral problems. Incorporating calm, relaxing activities into your child's day to balance the more physically demanding ones will help her maintain her energy levels and her good temper.

ACTIVITIES FOR OLDER CHILDREN

Once your child is settled at school, she may enjoy taking part in an after-school activity. Your local community center or library may have information on clubs, games, and activities available in your area. Think in terms of health and fitness rather than just organized games, and the range of activities to choose from is enormous, from soccer and tennis to ice skating and karate.

The more activities your child tries, the more likely she is to find something she enjoys doing. These trial periods can be frustrating for parents, and possibly expensive. To a certain extent you can avoid false starts by making sure your child is really eager and knows what's involved with the activity that interests her. You may love the idea of your daughter learning how to play tennis, especially if it's something you wish you had taken up when you were younger, but will she enjoy it? Ask her first and let her go along to watch a session before signing her up. This will also give you a chance to check out how well the activity is run. Do the children look as if they are having fun, as well as developing new skills? Are the coaches friendly and encouraging? Do they take into account each child's individual needs and abilities?

Children are also more likely to take part in a new activity if they

Set a good example – if your child sees you enjoying active pursuits, she is more likely to join in.

Make physical activity part of your family's everyday routine, like brushing teeth and eating a healthy diet.

Try to get your child outside for at least part of the day.

At least once a week try to do an activity together as a family, such as swimming or bicycling.

Take your toddler to a music and movement or toddler gymnastics class.

Encourage your older child to join an after-school activity class or club.

Help your child by teaching her basic skills such as hopping, jumping, skipping, throwing, and catching.

Invite friends over to play – active games are more fun with others.

Provide equipment for active fun such as a bike, jump rope, and balls.

Limit the amount of time your child spends in front of the TV and computer.

"...the more activities your child tries, the more likely she is to find something that she enjoys doing and will keep up"

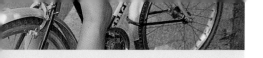

CHECK IT OUT

If your child is taking part in an organized activity or athletics outside school, you'll want to check out some things about the teacher or coach and how the activity is run.

Check that the teacher is properly trained and qualified.

Check that the activity is endorsed by a relevant organization.

Make sure the teacher is happy to adjust the activity to match your child's ability and needs.

Check that the teacher encourages fun and participation above winning.

Make sure that the playing environment is safe and that equipment is well maintained.

have a friend going with them. Speak to the parents of your child's friends and see if they might be interested in joining too. A possible bonus is that you may be able to share the responsibility for supervising the children and picking them up and dropping them off.

Your child's personality may be a factor in choosing a new activity. Children who are naturally athletic may flourish in a more competitive environment. If your child finds it hard to be assertive, a game such as soccer where she needs to be an active participant might become dispiriting. Activities such as swimming or dancing, where she can progress at her own speed might be a better choice.

Once your child has decided on an activity, be prepared to ease her in slowly. Some children may just want to sit and watch during the first session. A good coach will

come and have a friendly chat and make your child feel welcome, and then she will probably feel confident about joining in the following week. Don't pressure her. Instead, you should point out how much fun everyone else is having and reassure her that chances are good that she will enjoy herself too.

Once your child has started an activity, remember to give her a lot of praise and encouragement, particularly if she is learning a new skill. Keep the feedback positive and avoid pushing her too hard. Remember, the emphasis should be on having fun.

READY FOR ACTION

If your child has previously done very little activity, she should build up slowly. This is also important if your child has been ill or out of action for any other reason. Doing too much too soon could exhaust your child and she may simply get run down. Start instead by aiming for no more than half an hour of activity a day and gradually increase this over a period of time.

Your child will enjoy activities more if she is feeling energetic. Small children, especially, will tire quickly without regular rest and food. Take snacks for after school so your child has a chance to refuel before going on to her dance class or swimming lesson. Make sure she has breakfast before leaving for school in the morning and encourage her to have a good lunch before going on a long walk or bicycle ride.

Children burn up calories very quickly, so providing nutritious snacks, such as fruit, will help keep them going. When they are active, children also lose fluid rapidly and

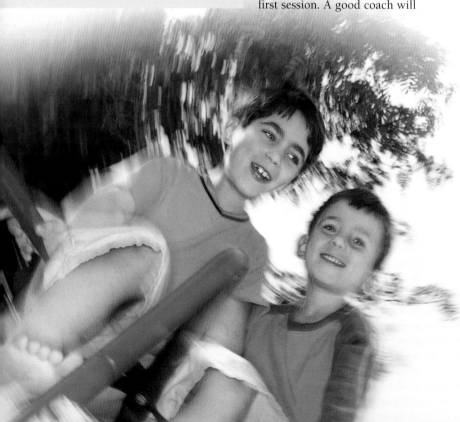

becoming dehydrated will make them irritable and lethargic. You should offer your child plenty to drink, preferably water or an electrolyte replenisher, during physical activities.

Growing children get tired easily, so having plenty of rest is important if they are to recharge their batteries properly. Between the ages of 5 and 11 children need at least 9 hours of sleep at night. Getting to sleep, however, may be a problem if they are overstimulated. Finish games such as dancing around the living room well before bedtime, so that your child can wind down.

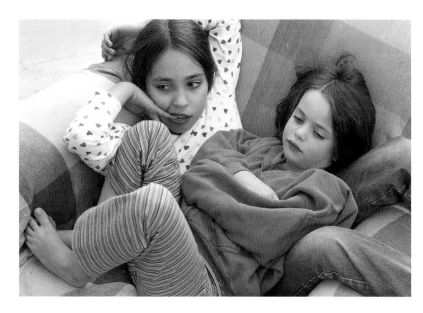

THE GREAT OUTDOORS

If you have a yard, you should make the most of it for your child. A jungle gym, swing, or even a rope hanging securely from a branch will encourage your child to be active outdoors. Playground equipment should be properly assembled on a level, energy-absorbent surface such as sand or bark, and securely anchored. Other activities that can get children moving outside include scooters, hula hoops, balls, bikes, and roller skates.

Don't forget the local park. It's free and can offer children great entertainment value. Play equipment can help younger children develop their strength and coordination. For older children, it can provide the space for them to kick a ball or play tag, soccer, or catch. You can take your child's friends with you and arrange a rotation with other parents for days when you can't supervise.

Although lazing on the beach can be very relaxing, active vacations can be invigorating and refreshing too.

There are also a lot of adventurous outdoor activity vacations available for families. A week-long vacation spent learning to canoe, sail, or ski could spark a lifelong interest for your child.

WATCH FOR BURN OUT

Encourage your child to try a range of different activities rather than specializing in just one at a young age. Many sports experts recognize that children who play one sport obsessively can become bored and burned out. Playing a variety of sports also helps develop different skills.

WALKING TO SCHOOL

If your child can walk to school you'll not only boost his physcial fitness but you will also help cut down on traffic congestion and pollution. Some schools have a "walking bus" program, led by volunteers. The "bus" operates along a route, picking up "passengers" before delivering them safely to school.

"...growing children get tired easily, so having plenty of rest is important for them to recharge their batteries...they need to wind down well before bedtime"

SLEEP

Sleep is essential for children. It stimulates growth, plays a crucial role in brain development, and affects how well your child manages everyday life. We all know that children need their sleep, and this need continues to be important through adolescence and even adulthood. Sleep is vital because it gives us the energy needed to function well and enjoy life.

> "...sleep is crucial for brain development, allowing your child to process new information"

WHY SLEEP IS IMPORTANT

Most parents will recognize that, without regular sleep, children may become bad tempered and difficult and find it hard to concentrate. Their appetites are affected, their immune systems are weakened, and they are more likely to pick up viruses and other infections.

For a child, sleep is also essential for growth. Newborns seem to sleep all the time. This is because they are developing physically at a great rate, and growth hormone is released and cells multiply fastest during sleep; as your child gets older, he will tend to grow in spurts, almost overnight sometimes, and may need extra sleep to compensate.

Sleep is crucial for your child's brain development, too. Newborns need about twice as much rapid eye movement (REM) sleep than adults. During the REM phase of the sleep cycle, the body is relaxed but the brain is very active. You may notice your baby's face twitch and eyelids flicker. Your sleeping baby is actually achieving a huge amount, processing and storing the mass of new information taken in during his waking hours.

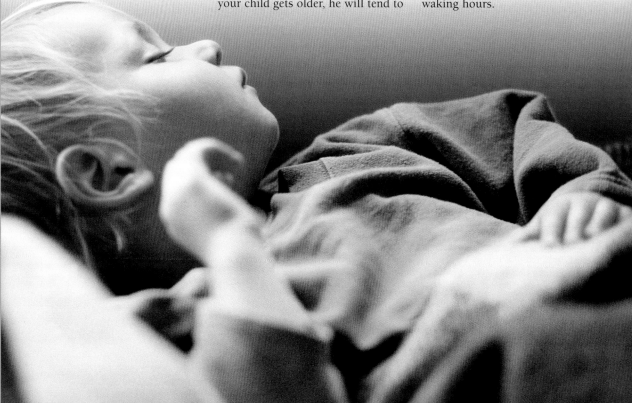

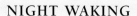

HOW MUCH SLEEP DO CHILDREN NEED?

Children vary in the amount of sleep they need, but there are guidelines. Your newborn probably will sleep 16–20 hours a day. This amount gradually decreases until, by 6 months, he is averaging 14 hours in a 24-hour period, including a couple of one- or two-hour daytime naps. By age 2, most toddlers sleep 10–13 hours in every 24, including a daytime nap that may vary from 20 minutes to a few hours. By the age of 3, sleep needs vary from 10–12 hours in every 24, and daytime naps may be only a happy memory.

As your child continues to develop, his sleep pattern will stay roughly within this range. Children starting school are often very tired for the first few weeks and will need extra sleep to compensate.

If you think your child may need more sleep, look at how well he manages during the day. A difficult, irritable child may need more sleep. Making bedtime half an hour earlier may make a big difference.

BEDTIME ROUTINES

Like many adults, children need a bedtime ritual. Follow the same routine every night and your child will quickly learn what's expected.

Bedtime could start with a relaxing bath followed by a story, a goodnight kiss, and then lights out. The key is to help your child unwind, so avoid boisterous bedtime games. It is preferable to put a child to bed while he is still awake. If he learns how to fall asleep on his own at bedtime – without being rocked or fed – he will learn that he can go back to sleep by himself if he wakes at night.

Even if your child is old enough to put himself to bed, he may still need help winding down. Activities such as watching TV or playing video games could be too stimulating just before bedtime. Encourage him to read or listen to soothing music instead.

DEALING WITH SLEEPLESSNESS IN OLDER CHILDREN

Older children can be prone to the occasional sleepless night. Tossing and turning only makes matters worse. It may be time to let your child stay up a little later so he can go to bed when he is truly tired. Otherwise, suggest that he read or listen to a story on tape. Letting him stay awake for a while and turn off the light when he's ready may help. Teenagers also tend to have a later sleep time, partly due to hormonal changes and partly because of evening homework, jobs, or social activities. They still need about 9 to 10 hours of sleep per night. Teens with insomnia should limit caffeine intake and consult their doctor if sleeping problems persist.

NIGHTMARES & NIGHT TERRORS

If your child wakes in the night distressed from a nightmare, reassure him that it was just a dream and dreams can't hurt. Tell him everyone has dreams and when he goes back to sleep it will be gone. Comfort him until he's ready to fall back to sleep. Night terrors are an extreme form of nightmare and, as with nightmares, they are no cause for concern unless your child has them frequently. Your child will appear to be awake with his eyes open and will be very scared. It's important to stay calm yourself. Don't try to wake him. He will soon settle down without waking and in the morning he will remember nothing about it.

NIGHT WAKING

For some children night waking continues to be a problem, which can last throughout the toddler years and beyond. Breaking the habit of your child needing you in the night can be emotionally and physically exhausting but may help everyone.

The process known as "controlled crying" (see p.31) can be as effective at breaking the night-waking pattern in children as it is in babies, although you may find that you need to be even more persistent with an older child. You could try the following things:

When your child wakes, avoid feeding or cuddling him or making a lot of noise.

Check that your child is safe, say a few comforting words, and then kiss him goodnight. If your child has come into your bed, take him back to his own bed right away.

If your child cries out again, don't go back immediately. He may need a chance to cry, stop crying, and then go back to sleep by himself.

Go back if the crying sounds more desperate, and repeat the sequence above.

You may have to do this repeatedly before your child finally falls sleep. But it's worth persevering now and for the next few nights. After a week or so, most children learn how to go back to sleep again on their own. Consult your doctor if sleeping problems persist.

HEALTHY EATING

OVER THE NEXT 10 YEARS YOUR CHILD WILL CONTINUE to grow and develop, but at different rates depending on his age. His diet will also change from being predominantly milk-based to including a wide variety of foods. The first five years in particular may involve a lot of trial and error, as your child learns to feed himself and becomes accustomed to new textures and flavors.

GOOD HABITS START EARLY

We all know how difficult it can be to break habits once they are formed, and this is especially true of dietary habits. So, although your child may seem a long way from adulthood, setting a good example now will make him more likely to eat a healthy diet in the future. Introducing your child to a healthy diet early in life is perhaps one of the best gifts you can ever give him.

A healthy diet does not simply involve eating the right balance of foods, but also takes into account the social and psychological aspects of eating. It has been shown that good eating habits, including aspects such as eating together regularly as a family, can enhance children's communication skills and language development.

WHAT IS A BALANCED DIET?

A balanced diet is one that includes foods that provide all the nutrients essential for growth and development. Canada's Food Guide is a very useful resource to help you decide on a healthy range of foods. You can obtain a copy from your doctor. Your child will achieve a balanced diet if he eats as wide a variety of foods as possible, including:
• 5–12 servings daily of Grain Products

• 5–10 servings daily of Vegetables and Fruit
• 2–4 servings daily of Milk Products
• 2–3 servings daily of Meat and Alternatives.

Note that the exact number of servings needed depends on the age and activity level of the child.

This model can be used by the whole family, but should be adapted for children under the age of 5 to include more carbohydrate-rich Grain Products and higher fat but nutritious foods, such as cheese, homogenized milk, and peanut butter. Young children need plenty of these foods to meet their energy and nutrient requirements. Energy (or calories) from fats or carbohydrates is essential to fuel the rapid growth and development that takes place in this age group. It is important to progress toward a healthy adult diet, but the diet of young children should not be too high in bulky fiber-rich foods or too low in fat. Low-fat products are also not recommended for children under the age of 2.

FEEDING YOUR PRESCHOOLER

To fuel the rapid growth that takes place during the preschool years, your child will need to consume adequate calories and nutrients. Their diet needs to be high in both

of these, but since young children have small stomachs, they cannot eat a great deal at one sitting. For this reason, offer your child small, frequent meals to ensure he receives adequate nutrition.

However, these early years are the right time to start influencing your child's eating habits. Toddlers and preschoolers are wholly dependent on their parents and caregivers for their food and they form their eating habits by copying the adults and siblings around them.

Eating a variety of foods can sometimes become an issue with a

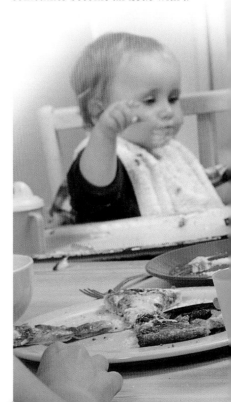

child, but it is less likely to be a problem if your attention is not focused entirely on him and what he is eating. Bringing the whole family together for mealtimes and making them social occasions can encourage your child to eat better.

Surveys have found that preschool-age children often do not consume adequate quantities of vitamins A and D. If your child has a poor or erratic appetite or if she follows a vegan diet, your doctor may recommend a daily supplement. Try to maximize the vitamins in regular meals.

EXERCISE IS IMPORTANT

Exercise is also important for good health. The increase in obesity in Canada is strongly associated with reduced activity levels. Children are becoming more obese partly because they spend more time playing with computers and video games and watching TV and less time being physically active. Activities don't have to mean expense. Visiting the park as often as possible and allowing your child to run around, and going swimming or on family walks, are good ways of keeping your child active. Encourage general activity

ORGANIC, GENETICALLY MODIFIED, AND IRRADIATED FOODS

Organic foods are produced with minimal use of pesticides and contain significantly lower levels of pesticide residue than food grown conventionally. Organically farmed animals are not given antibiotics or hormones routinely to prevent disease or promote growth. But there is no evidence to date to suggest that organic foods are either more nutritious or safer than nonorganic foods (although they are commonly believed to be so).

The extra cost of organic farming is reflected in the higher cost of organic products. Greater demand for organically farmed food may lead to lower prices for organic goods.

Genetic modification of food involves the transfer of desirable genes from one food to another. Genetically Modified (GM) food is often referred to as biotechnology-derived food. Health Canada conducts a thorough safety assessment of GM foods before they are allowed to enter the marketplace.

Irradiated food is exposed to low levels of radiation to delay ripening (thereby extending the shelf life) and kill molds, bacteria, and insects. Studies have shown that irradiated foods are safe for consumption. Health Canada allows radiation of certain foods (including flour, spices, potatoes, and onions) and requires labeling to indicate such processing.

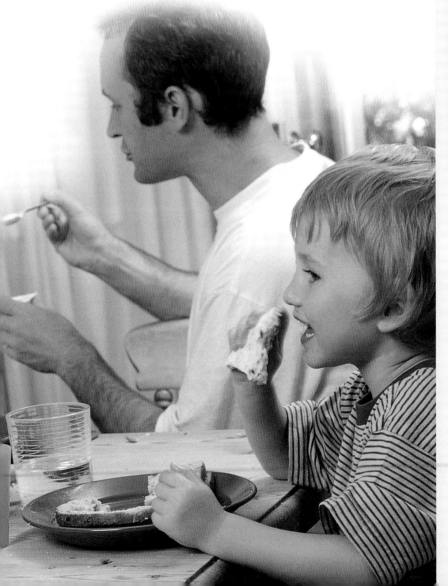

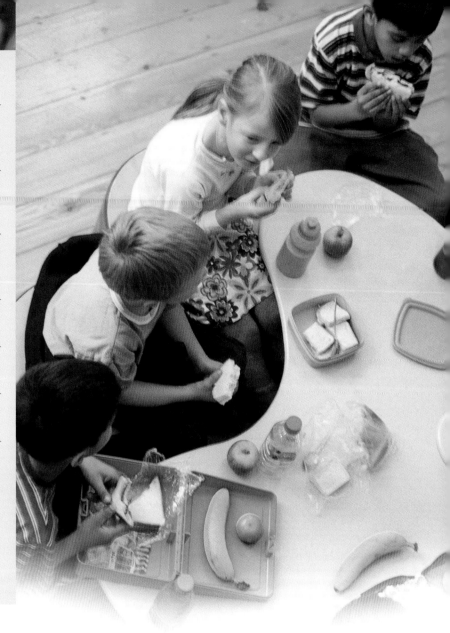

HEALTHY IDEAS FOR LUNCHBOXES

Hummus and carrot in wholegrain bread, banana, oatmeal cookie, yogurt drink or soya alternative

Ham and cheese sandwich using multi-grain bread, 2 clementines, slice of banana bread, water

Falafel in a pita pocket, low-fat yogurt or calcium- enriched soya alternative, fruit cup, cereal bar, fruit juice

Cheese sandwich, grapes, currant bun, yogurt, apple juice

Pasta salad, apple, carrot muffin, yogurt drink

Tuna salad in a tortilla, small box of raisins, lemon loaf, bottle of water

Bran muffin with a cheese stick, banana, chocolate pudding cup, juice box

with the family by having races or playing games such as soccer, baseball, or catch.

Your school-age child will have more opportunities for physical activity on the playground and in school sport activities, although these on their own may not provide sufficient exercise. Another way to increase your child's activity levels and his social skills is to introduce him to outdoor activities, scouting programs, or classes such as martial arts or swimming. You should make regular physical activity a part of your family's routine. This will not only help

prevent obesity and heart disease but will also develop strong bones and can improve mood and concentration in the short term. For more ideas on fitness activities, see p.104.

MOVING TOWARD ADULT EATING

From the age of about 5, your child will have finished the experimental period and should be eating pretty much the same foods as the rest of the family. From 5 years onward, there will be new challenges for you and your child, as he starts school and his social environment

begins to change. Meal patterns and activity levels will also change. Your child will begin to consume more adult-size portions of food at mealtimes as he becomes more active and there is less time for him to snack during the day.

Your child's growth will generally be gradual and steady. Once your child is school-age, you can start to introduce the sound dietary principles recommended for a healthy adult diet – eating low-fat, high-fiber foods, controlling weight within acceptable limits, and moderating salt intake. If you included a variety of beans, fruit, and vegetables and whole grains and bread in your child's diet during the preschool years, the transition to a healthy, more adult eating style will be smoother.

KEEPING A BALANCE

While it is important to help your child develop healthy eating habits, it is also important to remain realistic. Your older child will be introduced to new, and possibly what you consider "unhealthy," foods and eating habits by his new social circle and peers. There will also be more social occasions outside the home where you may have little influence over food choice. Children these days also have more spending power. This is where early teaching of good eating habits will influence your child to make healthy food choices on his own. Your child may also develop new food dislikes because of peer pressure. Remember that mealtimes should not become battlegrounds. You should continue to offer your child the same food as the rest of the family and make sure that mealtimes remain social occasions for everyone.

A GREAT SMILE GUARANTEED

Most school-age children have at least one cavity or filling, so it makes sense to develop good oral hygiene as well as dietary habits from as young an age as possible. Sugary foods and drinks contribute greatly to tooth decay in children and such foods also provide "empty" calories – calories that provide no nutrients. However, as parents we have to be realistic – it may be impossible to avoid all sweet foods. It is thought that we all have a tendency to like sweetness, possibly from when our

HEALTHY EATING FOR YOUR PRESCHOOL & SCHOOL-AGE CHILD

Tips for feeding toddlers and preschoolers

- Introduce any new foods gradually, no more than one every few days.
- Make your child's diet as varied and colorful as possible to encourage him to accept new foods and reduce the likelihood of bad eating habits.
- Provide small, frequent meals to accommodate your toddler's small stomach. Try 4–6 small meals a day.
- Whole milk should be given up to the age of 2. Low-fat milk, which is also lower in calories, may be introduced from 2 years onward if your child is eating well.
- Try to make mealtimes a family affair, with everyone sitting around the table.
- Dietary advice aimed at keeping adults healthy, such as eating high-fiber, low-fat food, is not appropriate for toddlers and preschoolers.
- Introduce fiber by serving whole-grain or whole-wheat bread, breakfast cereals, fruits, and vegetables.
- Encourage your child to eat five portions of fruit and vegetables a day. A rough guide for a portion of fruit for a toddler or preschooler would be a child-size handful – for instance, half a tangerine for a 2-year-old, half an apple for a 5-year-old.
- Make sure most of the foods your child eats come from each of the four main food groups, avoiding sugary or high-fat foods that do not provide many nutrients.
- Do not introduce peanut products into your child's diet before the age of 3 if there is a family history of allergy (eczema, asthma, allergic rhinitis, food allergies).
- Children younger than 4 years are at risk for choking on food cut into large chunks and firm, smooth foods such as nuts, raw vegetables, and hard candy, as well as on popcorn, hot dogs, and thick spreads such as peanut butter.

- If your child refuses a food, try reintroducing it later in a different form. For instance, carrots can be given raw, cooked, mashed, mixed with other foods, or cut into different shapes just for fun.
- Your child will have his own likes and dislikes. Respect these – you wouldn't want to be forced to eat a food you dislike.
- Make sure your child is drinking enough fluids, mostly milk or water – 6–8 drinks a day is a rough guide.
- Keep candy, chocolates, and chips to a minimum.

Tips for feeding 5–11 year olds

- Make sure your child eats regular meals, especially breakfast (see p.118).
- Ensure that he eats from the food groups (see p.112) as outlined by Canada's Food Guide.
- Provide plenty of carbohydrate-rich bread, rice, pasta, and cereals.
- Try to get your child to eat five portions of fruit and vegetables daily. A portion is one apple, pear, or peach; two tangerines or plums; a handful of grapes; a small bowl (about 100g/4oz) of canned fruit in natural juice; 1 small side salad; 2 tablespoons of cooked vegetables.
- Serve lean meats, fish (especially oily fish, such as salmon or mackerel, which are rich sources of omega-3 fatty acids), beans, and legumes.
- Low-fat or fat-free dairy products should now be used as your child's main source of calcium.
- Avoid using too much oil or butter in your cooking.
- Do not add salt to food at the table, and minimize the use of salt when cooking.
- Keep candy, chocolate, and sweet drinks to a minimum.

PROTECTING YOUR CHILD'S TEETH

Good dental health is closely linked to a good diet. Along with regular trips to the dentist, there are many ways to protect your child's teeth from decay.

Carbonated, sugary drinks should be avoided. The acid and sugar in these drinks damage teeth. Sugar-free diet drinks are not intended for young children either. They contain artificial sweeteners, such as aspartame, which should be consumed in moderation.

Limit daily juice intake to small amounts of 100% juice as part of a meal or snack. Limit children ages 1–6 years to 120–180 ml (4–6 fl.oz) of juice and older children to 240–360 ml (8–12 fl.oz). Frequent exposure to the acid and sugar in juice can damage the teeth. Dilute juice with water if your child often drinks juice.

Introduce your child to a training cup as soon as he is ready. Phase out bottlefeeding from the age of 8–12 months. Breastfed babies may skip feeding from bottles entirely. Don't let your baby fall asleep with a bottle or while breastfeeding. Wipe his gums and/or teeth using soft gauze, a washcloth, or an infant toothbrush and plain water before bedtime.

Teach your child to brush his teeth as soon as possible. Make this fun so that it becomes a lifelong habit. You will have to do most of the work at first, but your child should be able to brush his teeth alone by the age of 6 or 7.

Your child should have a comprehensive dental examination by a dentist in his early toddler years, or even sooner if there are any dental problems.

ancestors used sweetness to distinguish ripe fruits from unripe, decayed, or poisonous fruits, which were bitter or sour. Breastmilk is also naturally sweet. However, we can minimize the damage that sweet foods can cause. Studies show that it is the frequency and not the quantity of sugar consumed that does most damage to teeth, so when a sugary food is eaten, it should be with meals and not between them.

IS MY CHILD DRINKING ENOUGH?

Fluids are essential to prevent dehydration, of which thirst is a very early sign. Children have a greater requirement for fluids than adults due to the greater fluid losses through their relatively large surface area. Fluid requirements are affected by a child's activity, the weather, and whether he has a fever, but the average requirements are 6–8 drinks a day. The amount taken in a drink will increase with age. An average drink for a 1- to 3-year-old is about 150 ml (5 oz), while an average drink for a 10-year-old is about 250 ml (9 oz).

Water should always be the first choice for drinks. Small, frequent

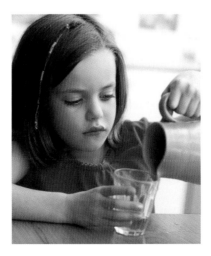

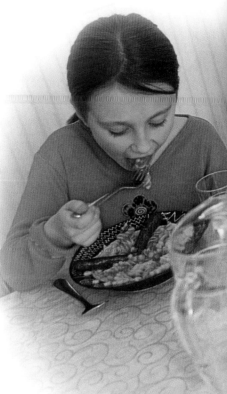

sips of water are recommended with and between meals. Drinks containing caffeine or sugar are not recommended, since these can actually increase fluid requirements. A simple but useful guide to whether your child is drinking enough is the color of his urine. The darker it is, the more dehydrated he is. Urine should be pale yellow to almost colorless, except first thing in the morning, when it is darker from being concentrated overnight.

PICKY EATERS

Your child may like and dislike certain foods at different times. If he refuses a new food, you can introduce it again later in a different form. However, if he repeatedly shows a dislike for a specific food, offer an alternative – we all have our own likes and dislikes. If your child consistently refuses a particular

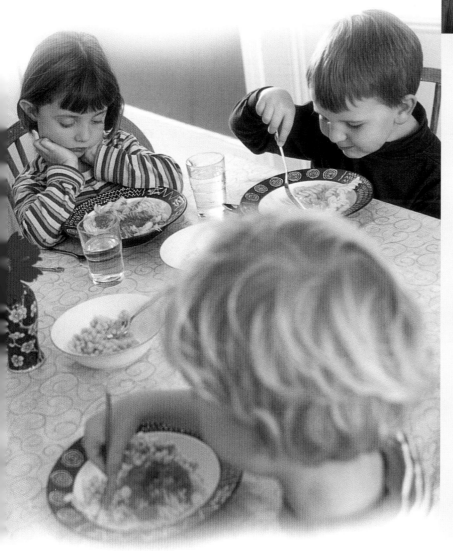

COMMON REASONS WHY A CHILD MAY NOT EAT

Illness or fever. If your child is coming down with, or recovering from, a cold or other illness, he may not want food. This is to be expected; his appetite will return later.

Snacking between meals, especially close to mealtimes. Your child will eat better at mealtimes if you avoid snacks or keep them small.

Drinks. Children's stomachs are smaller than adults', so drinking large quantities of milk or anything else can fill them up.

Constipation. Constipation may be the result of too little fiber and/or too little fluid. Increase fiber intake by giving fruits, vegetables, grains, and cereals. If your child's urine is not very pale yellow in color, encourage more drinking (plain water is best).

Be reassured that, with good guidance, most children will eventually form healthy eating habits.

vegetable or fruit, suggest another one. If he won't eat cheese, try giving him yogurt instead. Try serving a food again later, since it may take many attempts before he likes it. You can also try to serve a food you know your child enjoys with one she has refused in the past.

It is also not unusual for children to have erratic eating patterns at some point in their development. On some days a child may eat everything on his plate and on other days eat very little or refuse a meal entirely. Such erratic eating may reflect a child's growth spurts and/or his activity levels on that day. Some studies have shown that erratic eating patterns do not lead to poor overall food intake.

Children may also pick up on stresses around the home and may learn to use mealtimes as a battleground. As distressing as this may be, do not make a fuss and avoid focusing your attention entirely on your child's refusal to eat or the small quantity that has been consumed. If your child refuses to eat a meal, just remove his plate after the whole family has finished eating. Do not offer your child a complete alternative. Try to remain calm and encourage conversation among other members of the family. Your child will eat at the next mealtime when he is hungry. If he asks for a snack before the next mealtime, offer leftovers from the last meal, fruit, or a glass of water.

It is important that you remain consistent, so do not give in to demands for additional snacks.

If you feel your child is not growing adequately (see p.70), you should get professional advice from your doctor, who may refer you to a nutritionist.

THE VEGETARIAN CHILD

A child can grow normally following a vegetarian diet, if it is well balanced. Millions of people throughout the world are perfectly healthy and strong on a vegetarian diet. Vegetarian alternatives are now widely available in all major supermarkets as well as health food stores, and recipe ideas are plentiful. In addition, some studies show that

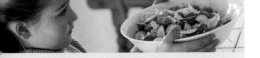

ARE VEGAN DIETS SAFE FOR CHILDREN?

Vegan diets are strictly vegetarian and contain no animal products such as dairy products, eggs, meat, or seafood. Having a child on a vegan diet requires much attention to detail. As tofu, textured vegetable protein, and calcium-enriched soy drinks become more widely available, the variety and quality of vegan diets is improving. But such diets do lead to a high fiber intake, so take care when planning meals for children under the age of 5. A high-fiber diet will fill a child up quickly without providing adequate calories and nutrients, so growth may be affected. Consult your doctor to ensure that your child receives adequate nutrition on a vegan diet.

To make sure a vegan child's diet contains enough energy and nutrients, choose fat- and nutrient-dense foods. These include:

• Nut butters, such as peanut butter (avoid these until at least 3 years if there is a family history of asthma, eczema, allergic rhinitis, or food allergies), almond butter
• Seed paste (tahini)
• Hummus, made from tahini and mashed chickpeas
• Avocados, which are also an excellent source of essential fatty acids
• Margarine or oils: use liberally when preparing bean and lentil dishes

Vitamin B$_{12}$, which is essential for the formation of healthy red blood cells, also is often low in vegan diets. Soy products, fortified cereals, and some fortified soy drinks are good sources of vitamin B$_{12}$. Standard soy drinks are low in fat, so it may be best for to continue with infant soy formula until your child is 2 years old. Discuss these issues with your doctor. Fortified soy drinks can be introduced from 2 years.

children brought up on a vegetarian diet consume more fruit and vegetables and are less likely to suffer from diseases such as obesity, bowel cancer, and heart disease as adults. The most important thing for vegetarian children is to keep their diet varied and make sure the fiber content of the diet is not too high, especially in children under the age of 5. Low-fat diets should be avoided in children under 2 years of age.

Iron and vegetarian diets

The body does not absorb iron from vegetable sources as well as it absorbs iron from meat sources. Vitamin C helps the absorption of iron, so foods rich in vitamin C should be part of your child's meals. These could be in the form of fruit or vegetable juice, fresh vegetables (carrots, tomatoes), or fruit.

Consult your doctor to ensure your child's diet contains an adequate amount of protein. Try to include a mixture of vegetable sources, tofu, textured vegetable protein, beans and legumes, dairy products, calcium-enriched soy dairy alternatives, eggs, nuts, and seeds to provide the protein he needs.

MAKE BREAKFAST A FAMILY AFFAIR

For most of us, breakfast is the most important meal of the day. It is usually 12–14 hours since we last ate and our blood sugar levels in the morning are low. It is especially important that children start the day with a good portion of starchy carbohydrate. This helps replenish energy reserves and keeps blood sugar levels from dropping mid-morning, helping concentration in school.

It is best to avoid giving your children heavily sugared cereals.

Good alternatives include oatmeal and other oat cereals, wheat or rice cereals, bran flakes, and granola (with no added sugar). Look at the nutritional label on the package and choose brands with less than 20g of sugar per 100g of cereal. You may want to add some berries or chopped fruits such as bananas.

DOES MY CHILD NEED SUPPLEMENTS?

Your child's vitamin and mineral requirements can all be met from food alone. As much as possible, try to maximize the natural vitamins in your child's regular meals. Milk is the single best source of vitamins in the diet. The more varied your child's diet, the more likely he is to be getting a variety of vitamins and minerals. Research shows that vitamins and minerals in isolation do not benefit health as much as naturally-occuring vitamins and minerals consumed as food. However, if your child has a poor or erratic appetite or if she follows a vegan diet, your doctor may

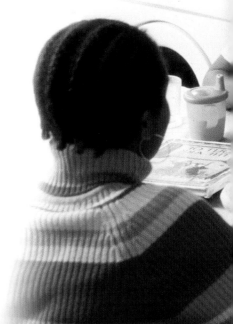

recommend a daily vitamin supplement. There is no reason for your child to take supplements over and above the recommendations. In fact, overconsumption of one specific vitamin or mineral can prevent absorption of another, and high intakes of certain vitamins and minerals can be toxic to the body. It is important not to introduce any vitamin or mineral supplements into your child's diet without consulting your doctor.

Vitamin D is necessary for healthy bone development, and the action of sunlight on the skin provides the majority of our vitamin D requirement. However, this effect may be blocked by sunscreen, which is important for preventing sun damage to the skin. People with low exposure to sunlight are at risk of having low vitamin D levels. These include people who are housebound or in the hospital for long periods of time, people with darker skin, and people from ethnic groups who do not expose much of their skin to sunlight. In these circumstances, adequate dietary intake of vitamin D

"Breakfast is the most important meal of the day."

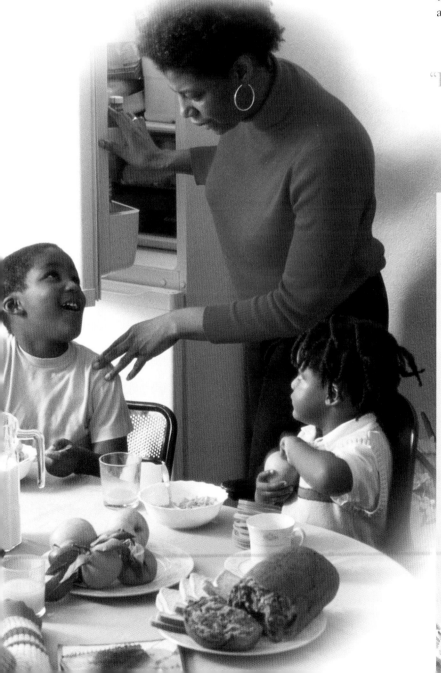

CHILD-SIZE PORTIONS AND HEALTHY BREAKFAST

For youngsters, adult-size servings can be overwhelming.
In this era of oversized portions, it is important to give children appropriate servings of food. Serve one-fourth to one-third of an adult portion size, or one tablespoon of food for each year of the child's age. Give your child less than you think he will eat, and let him ask for more if he is still hungry.

There is a wide range of healthy breakfast ideas.
Traditional breakfast foods, such as cereal, fruit, eggs, yogurt, bagels, and muffins, are appropriate choices, but some children prefer leftover dinner foods.

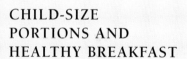

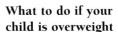

"...introducing your child to a healthy diet early in life is perhaps one of the best gifts you can ever give him"

is essential. Children will obtain the recommended amount of vitamin D by drinking 500 ml (16 oz) of milk per day. Ask your doctor or your nutritionist if you are concerned that your child is not getting an adequate amount of vitamin D.

OBESITY AND YOUR CHILD

North America has one of the highest incidences of obesity in the world, with the prevalence of obesity in children and adolescents increasing each year. The situation is escalating, and government health officials are taking it seriously. Obesity is an important health issue because it increases the risk of premature death, diabetes, and heart disease, as well as severe back pain and other joint problems.

Is it all in the genes?

There is some truth in the idea that obesity is due to genes – genetic factors do play a part. Children with parents who are both obese have an 80 percent chance of becoming obese, compared to a 20 percent chance if both parents are slim.

However, research shows that an unhealthy lifestyle is a major risk factor for obesity. Obese parents are more likely to be less active and consume high-calorie, energy-dense foods, passing these bad habits on to their children, who in turn become obese. And it is not just the type of foods children eat but also their activity levels that determine whether they will be overweight. Obesity in childhood needs to be taken seriously and tackled. Beyond the physical problems it causes, it can also cause psychosocial problems, including depression and loss of self-esteem. Overweight children may be teased, bullied, and socially excluded.

What to do if your child is overweight

Children develop at different rates, so other children the same age as your child may be bigger or smaller, or at a different stage of physical maturity. Your child will be weighed and measured during regular checks with the doctor., and the readings can be plotted on a growth chart to follow your child's height and weight over time. You can plot your child's chart at home, too.

The curved lines on a growth chart represent percentiles. A percentile is based on a scale of 100. If your child is in the 50th percentile, half the children his age are bigger and half are the same size or smaller. On a growth chart, these lines indicate expected patterns of weight gain and height growth. The ideal situation is when height and weight percentiles are about the same, but the percentiles may differ depending on your child's build. Children whose weight percentile is much higher than their height percentile (for example, who are in the 95th percentile for weight and the 50th percentile for height) are overweight or possibly obese.

Treating obese and overweight children is different from treating obese and overweight adults. Using a weight-loss regimen intended for adults may compromise your child's growth and development. Dietary restrictions should be supervised by your doctor and nutritionist. The key to success is a change in lifestyle, and this means appropriate dietary changes together with increased exercise. Also, your child must be motivated or efforts are unlikely to be successful.

It is important to help prevent your child from becoming overweight, but if your child is

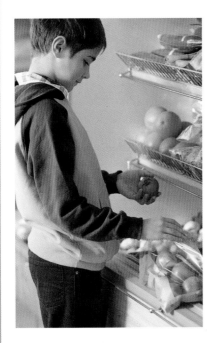

overweight and not obese, one goal may be to help your child maintain a static weight so he becomes leaner as he grows in height. If a child is obese, actual weight loss may be needed, but it is essential that you seek professional advice before attempting this. Very low-calorie diets and any diet resulting in excessive and fast weight loss in children may be dangerous and should not be used. The diets of children under 5 years old are easier to change, because you have greater control over food choices. Older children will be eating and spending more time away from home, so the child may need extra support and instruction to follow the diet. At this age, it is important that the child himself wants to do something about his weight. The whole family may need to provide support for the child and improve any unhealthy eating and activity habits, too. A sensible, balanced approach toward food and weight has to be adopted, though, or an affected child could develop an eating disorder.

EATING DISORDERS

Eating disorders include problems such as anorexia, which is deliberate self-starvation, and bulimia, which is a tendency to binge on food and then purge the body through vomiting or laxatives. Although eating disorders are uncommon in young children and children of grade-school age, children in both of these age groups are becoming increasingly aware of body image and dieting.

You can help prevent your child from developing an eating disorder by emphasizing the importance of a healthy diet and exercise from an early age, and by setting a good example for your child by eating

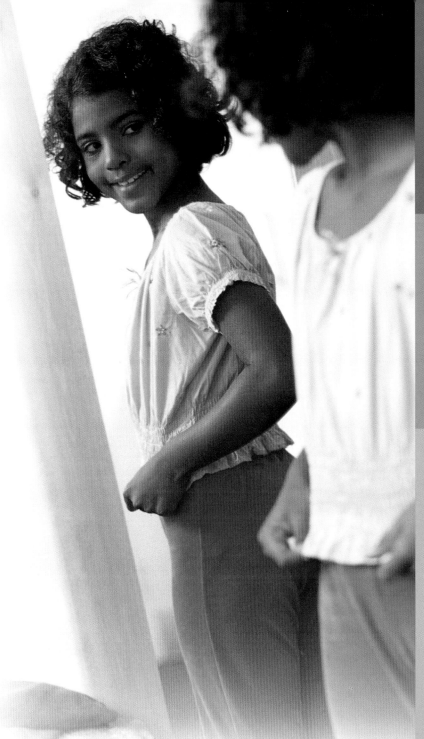

healthily and exercising yourself. If you are worried about your own weight or are dieting, avoid showing your concern in front of your child, who may pick up on your anxieties.

Some warning signs of eating disorders include weight loss, irritability, and distorted ideas about body size. Children who

have perfectionist tendencies and children who perceive that they are under a great deal of pressure to succeed may be more susceptible to eating disorders. If you are concerned that your child may be developing an eating disorder, you should see your doctor for advice as soon as possible.

GROWING
INDEPENDENCE

A S CHILDREN DEVELOP, THEY WANT TO DO THINGS FOR THEMSELVES. It's part of growing up and parents need to encourage a child's independence. You can do this by helping your child practice new skills, with help at first. As your child grows older, encouraging him to do things on his own, such as homework or getting ready for school, will help him develop a sense of responsibility.

> "A sense of self-esteem is essential for a child to develop independence."

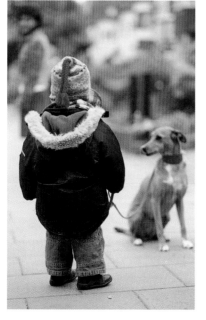

STAGES OF DEVELOPMENT

Much of what a child can do depends on his stage of mental and physical development, which in turn depends on the growth and maturation of his brain, nerves, bones, and muscles. The brain, which controls the body through the peripheral nervous system, develops particularly rapidly during the first two years of life. A child gains control of his head, then his limbs and trunk, and finally achieves fine control of his fingers. This means he can perform more delicate tasks, such as holding a pencil and writing. As his nervous system continues to mature, your child becomes able to control the nerves supplying his bladder and bowel.

Complex interconnections in the nervous system occur with rapid learning of all kinds of skills during childhood. Bones and muscles also lengthen and become stronger in this period. Later on, during puberty, sexual maturation begins.

How you can help

How can you support and help your child as he develops, encouraging his independence? In the beginning, it's important to learn to pick up on the signals your child gives you that

he is ready to do things by himself. For instance, when your baby reaches out for something, try to let him get it himself; don't hand it to him right away. Give him a spoon and let him try feeding himself. Give toddlers simple choices to help them feel in control. Would your child like an apple or a pear, or a red or yellow toothbrush?

As soon as he has the manual dexterity, give your child a brush to hold and show him how to brush his hair. Let him try brushing his teeth, although you'll still need to help until he is 6 or 7 years of age. At age 3, he might be able to wash his face and brush his hair with a little help. At age 4, he'll probably be able to dress himself but may need help with buttons.

When he's learning something, like tying his shoes, give him the time he needs. Whatever he's doing, let him perform the task himself. This will give him the message that you are confident in his abilities. Only offer help if he really needs it.

BUILDING YOUR CHILD'S SELF-ESTEEM

A sense of self-esteem is essential for a child to develop independence. Children develop self-esteem

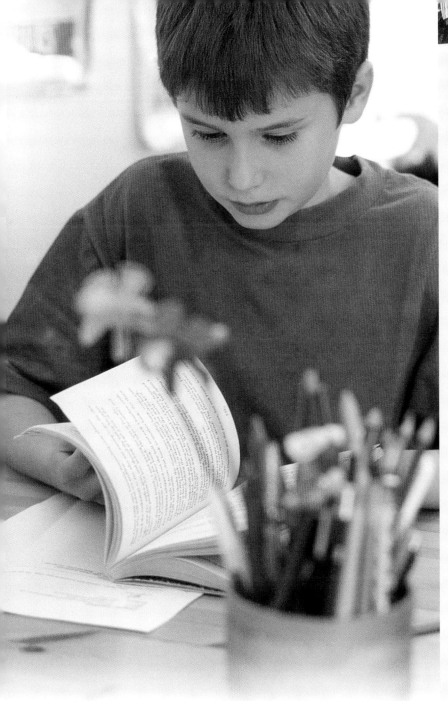

PHYSICAL INDEPENDENCE

As a child grows older, he'll want more physical independence. He might want to go to a store, walk to a friend's house, or go to the park without you. This is a worry for many parents. Traffic has increased, making streets more dangerous, and well-publicized cases of child abduction make the fear of this, however rarely it happens, very real. Children need to learn the skills to be able to take care of themselves, so start at an early age teaching them about safety issues. Remember, most children do not have the necessary skills to handle traffic situations until at least 10 years of age. Other factors such as traffic patterns, location, and your child's maturity and distractibility levels should also be considered in your decisions about safety and independence.

It is important to balance structured activities with independent play. It's very easy to pack a child's life full of activities, but it's important to get the balance right. Your child needs time alone for quiet and unstructured play.

Allowing children some private space as they get older also helps reinforce self-respect. Not all children can have or want a room of their own, but it's helpful if they have at least one area they can think of as theirs alone.

through being loved and appreciated by their parents. They need love consistently and unconditionally in order to feel valued. Knowing that he is loved and that his opinions and thoughts matter to you will make your child feel secure and help develop his confidence.

You don't need to organize a lot of special outings or buy presents to let your child know you care about him. Spending time doing

something simple together, like taking the dog for a walk, talking to your child and listening to what he has to say, and letting him know you enjoy his company, will all help him feel special.

You should also tell your child you love him and explain why. For instance, you could say "I love the way you kiss your sister when she's feeling upset." Notice things your child does without being asked and comment positively on them; for instance, "Thank you for putting your toys away, you've done a good job." Give specific compliments, rather than just general praise, to reinforce the desired behavior.

Praise is just as important for older children, whether they've done well at school, have been helpful around the house, or have simply been thoughtful to someone.

Encouraging your child's interests

Working together to discover your child's strengths and areas of interest will not only boost his confidence but also help him get to know himself a little better. If he is not interested in a hobby or sports that you are passionate about, it can be disappointing for you but it may be best to follow your child's lead in this. Listening, and making it clear to him that you have taken in and understood what he is saying, is important. You don't always have to agree with him but the fact that you are taking his thoughts and feelings seriously will help him develop confidence in his opinions. You will sometimes need to give criticism, but if this is done constructively it can be effective. Pick your time carefully and avoid offering criticism in front of friends or siblings or when he is hungry or tired. Try to start with a positive comment such as "You are usually really good at practicing your reading, but in the last few days…"

Developing physical skills

Having a good range of physical skills will help your child feel confident. If he can run, ride a bike, climb a tree, and generally have the opportunity to be physically adventurous, he will develop confidence in his own abilities. In the first five years, there is little difference between boys and girls in terms of their growth and physical shape. But girls may be better at games that involve precision and judgment, such as hopscotch and running short distances, while boys

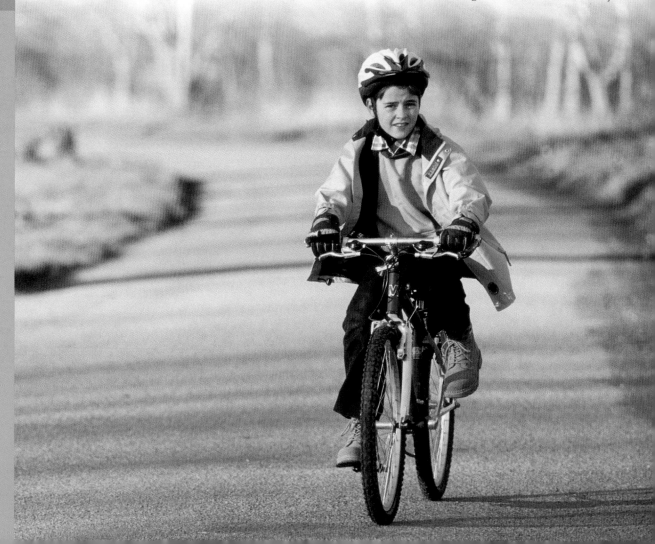

may prefer activities such as throwing and catching and may be stronger than girls.

If your child shows an interest in a particular activity, try to encourage him, since this will help his confidence as well as his physical fitness. Most children find at least one physical activity they enjoy, and there are many available, such as soccer, swimming, bicycling, dancing, gymnastics, and karate.

Encouraging your child's skills in other areas will also help give him a sense of worth. See what he enjoys, whether it's learning a musical instrument, drawing, or making or collecting things. Give plenty of praise and let him know you think he's good at his chosen activity.

Children learn by example, and parents are their most influential role models in the early years. This means that your own self-esteem is important too. Making time for yourself is often difficult, especially when children are very young. But if you can find time for your own activities, whether it's playing a musical instrument or a game of tennis, your children will benefit.

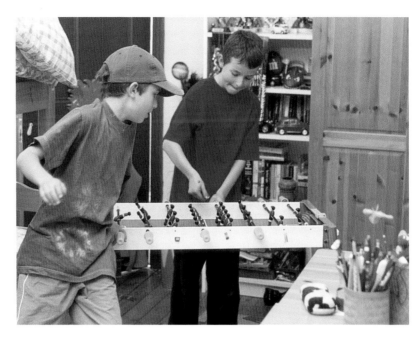

STRIKING A BALANCE BETWEEN INDEPENDENCE & RULES

As your child grows and becomes more independent, he will need to know the rules and boundaries that you place on his behavior. Abiding by rules is an important part of being able to live in a community. For families, rules are important so that everyone can live comfortably together under one roof. Even babies need to learn the meaning of "no" and "yes." Children need rules, because when you provide rules, they have a clear idea of what's expected of them.

When children are young, rules can be very simple, outlining the behavior you would like from them. As your children grow up, some rules can be adjusted, but you can stick with the basic principles. Involving your child in reviewing rules will help him understand why they exist.

Within this framework of rules, your child will need to know that his opinion does count. Encouraging him to develop his views and opinions will help him understand himself better and increase his confidence. Discuss what happened at school today, what he enjoyed, what he didn't, and why. As your child grows older you can widen this to include more abstract ideas, such as politics or global issues.

Also, you should try to involve your child in family decisions as much as possible. Some families find that setting aside a regular time and place to talk is a good way to discuss issues together. For others this approach may be too formal, and

"...growing with your child means trusting him and respecting his decisions on issues such as choosing friends"

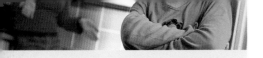

DISAGREEING WITH AN OLDER CHILD

There will be times when you feel your child's decision is the wrong one. With older children, pick a good moment and discuss your views with him. Give him the chance to share his decision and listen carefully to his views. Be prepared to explain the reasons why his choice isn't a good idea in clear terms he will understand.

By the age of 11, a child who has been given practice in decision-making feels confident in his own abilities and has a good sense of who he is. He will be well prepared for the next phase of his life – adolescence.

just spending time doing an everyday activity, such as driving in the car, can provide enough good time to talk.

You don't always need to agree with one another; in fact arguments and disagreements are inevitable and an important part of family life. They provide a child with a safe opportunity to experiment with making his views known and standing up for his beliefs. They also help prepare him for life outside the family, where people often disagree. If you feel you need to get your children talking more, try offering another perspective to facilitate the discussion.

BEHAVIOR & ROUTINE

Young children like routine because it makes them feel feel secure. At an early age, a bedtime routine can help

your baby settle down. A bedtime routine can be helpful for an older child as well.

As children grow up, families often find it helpful to develop a routine for getting things done. If your children know what to do and when to do it on a daily basis it will help you get them out the door on time in the morning.

Children also need to learn how to behave appropriately. If they don't, they'll find it hard to get along with friends and cooperate, both of which are important at school. Discipline isn't really about punishment. It's more about teaching your child how to behave so that he eventually learns how to control his own behavior.

There are some basic principles of discipline that most people agree on. For instance, most families encourage their children to be truthful and polite, rather than rude or aggressive. The first step in achieving good discipline is to make sure that your child feels secure and loved and receives plenty of attention when he is behaving well. You must also watch your own behavior and make sure that you are setting the right example; children learn from their parents.

Discipline needs to be consistent from both parents and others involved in the care of a child. If your child lives between two homes, ensure that everyone's following the same rules. Make sure your child understands what's expected of him.

Dealing with problem behavior

Setting firm guidelines about the behavior you expect will give your child a clear idea of what is acceptable and what isn't. Be consistent in how you apply the rules. If you ignore them one day

"...if children don't learn how to behave, they'll find it hard to get along with friends and cooperate with others"

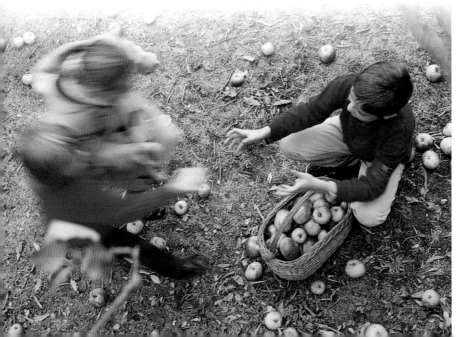

and impose them the next, he can become confused. Be prepared to give an ultimatum then quick, clear consequences. Conversely, remember to acknowledge your child's good behavior by giving him positive reinforcement, such as praise or a special activity or treat as a reward.

When your child behaves badly, let him know you disapprove of his behavior but not of him personally. For example if he hits someone, make it clear it's not acceptable by saying that he has hurt the other child, not that he is a bad boy.

It's never a good idea to hit your child. Not only does this give a child the message that physical violence is acceptable, but there is a wealth of research to show it does nothing to help children learn to improve their behavior. Other strategies, such as withholding treats or taking a "time out," work better.

Difficult behavior can make it hard for you and your child to get along. It's important to spend time having fun, so plan activities into your lives, whether it's a visit to the park after school or reading a book together before bed. If you are having trouble handling your child's behavior, you should talk to your doctor.

GROWING WITH YOUR CHILD

Growing with your child means recognizing his capabilities and encouraging him to test them at each different stage. This encouragement will help him improve his sense of independence and self-reliance. For young children, it could mean encouraging personal skills, such as dressing. For older children, it could mean respecting their decisions on issues such as choosing friends.

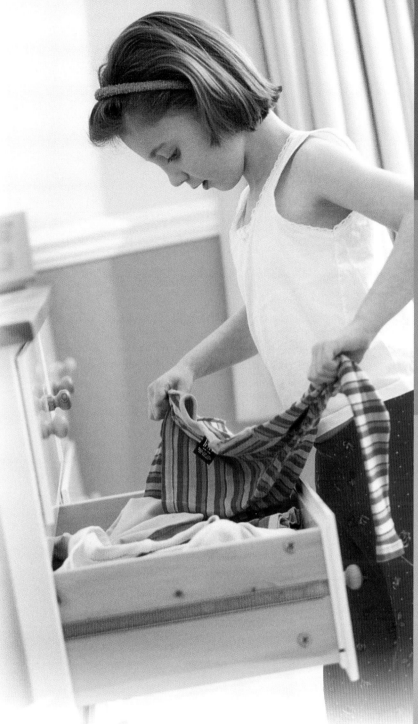

"...encouraging decision-making skills, such as choosing clothes, can help children develop self-reliance"

EMOTIONAL
DEVELOPMENT

O NE OF THE MOST IMPORTANT SKILLS you can help your child develop is
his ability to express his emotions in a clear, appropriate way. If you
do this, it will serve him well as he grows older. Learning to express his
feelings clearly and without aggression will help his emotional development
and will help others understand why he feels as he does.

HELPING YOUR CHILD EXPRESS HIS FEELINGS

It isn't always easy for a child to
express himself, and it may be
something boys find harder than
girls. If your child expresses himself
too aggressively or loudly, he may
be reprimanded. If he's too quiet,
he may be ignored. With your help,
your child can learn to assert himself
in an appropriate way.

The first step is to put names to
different emotions. You can start by
naming positive as well as negative
feelings in everyday conversation.

It might be tempting to avoid talking
about feelings of unhappiness or
anger, but it's important for a child
to recognize these feelings and learn
how to deal with them. You could
say "I can see you are feeling angry
because Tom has taken away your
book," or "You look happy today.
Is that because we're going to go
to grandma's house?"

As your child's vocabulary
improves, encourage him to describe
his own emotions. You could say:
"You look unhappy. Perhaps you're
cranky or tired – how are you

feeling?" Asking open questions
such as "what do you think
about?…" or "how did you feel
when?…" can help this process.

You will need to give your child
guidance about the best way to
express his feelings. For instance,
being angry is fine, but hitting
someone because you're angry is
not. Suggest alternative strategies,
such as counting to ten before
saying something when you're angry,
or walking away from the situation
until you feel in control again. How
you model your own expressed
feelings has a strong impact on
your child's ability to do likewise.

DEALING WITH TANTRUMS

Many children go through the
"terrible twos." Around this age,
a child's intellectual and cognitive
abilities are developing fast.
Children start to realize they are
separate beings and are becoming
increasingly independent. In short,
they begin to assert themselves.

A tantrum is more likely to
happen if a child is hungry, tired,
bored, or overstimulated. He may be
frustrated at his own limitations if,
for example, he can't fasten buttons
on his shirt, or if he wants to tell
you something but lacks the verbal

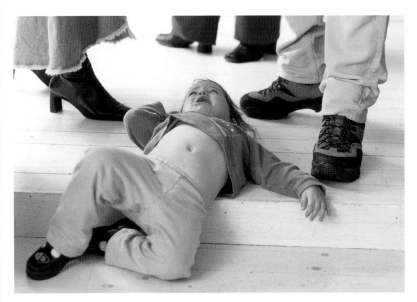

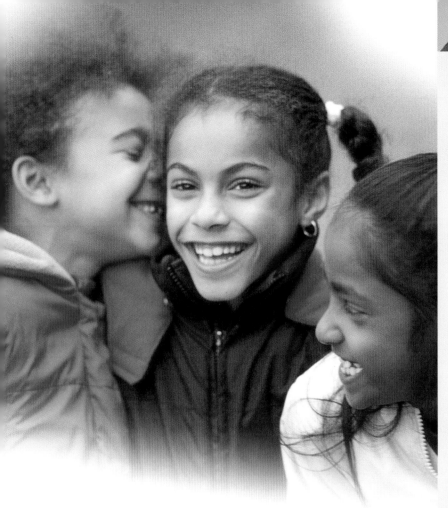

It's perfectly normal for a young child to cry when he's left with someone else or at child care, preschool, or even school for the first time. This can be upsetting for parents but in most cases it doesn't take long for a child to be comforted and enjoy his day. Remember that being left with another trustworthy person helps your child learn to form new relationships and develop social skills. Preparation is important. If your child is starting preschool, visit it together beforehand and meet his teachers. Talk positively about what fun he'll have. Read books together about starting preschool.

When you leave, kiss him and tell him you are going and when you'll be back in terms he understands, for instance "I'll be back before lunch." Wave and walk away. Don't be tempted to go back, even if he's crying. This may reinforce his tears. It will help if he has someone nearby to comfort him. Most children settle in after a few weeks but if your child consistently cries when you leave, try standing outside and listen for a few minutes to reassure yourself that his crying stops. Children may also cry when you pick them up. This doesn't mean they haven't enjoyed their day. Until the age of 3 or 4, a child will often feel a rush of overwhelming emotion that results in tears when he sees his parents again. Check with his caregiver or teacher to make sure that he's been fine. Showing your child that you feel confident about leaving him will help him feel confident too.

After age 5 or 6, separation anxiety is much less common. If by age 7 your child is still reluctant to go to school, it could indicate a problem. Talk to your child's teacher or your doctor.

---

skills to do so. He may be angry at being thwarted in some way; for example, you may have said "no" to a cookie before lunch.

When a tantrum does happen, it's important for you to try to remain calm during the outburst. Make sure the environment is safe, and wait for the tantrum to end. The purpose of your child having a tantrum is to get what he wants. If you give in, he will learn he can get his own way by having a tantrum again.

Your reactions

There's no point in trying to reason or argue when your child has a tantrum. It's also important not to laugh, even if the reason for the tantrum seems ridiculous – the anger and frustration that triggered it are genuine. Remind yourself what the tantrum is about, for instance, "This is because I said no to a cookie." Your child will get a reassuring message that you are in control.

Occasionally, a child will hold his breath during a tantrum. These breath-holding spells can be frightening for parents. Stay calm and don't panic or your child may panic too. If he holds his breath for long enough, he may even faint briefly. If this happens, your child will start breathing again naturally. For this reason, breath-holding is not harmful.

Distraction and avoidance techniques

Sometimes it's possible to distract a child out of a tantrum. It might be worth offering a favorite book

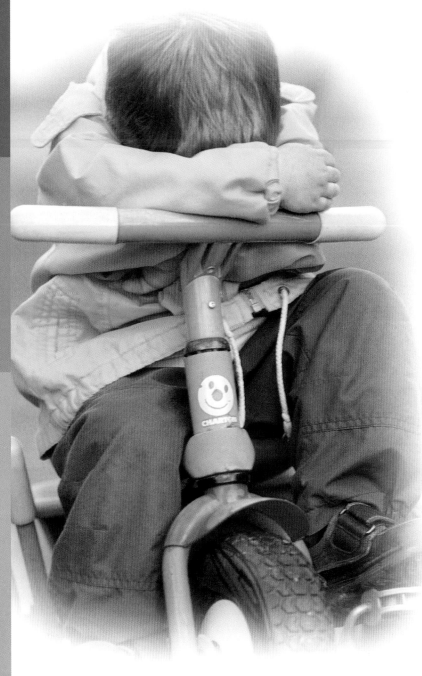

or toy or just talking calmly and quietly. There might be something you say that catches his attention.

Give your child attention once he has calmed down. There's no point in admonishing him. Join him in something he enjoys and won't find frustrating, such as looking at a book together or playing a game. He will probably appreciate cuddling to remind him of your continuing love.

Averting a tantrum is better than dealing with one and there are some approaches that may help. Give your child plenty of opportunities to let off steam by running around the yard or in the park, or even playing noisily in the house if it's raining. Make sure he has a regular routine of daytime naps, bath, and bedtime. Avoid long stretches without food by carrying snacks when you go out. Don't wait until his behavior deteriorates before you offer them. Providing simple choices, such as letting him choose what kind of sandwich he'd like at lunch, can help your child feel in control and may reduce the chance of a tantrum.

If you work outside the home, do not feel you have to provide something exciting when you get home. Just being there and quietly reading a book or watching a video together is important to your child.

It may be useful to keep a record of your child's tantrums. This will help clarify when they are most likely to occur and what provokes them. You could then try to avoid these situations.

Be reassured that children eventually grow out of tantrums. See your doctor if your child has more than a few temper tantrums every day, if they continue regularly after the age of 4, or if you feel you can't handle them. Extra support may be needed.

"When a tantrum does happen, it's important for you to try to remain calm during the outburst."

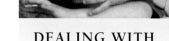

HELPING ANXIOUS CHILDREN

It's very common for babies and young children to be afraid of things. Fear of water, loud noises, and new places are some of the most common fears at this stage.

These fears make sense. Your baby is learning about the world, and fear is a natural protective response that prepares the body to flee or face what is threatening.

You may be able to help. If your child is afraid of water, he may feel safer in a baby bath placed in the bathtub. Encourage him to splash and introduce toys. At other times, for example if there's a loud noise, you cannot do much but be there; giving him a hug will reassure him.

Children develop powerful imaginations at around the age of 3 or 4, and very often have fears that seem puzzling to adults. Tigers and lions in the backyard, monsters in the closet, the dark, a loud noise such as a lawnmower, and even the sound of the wind can frighten them. These fears may be a way of giving shape to feelings of anxiety at a time of change in the child's life, such as starting a preschool, or when a new sibling arrives.

It's important not to dismiss your child's fears, which for him are very real. Reassure him that you take his fears seriously by gently asking why he is worried. Children have funny ideas about things, which you could correct. If he is afraid of a particular object, introduce it gradually. For example, if he dislikes the vacuum cleaner, prepare him by telling him that you are going to vacuum but he can stay in the next room.

It helps if there's someone else with him to give comfort; remember to praise him for being brave. If it's something more intangible that's

frightening him, such as the dark, use a night-light and leave a light on all night outside his room. Reassure him that you are close by.

Many children instinctively work through their fears through play. If your child enjoys drawing, provide crayons and paper to allow him to express his feelings in this way. Don't worry if he doesn't seem to reveal anything you think is significant.

Very occasionally there may be a medical reason behind a child's fear. For instance, if he seems upset by loud noises or runs away if he hears anything loud, it's worth a visit to your doctor.

Preadolescent anxieties

It is a normal part of mental development for preadolescent children to develop anxieties about specific things. This process will eventually help them understand and cope with events and concerns that may be out of their control. There is also some evidence to suggest a genetic component to the development of anxieties. Anxiety can also be learned from other people around you.

Certain life events can also play a role in triggering anxious feelings and behavior. Try to determine if

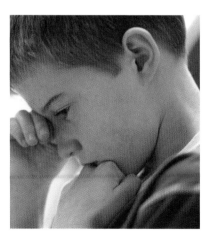

DEALING WITH MOOD SWINGS

Once past the "terrible twos," young children are rarely moody and irritable for long. If they are, there is usually a good reason for it.

Hunger, fatigue, and thirst can affect children. Making sure that your child has eaten enough and isn't overtired or thirsty can help alleviate moodiness. Keeping a few healthy snacks, such as raisins or granola bars, and a bottle of water on hand when you're out can help prevent any sudden deterioration in mood.

If your child becomes moody and hunger or fatigue do not seem to be the problem, explore whether there's a problem at child care or school, or with friends. Or have there been any changes in your family or routine he feels unhappy about? For some children, depression (*see below*) can cause a range of symptoms, including mood swings.

As puberty approaches, your child will be exposed to hormonal changes that could make him feel moody. Although adolescence usually starts at around 10 for girls and 12 for boys, the hormonal changes responsible for initiating the process begin some years earlier. Your child himself may not understand why he feels the way he does or be able to explain his feelings clearly. Consequently, this can be a difficult time for the whole family.

If your child seems so moody and unhappy that it is interfering with normal activities, it may be about more than adolescence. He may be depressed. If you think this might be the case with your child, ask your doctor for advice. Help can then be arranged if it is necessary.

"...it's very common for children to be shy, but with support and encouragement most are able to overcome it"

there is a pattern to your child's fears. If he is afraid of taking the bus, does he feel the same about other forms of transportation? Is there any occasion when he can manage to travel? It is also worth exploring whether his fears could be masking something else. For example, are there any problems at school or with bullying (*see p.151*)?

Most fears pass in time, and with your encouragement your child should grow out of them. If you feel he would benefit from further support, consult a doctor or child psychologist. Effective interventions available can help children overcome their fears.

HELPING SHY CHILDREN
It's very common for young children to be shy. With plenty of support and encouragement, most children can learn to overcome it. The key is

to build confidence and self-esteem. Choose games and puzzles you know he'll be able to do and give plenty of praise when he does them. Involve him in activities with tangible results such as cooking. Notice little things he does without being asked, such as tidying up. Explain things in advance. Every night talk through what he'll be doing the next day.

If he's being cared for by someone else give him a clear idea of when you'll be back, for instance after lunch or before dinner.

If your child is starting school, inform his teacher about his shy nature and ask to be notified if he's not talking to anyone at school after the first few weeks. He may need extra help. It's important that he can communicate effectively to develop relationships with teachers and children as well as for learning.

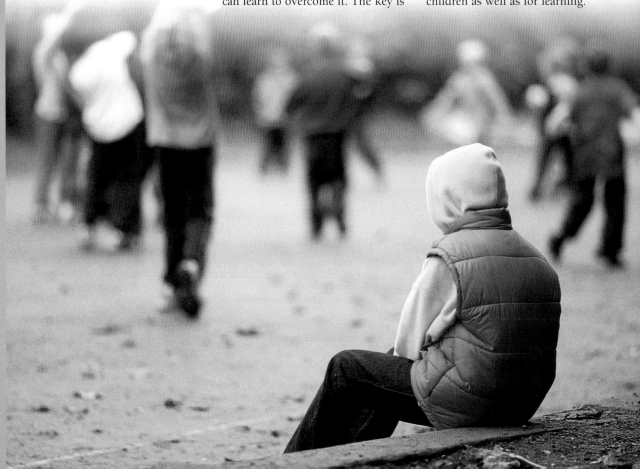

BEHAVIORAL PROBLEMS

Behavioral problems often start in early life, although they can affect children of any age. Tantrums, biting, hitting, or kicking are usually a temporary part of normal development. An older child might cheat, steal, or lie, refuse to follow rules, or get involved in fights.

If problems are dealt with promptly and appropriately, they can usually be resolved fairly rapidly. But sometimes these antisocial behaviors can be more serious. A child might develop a hostile attitude, be consistently disobedient and defiant, or lie or steal without any sign of remorse or guilt. Refusal to follow rules might lead to breaking the law. This is known as a conduct disorder.

There are some predisposing factors. A child who has always had a difficult temperament, is depressed, or has been bullied or abused may be more prone to developing a conduct disorder. Children who are hyperactive have problems with self-control, paying attention, and following rules. A child with learning and reading difficulties who is not receiving the appropriate help can find it difficult to understand and take part in school, which may lead to boredom and misbehavior.

Conversely, a bright child who is not being challenged enough by his schoolwork may also misbehave. Parents who feel overwhelmed by problems with their child's behavior may also feel exhausted or depressed and find it hard to cope.

What can help? Giving your child attention and praise when he is behaving well from an early age will give him a clear message about the sort of behavior you appreciate. Giving him your attention when your child is behaving badly, even

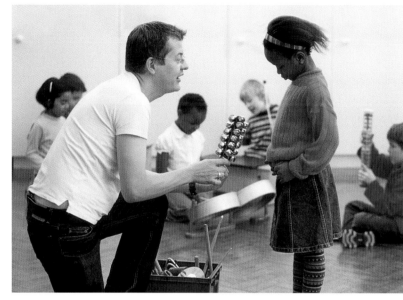

if it's in the form of being lectured, can give your child the message that he gets attention when he breaks rules. Being firm about rules, and fair and consistent in the way they are applied, will help him learn that rules are important.

If you are concerned about your child's behavior at home, talk to your child's teacher to see if he is having problems at school. Extra help at school may be necessary. You may need advice from the principal, school nurse, counselor, or psychologist.

If serious problems continue, it is worth asking your doctor for advice. A referral to a specialist in child mental health might be needed. Specialists can help find out what is causing the problem and suggest ways of improving behavior.

Telling lies

Very young children rarely lie. However, at about age 3 or 4, children often can't separate fantasy from reality and might genuinely believe in something they've dreamed about or made up. What

"...if behavioral problems are noticed early and are dealt with promptly and appropriately, they can usually be resolved rapidly"

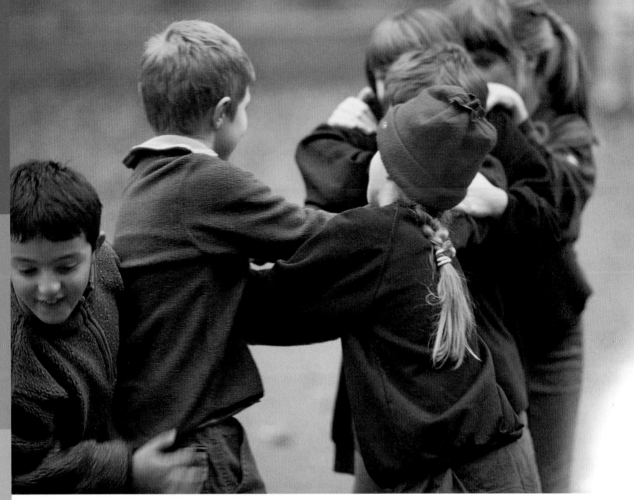

"...for most children, being the winner is much more important than playing by the rules, but it's important to teach your child about playing fairly"

seems like a lie to you might be something they think is really true. As your child grows older and becomes able to distinguish fantasy from reality, he might tell lies to protect himself after a small offense, to impress other children, or to please you.

Talk to your children about the importance of telling the truth. You could tell the story of the boy who cried "wolf," whose lies led others not to believe him when he finally told the truth.

Praise your child when he tells the truth. If he is recounting what is obviously a tall tale, talk about what's real and what's not. If you see your child doing something wrong, such as pinching his sister, and he then denies it, let him know you saw what he did. On the other hand, if you didn't actually see what happened and are just suspicious,

check the story carefully; he might be telling the truth. It also helps to set the right example for your child by not telling white lies yourself.

Cheating

For many children, being the winner may be much more important than playing by the rules. It's important to teach your child about playing fairly. If you let him get away with cheating, he will get the message that it's acceptable to win by devious means rather than by luck or merit.

Whatever game your child is playing, make sure everyone knows the rules in advance. Explain that it's much better to stick to the rules, and encourage your child to think about how he would feel if someone cheated on him. If you see cheating happening, stop the game. With young children, it might help having an adult on each side at first.

If an older child is cheating at school, talk to him and also to his teacher. He may need extra help.

Cruelty

When a toddler hurts or teases a person or an animal, it is rarely intentional; your child does not have the level of understanding to allow him to empathize with others. But sometimes this kind of behavior can develop into a habit if a child sees it as a way of getting attention.

If your child engages in cruel behavior, tell him "no" very clearly and move him away from whatever or whomever he has hurt. Ignore him for a minute or two while you attend to the "victim." This sends a clear message that hurting others is not appropriate and will not get him your attention.

When an older child acts cruelly, it's more serious, since an older child fully understands what he is doing. If you suspect that your child is being cruel by bullying another child, whether on his own or as part of a group, you need to act right away (*see p.151*).

When older children are cruel to animals it can be a sign of emotional disturbance. Your child may need extra help; talk to your doctor.

Stealing

A young child who takes something will probably not realize that it's wrong. If your child has taken something, it's best if he goes with you to return it, explaining that it was taken by accident. Tell him that taking things upsets people.

When a school-age child steals, it's important to establish the facts. Keep calm, and keep in mind that it's not uncommon for a child to steal something at least once. Discuss how to remedy the situation, suggesting that he return the property and apologize himself.

Repeated stealing may indicate a deeper problem. Try talking to him or suggest he talks to someone else he can trust, such as a family friend or mental health professional.

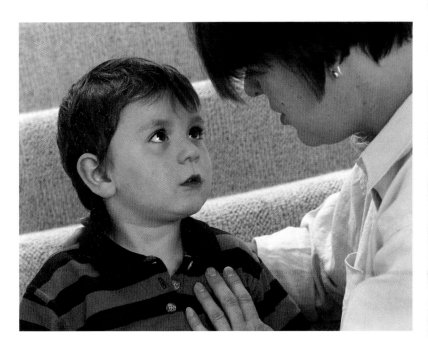

AGGRESSION

Biting, hitting, pinching, and hair-pulling are fairly common among preschool children and are rarely done with a full understanding of how much these behaviors hurt others. Children usually grow out of these behaviors, but sometimes they can develop into habits and it's best to stop them before they do.

If your child bites you, move away from him to show that he has hurt you, and say "No biting. It hurts." If he has bitten another child, remove him firmly, say "no," and give your attention to the other child for a couple of minutes.

School-age children occasionally bite, but it's usually done with the knowledge of how much it hurts others and in the context of fighting. The same goes for hitting, pinching, and hair-pulling.

When a child has outbursts of temper and hits someone, you need to intervene. It could be happening because your child needs an outlet for feelings of anger or aggression. Acknowledge his anger, but make it clear what the boundaries are for acceptable and unacceptable behavior. Suggest alternative strategies for dealing with anger. Your child might find doing a physical activity helpful, such as playing soccer, dancing, singing, or even shouting into a pillow.

Alternatively, if your child is aggressive toward a sibling, suggest that he comes to talk to you whenever he feels angry rather than hitting. If the problem persists, find out whether he's worried about anything. A problem at school or with friends may be behind his aggression.

SOCIAL DEVELOPMENT

IN THE TODDLER AND PRESCHOOL YEARS, you will be your child's main role model. He will pick up many ideas and attitudes about people and relationships from you. After your child starts school, his peer group will have increasing influence on his thinking. Interaction with peers is important for his development, but it is even more important that he have a strong sense of his own values and identity.

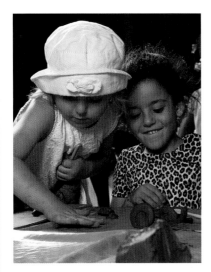

LEARNING ABOUT VALUES

Most children have a strong sense of what is fair and what isn't. Even young children are more morally sophisticated than we might assume. Ask any 4-year-old a question such as "which is worse, hitting someone or sticking your tongue out at them?" Most will reply that hitting is worse.

Parents can do a lot to help their child develop his own moral judgment. The way parents approach this can powerfully influence the way their child develops and the sort of person he becomes. Defining your own family values is a good first step. Make it clear what you consider to be right and wrong and discuss this openly.

The best way to teach your child good values is by example. How closely and how well you live by what you say will determine how your child views your values. For example, if you impress upon your child that he should always tell the truth, make sure you always do this too. It may be convenient for you to sometimes tell white lies (such as "tell her I'm not here"), but for your child, who may overhear, this may be confusing.

As your child grows, continue to be open about your own values. It will give him the opportunity to challenge them. Some families like to have regular meeting times when they can discuss issues. These discussions could take place at a particular meal, for instance, although it may be easier to approach things a little less formally.

As your child develops, he will feel valued if he can see that what he does and how he behaves give you pleasure. It's important to make

"...friendships are very important in a child's life and your child's peer group becomes increasingly influential as he grows up"

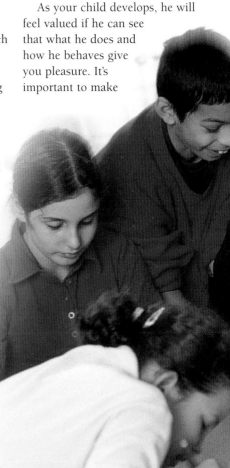

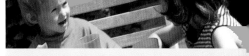

it very clear to your child which actions and behaviors make you happy. This feedback will give him a clear idea of what you expect from him.

LEARNING ABOUT TOLERANCE

Children may encounter certain treatment in their daily lives, either preferential or discriminatory, based on their gender, young age, race, or other qualities, and they may also notice others being treated a certain way because of their traits. The racial and ethnic composition of our country is rapidly changing, and children are also being exposed to different cultures of the world through the media. As a result, it is important for children to understand and value the diversity of people who are different from them.

As a parent, you can take the opportunity to bring diversity into your life and expose your child to people of different races and cultures. Try to socialize with friends from different backgrounds and participate in various cultural events and celebrations. Help your child understand that there are more similarities than differences among people.

Whenever possible, dispel stereotypes you may encounter. Discuss diversity and prejudice with your child, making it clear that discrimination in any form is unacceptable. Most importantly,

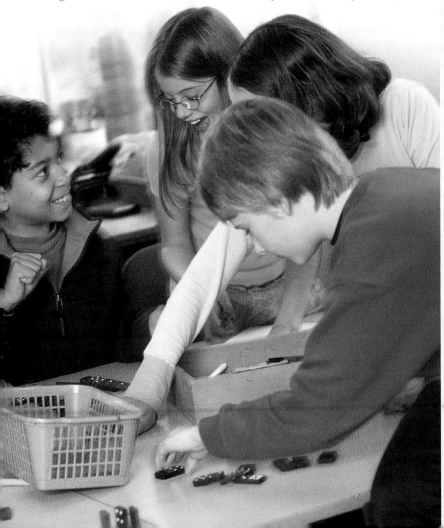

EMOTIONAL LITERACY

It is important for children to be "literate" in understanding emotions – their own as well as those of others – to enable successful interactions in the future.

From an early age, name emotions so that your child learns to recognize them. For example, you could say, "Your sister is crying because she's feeling sad." As your child develops, start naming emotions in response to actions. You could say, "You've drawn me a great picture and that makes me happy"; or, "You've taken away your brother's toy and he's upset. Please give it back and play with something else."

As your child grows up he may still need reminding about other people's feelings. You may need to point out to your 11-year-old when he upsets someone. Helping your child recognize and take responsibility for his actions and feelings is important.

It will help if your child can acknowledge his feelings in a positive way. You could start this process from an early age. For instance, if your 2-year-old trips over a step and hurts himself, don't try to absolve your child of any responsibility by saying, "Naughty step." Give your child a hug and remind him that people sometimes trip, and it's good to look where he's going.

With your older child, you may find yourself getting blamed for all kinds of things. For example, your child may say, "You make me go to school." Refuse to accept the blame. You could reply by saying something like, "All children need to go to school but you don't sound very happy about it today. Is there something you are upset about?"

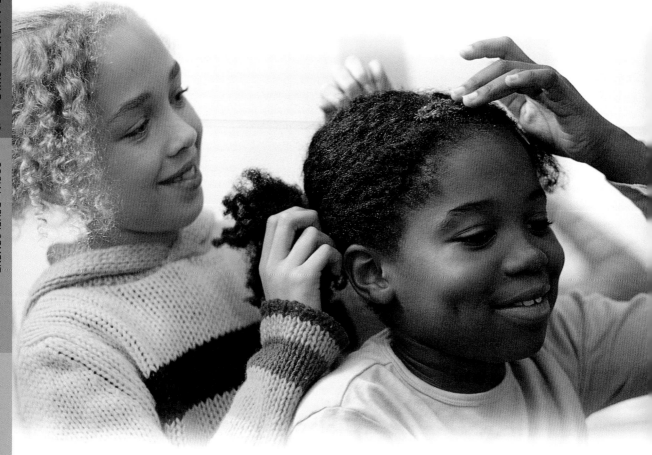

"...exposing your child to a range of different tastes and images from an early age can help prepare her for the diverse world in which she lives"

your child will need to see you demonstrate your own attitude of tolerance in your words and actions.

Exposing your children to a range of different tastes, images, and musical sounds from an early age can help prepare them for the diverse world in which they live. When children start learning the names of different foods, you could start explaining which countries they're from (with the help of a children's map).

Check your child's play materials. It may be a good idea to include black, brown, and white dolls and action figures that come in both genders and in a variety of roles, in order to encourage a positive attitude to different skin colors and genders at a later age.

With such a simple, positive approach, you'll be helping to lay the foundation for your child's respect for different countries and for people whose heritage is linked to those countries.

Another very important starting point is allowing your child to socialize and interact with people from other races, cultures, or religions. This helps challenge perceptions of what is "different," since it often reveals that, essentially, we are very similar. In places where there are few children from other racial backgrounds, you may want to use various media selectively to raise your child's awareness. These days many children's books and programs include cartoon characters and children of different heritages.

Tolerance at school

Intolerance needs to be addressed in school by teaching understanding and cooperation among people in addition to academic skills. Prejudice from home may surface in the classroom, in the playground, and on the way to school.

Schools need to work very hard on this issue because what children learn at a young age can be retained throughout life. Your child's school should have a tolerance policy. This should set out clearly how the school tackles any form of racism. Check to see if it could be improved and if you think it can, discuss your ideas with the school's principal. Ask whether the school celebrates ethnic holidays and whether they invite diverse speakers to address the school.

Once your child has started school, there is a great deal you can do to reinforce the tolerance message. Invite parents and children from different ethnic groups into your home, and make an effort to pronounce any unfamiliar names correctly. Make sure your child's reading materials depict characters from all backgrounds and show people in a variety of real roles rather than in one category that is linked stereotypically to a particular ethnic heritage.

Acknowledge that cultures from around the world have contributed to advances in knowledge, inventions, nutrition, and clothing. Let your child know that people from all backgrounds have contributed to Canada's wealth, health, and safety. Highlight that in Canada, mixed relationships and children of dual or multiple ethnicity are common. Above all, monitor what your child hears and understands, and be aware of your child's attitudes and those of her friends and classmates. Look out for any negative attitudes and views from your child, which you could challenge. Put older, more racist or sexist TV programs into an historical context, and talk about why they are wrong.

ANTISOCIAL BEHAVIOR

No child is perfect. All children try out various forms of challenging behavior at some point, whether it's being rude, disobedient, or aggressive or ruining or breaking something that's precious to someone else. The way you tackle challenging behavior will have a big influence on whether or not your child chooses to repeat it. It takes time for children to learn how to behave in a socially acceptable way, but with help from parents and teachers, most learn fairly quickly.

Most young children reserve their worst behavior for their parents or caregivers. It's a way to test their boundaries in the environment where they feel most secure.

"...it takes time for children to learn how to behave in a socially acceptable way, but with help from parents and teachers, most learn fairly quickly"

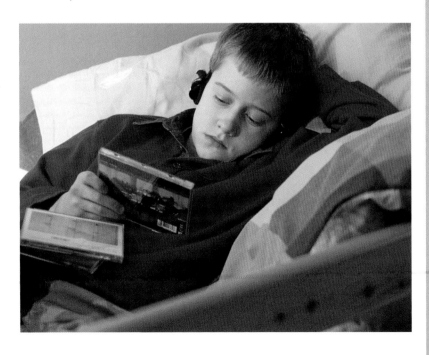

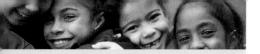

YOUR CHILD'S PEER GROUP

Friendships are very important in a child's life and a child's peer group becomes increasingly influential as he grows up.

One reason that the peer group is so important to children is that it provides the context in which they can begin experimenting with different behaviors in social situations. By doing this, children are learning important lessons about negotiation and cooperation and how to deal with conflict and competition without adults present to advise or intervene.

There are different patterns to friendships. Some children have a lot of friends. Others prefer to have one or two close friendships. If you feel that your child is not making friends, there are several things you can do to encourage friendships (see p.150).

Friendships sometimes hit a rocky patch, and your child's "best" friend may change on a regular basis. These things are normal and are not usually anything to worry about, unless your child seems overly concerned or upset.

Children are usually eager to "fit in" and be just like their friends. It's important that you encourage your child to start thinking about, valuing, and expressing his own opinions and judgments in the years before adolescence. If you do this, it will help him form an idea of who he is and have the ability to express his opinions, which may help him resist being overly influenced by others.

When your child starts school, the school will have behavior codes and rules that he will be taught and will need to adhere to, or risk being reprimanded. Before your child goes to school, it will help if you introduce some simple rules for the way you expect him to behave at home. Without overburdening him, setting down a few simple rules, such as not taking his brother's toys without permission, will help him get used to obeying rules and to the idea that rules can help make life easier for everyone.

Make sure you set a good example yourself and be consistent in your own behavior. There's no point having a "no swearing" rule if you swear in front of your child.

It also helps if you involve your child in the rule-making process. Make sure he agrees to the rules and understands what they involve.

Dealing with rudeness or disrespect

If your child is rude or disrespectful, you should ask him to stop these actions immediately and give him the chance to alter his behavior with a warning of quick, clear consequences. For example, you could say to your child: "If you continue doing that, you can't play your computer game today." This strategy will work better than a long-term threat, such as saying a child won't receive a certain present for his birthday, which will almost certainly be forgotten by the time the event comes around.

It is essential that you carry out your punishment if the behavior recurs. This is not always easy to do, but empty threats will only undermine your authority and can actually make your child's behavior worse over time.

It can be difficult to keep calm when your child seems to be behaving badly deliberately. Getting angry won't help, though. Respond to his behavior quickly, for example by sending him to his room for a few minutes immediately. This can help everyone feel calmer.

WHEN BEHAVIOR BECOMES A PROBLEM

Some children might have a pattern of persistently bad behavior for weeks or months. Their behavior breaks the rules of what's acceptable at home, at school, and in their community, and can be difficult for parents to handle. This type of behavior is known as a conduct disorder (see p.301).

A child is more likely to develop a conduct disorder if he has a difficult temperament, has problems with reading or writing, has been abused or bullied, or has some form of hyperactivity, which makes it difficult for him to concentrate and follow rules.

In some cases, children with behavior disorders grow out of them as they get older, and their behavior improves. But some of those affected unfortunately don't. If a conduct disorder isn't tackled early, a child is at risk of getting involved in fights, developing an aggressive attitude, and becoming hostile and defiant as he gets older. He might lie or steal without feeling any guilt.

Teenagers with conduct disorders can get involved in criminal behavior and then in trouble with the law. They sometimes start taking risks with their own health and safety, for instance by joyriding or taking illegal drugs.

This kind of behavior can put tremendous strain on the whole family. At school, a child might find

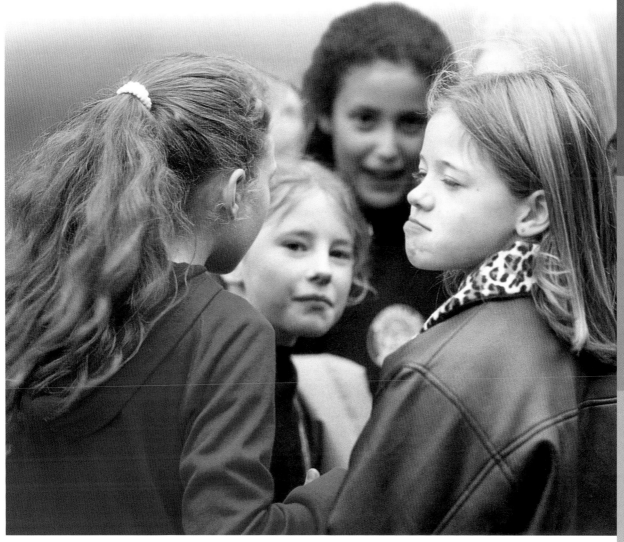

it hard to make friends because he is rude and aggressive. Even though the child may be bright, he may cause problems in class and be asked to leave. A child with a conduct disorder may be troublesome, but inside he may feel worthless and may not know how to change for the better.

How you can help

Parents can help improve the situation. Providing clear, fair, and consistent discipline will help improve a child's behavior, as will praise and rewards when the child behaves well or improves his behavior. But parents don't need to struggle with their child's behavior on their own. If you are concerned about your child's behavior, it is worth discussing it with his teacher. Extra input may be needed. You may also benefit from advice from your doctor or school psychologist.

If serious problems with your child's behavior continues, see your doctor. You may need to seek more specialized help as well, and your doctor may refer you to a child and adolescent mental health specialist in your area. A specialist can help by identifying any causes for your child's problems, giving practical advice on how you can manage your child's difficult behavior, and suggesting strategies for how it could be improved.

"...with their peers, children begin to experiment with different behaviors in social situations"

LIVING WITH CHRONIC
ILLNESS & DISABILITY

IN TERMS OF PHYSICAL WELL-BEING, MOST CHILDREN ARE HEALTHY. Their illnesses, while frequent, are mild and short-lived. Some children, however, suffer from chronic illnesses or health impairments, and these children and their families face the challenging task of adjusting to daily life with the special needs and medical issues that go along with such a condition.

INITIAL REACTIONS

Some children may have a medical condition that has been detected prenatally, such as a heart abnormality discovered on an ultrasound or Down syndrome diagnosed through genetic testing. For other children, the problem is diagnosed after birth or develops later in life.

For many parents, the news that their child has a disability or chronic disease may be unexpected and possibly devastating. Many families feel a sense of powerlessness and apprehension about facing a future filled with unknowns. A first step in coping with your child's special needs is to find out as much information as you can about the condition and its care. Knowledge is empowering and can help guide you through the potentially complicated process of dealing with the health care system.

Another important key is to work closely with your doctor, who can coordinate your child's medical care, which may include visits to different specialists and other members of the health care team. Make sure this doctor is familiar with your child and his condition as well as the available services in your area.

It is important that you should feel comfortable collaborating with this coordinating doctor. Be sure to find out how best to contact him or her, or a covering doctor, when you have questions or in case of an emergency. Consider your family to be partners with your medical care team and share the responsibility for your child's well-being by making decisions together.

LEARNING TO COPE

Most families learn to cope very well, and often discover a courage and inner strength that they didn't know they possessed. For others, it remains a struggle, but they should not be embarrassed or feel as though they have failed if they need to ask for more help.

Parents who cope best often say they find it helpful to focus on one problem at a time, rather than letting themselves become overwhelmed by the situation. Be positive about small achievements, and prepare for disappointments as well as successes. For instance, if you are trying out a new treatment for your child, be realistic and don't raise your hopes too soon.

Most people you meet will have no experience of a child with disability or illness and won't know how to react. It's almost inevitable that some will say the wrong thing, which can be upsetting. Make it clear that although your child has a disability or a health condition, he is valued no less as a human being. Demonstrate that he has the right to

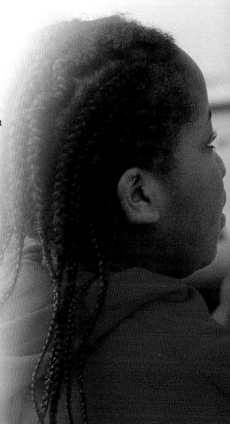

love and understanding, and that you value his individuality. Try to be positive. Others are then more likely to follow your lead.

HELPING YOUR CHILD COPE

Children with chronic diseases often deal with more stress than other youngsters. You can help your child cope with this stress by keeping him informed about the condition and the treatment, building his self-esteem, and helping him lead as normal a life as possible.

Your child's knowledge of his condition and his involvement in his treatment depends on the particular condition and his level of development. The type and amount of information you convey to your child should be appropriate for your child's age and developmental stage. Find out what your child does and does not know and inform him what to expect at an upcoming doctor's appointment or hospital visit.

Remember that as children grow older, they are increasingly able to understand their condition and assume responsibility for their own care. Periodically assess what your child understands of his condition, fill in the gaps, and correct any

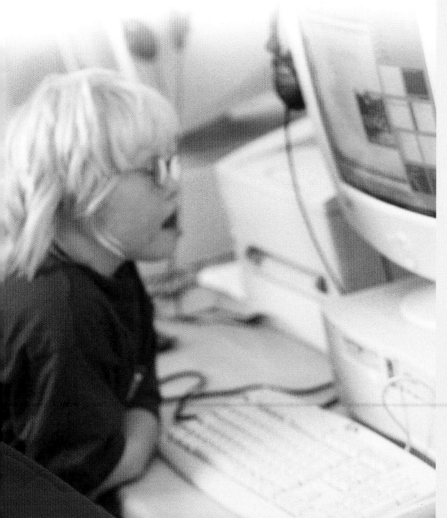

HEALTH IN DISABILITY

You and your child may find specific help, support, and advice useful. Your doctor or specialist can refer you to a range of medical, nursing, and other services. These may include:

A pediatric nurse to help with practical tasks involved in caring for a child at home, such as changing dressings or giving injections.

An occupational therapist to help your child manage daily tasks, such as dressing and going to the bathroom. He or she can also give advice on, and sometimes arrange for you to be supplied with, aids and adaptations for your home.

A physiotherapist to provide treatment to relieve pain and increase mobility. He or she can also advise on things like how to lift your child.

A psychiatric nurse to give you advice if your child has mental health problems and sometimes to give a child medication.

A speech therapist to help children with language or communication disorders.

A child development center to assess your child's needs and organize therapy if necessary.

A stroller or wheelchair if your child has serious walking difficulties.

Remember that routine issues such as immunizations, dental care, injury prevention, good nutrition, and regular exercise are important for your child, just as they are for children without a chronic condition.

misperceptions. Emphasize your child's strengths – the things he can do despite the condition. Whenever possible, try to give him choices in dealing with his condition, such as choosing from which arm to have blood drawn, so that he has control of some aspects of the situation. He may feel less alone if he has the opportunity to spend time with other children with a chronic illness.

Encourage your child to lead as normal a life as possible, both at home and at school. Have him keep up with schoolwork, form friendships, and participate in the same activities as other children his age whenever possible, but keep his limitations in mind and have realistic expectations. Unnecessary restriction of activities can reduce your child's enjoyment of life and interfere with forming friendships.

You and your child may feel sad or overwhelmed, and such feelings may come and go for both of you. This is normal and healthy, but if these feelings begin to interfere with daily life, talk to your doctor. Counseling may be recommended for your child or the entire family.

HELPING BROTHERS & SISTERS COPE

When parents must pay extra attention to a child who is ill, brothers and sisters may feel neglected. They may be resentful that family days out are limited and infrequent. At school they may be teased, and at home they might have difficulty completing homework and may have their sleep disturbed. They might also have difficulty coping with the stresses of having a sibling with a chronic health problem.

Keep your other children informed about their sibling's condition and answer their questions. Encourage them to take pride in helping their sibling however they can. Participating in their sibling's care can teach them empathy, responsibility, adaptability, and creativity. Try to establish a balance between the needs of your child with special needs and your

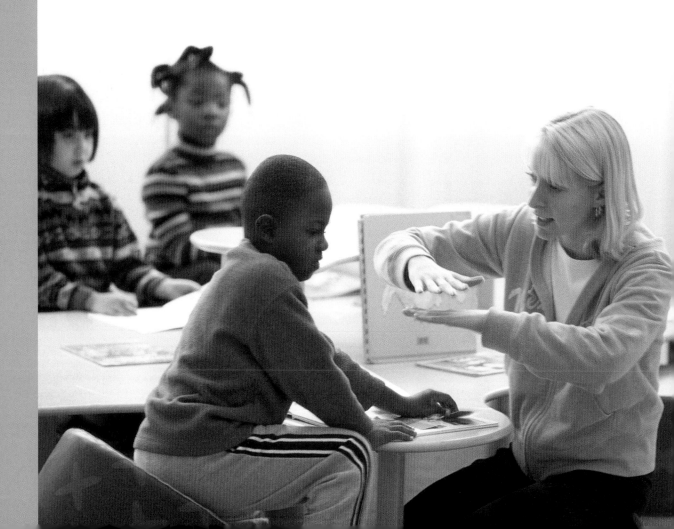

other children. Set aside a special time regularly to spend time with each child individually.

SUPPORT FOR INFANTS AND TODDLERS

Early intervention services help children with developmental delays or disabilities. The provincial and territorial governments are each responsible for providing social services to their citizens. In 2001 the federal government committed a substantial amount of funding, over five years, to support the provincial and territorial governments enabling them to build on and complement existing programs and services for children and their families. With the exception of Quebec, each province or territory is using its share of the money to provide its own resources under a common set of initiatives. These initiatives include the national child benefit and the early childhood development initiative. For example, British Columbia's early childhood development initiative includes an infant development program that provides home-based services to infants up to age three who are at risk of developmental delay or who have a developmental disability. For more information on available programs, contact the ministry responsible for social services in your province or territory.

EDUCATION & DISABILITY

It is recognized that some students have special needs that require additional supports beyond those ordinarily received in the school setting. The Education Act (or School Act) in each province or territory requires school boards to provide these exceptional students with special education programs and services that are appropriate to meet their needs. Consult with your provincial or territorial ministry of education to determine the eligibility requirements and what programs and services are available in your area. Your doctor, teacher and other school personnel will likely work together to ensure your child gets the education he needs.

If your child has a medical condition, let the teacher and principal know. Find out the school's medication policy and give them instructions in writing regarding medication names, dosages, and times to be given.

Be sure to provide the school with emergency contact information for parents or caregivers as well as for your child's doctor. Special precautions, dietary requirements, or transportation needs should also be provided. You should notify the school of any changes in your child's routine, including changes in medication dosages.

"Keep your other children informed about their sibling's condition… Participating in their sibling's care can teach them empathy, responsibility, adaptability, and creativity."

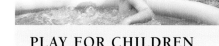

PLAY FOR CHILDREN WITH DISABILITIES

Play has an important role in the development of all children, whatever their abilities. In addition to promoting motor development and creativity, it also offers a valuable way for your child to socialize with other children. For children with disabilities, play opportunities in the community can be limited. However, the situation is improving, and many organizations are working hard to make more opportunities available.

If your child has a medical condition or special needs, think about the type of activities that may interest him. For example, he might enjoy attending a camp or class for children with similar conditions. Your school's special education department may have special play programs and may be a good source of information about other activities.

To find out what play facilities and other opportunities exist in your area you could try contacting the following places:

- Local community center or children's hospital
- Your local library (these often have year-round activities for children)
- Specific local play facilities, such as playgrounds, amusement parks, community recreation centers, and swimming pools
- National organizations that serve children with disabilities (many of these organizations have local chapters)

STARTING SCHOOL

GOING TO SCHOOL IS ABOUT MUCH MORE THAN academic achievement. It's the main way children socialize and is an important step for them in becoming more independent and well-rounded. Your child will fit into school life better if he has acquired some everyday skills and the basics of how to behave. These include going to the bathroom by himself and knowing how to listen and take turns.

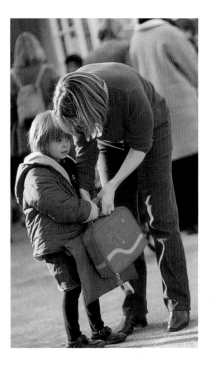

PREPARING YOUR CHILD FOR SCHOOL

The best way to prepare your child for school is to start early. The most important factor in determining a child's academic success lies in language acquisition. Reading regularly to your child from infancy on will increase his comprehension and vocabulary and can be fun for you both. Set aside a special time for reading to your child, perhaps before he goes to bed. You can continue this practice as he grows older.

Going to child care or preschool can also prepare your child for school. Make sure the one you choose focuses on play rather than on strictly academic learning. The most important lessons your child should be learning at this point are about getting along with others, and this should be fun.

Visiting the school

Once your child is enrolled at school, start talking to him about it. There are many books about starting school that you and your child can read together. Most schools offer visits before classes start to give your child the opportunity to look around his classroom, meet his teacher, see where the bathrooms and cafeteria are, and see where he will put his belongings.

Find out about the school's routine so you can talk with your child about what will be happening and when. The school should also give you the opportunity to ask questions or discuss any issues relating specifically to your child. If he has a problem, such as an allergy or a medical condition, let both the teacher and the principal know verbally and in writing. If relevant, you should also ask about the school's policy regarding bringing in prescribed medications, such as asthma inhalers and epinephrine injections for serious allergies.

First days

The night before your child's first day, get everything ready so that he feels well prepared. Lay his clothes out and have his bag packed. It's a good idea to do this together every night for the first few weeks so that the mornings go more smoothly. From then on, encourage him to prepare for the next day. For example, if he has been asked to bring something in, encourage him to choose the item the night before and put it where he won't forget it.

Your own approach to school is important. If you have a positive attitude and tell your child you know he can manage, he will feel more confident. If you're visibly upset when he goes, he may feel

> "Your own approach to school is important. If you have a positive attitude…he will feel more confident."

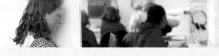

discouraged and believe that you don't think he'll do well.

Be sensitive to your child's behavior during the first few weeks at school. It is very important that he's making friends. Inviting one or two of the children he seems to like to your house after school may help them bond.

After school, don't worry if he doesn't talk about his day right away. He might start chatting about something, or singing a particular song he's learned, later on. Give him a chance to unwind at home and then you can casually ask a few questions about his day.

ACHIEVEMENT & YOUR CHILD

There may be occasions when you become concerned about your child's progress. For instance, if he's not reading fluently by age 7 or 8, you should discuss his progress with his teacher.

CHILDREN WITH SPECIAL EDUCATIONAL NEEDS

If you feel your child is generally falling behind at school, or if he has a problem with a specific subject such as reading, you should seek professional advice. Ask your doctor to check for physical problems that could be making school hard for him, such as vision or hearing difficulties. If your child is having trouble with linguistic skills, he may be referred to a speech and language therapist. Your child may also benefit from a full educational assessment to pinpoint areas of difficulty; a plan to help him achieve his potential may then be drawn up. See your school's principal to find out your next steps and arrange a meeting with your school's special needs coordinator.

Your child has the right to receive an appropriate education. The Education Act (or School Act) in each province or territory requires school boards to provide exceptional students with special education programs and services that are appropriate to meet their needs.

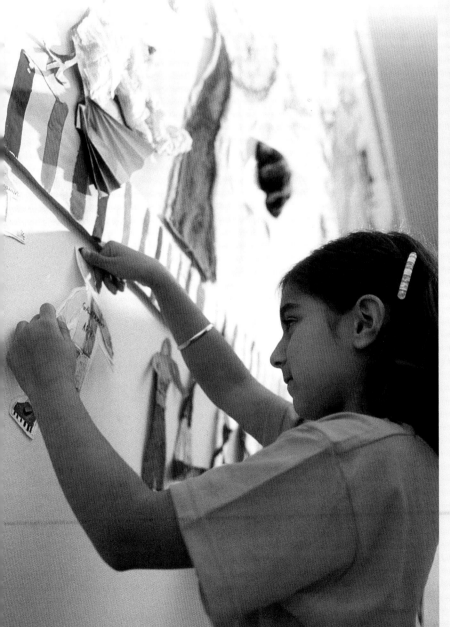

"You should focus on the things he can do and seems to enjoy, and give him plenty of praise and encouragement."

It's worth remembering that most children are of average ability and it's the exception rather than the rule to be above or below average. It's also worth keeping in mind that girls initially tend to do better than boys at school. They generally have better language skills and may continue to perform better linguistically than boys for several years. Boys seem to catch up to girls after that.

For children of high-achiever parents, life at school can be especially difficult. They may not be as academically able as their parents, and they may feel that the standards their parents have set for them are too high. Children, like adults, can become stressed if they are persistently asked to perform beyond their capability.

During the first few years at school, if your child is a good talker and listener and knows basic mathematics, there should be nothing to worry about academically. Nonetheless, you may find it

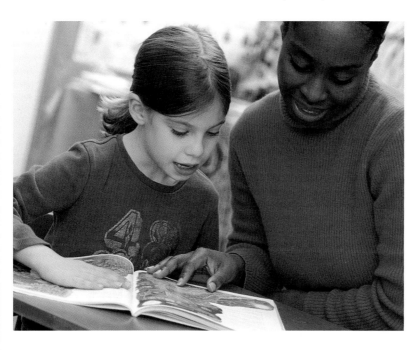

difficult to avoid comparing him with other children. Some children will be better at drawing, reading, or writing while others will be better at class discussion or sports. You should focus on the things your child can do and seems to enjoy, and give him plenty of praise and encouragement. Letting your child know that you recognize his strengths will give him the message that you value him.

However, it's important to get the right balance between playing on your child's strengths and encouraging him in areas where he may be weak. If you feel your child is not achieving to the best of his ability, trust your instincts. As his parent, you know him best. Young children are not usually lazy at school and there is often a good reason for any problem. It may be that your child has a specific concern, which could be about something very simple. It could be that he does not relate well to his teacher, or he may have general or specific learning disabilities. Ask your child's teacher for help.

If you feel your child would benefit from being a little more challenged than he is at school, look for activities you could do together at home. Slightly more difficult books may help develop his language skills. Simple board games can help improve his counting skills and also help him learn about taking turns. Card games are also good for adding and counting.

You can bring math into everyday life by teaching your child how to use money, and by involving him in activities that require counting and measuring, such as measuring ingredients for cooking. Learning in this way can reinforce lessons found in school books.

IF YOUR CHILD REFUSES TO GO TO SCHOOL

Your child will probably be going to school for a full day by about the age of 6. However, it can take a young child several months to settle into a school routine. Take it slowly and don't expect too much to begin with, and your child should gain confidence quickly.

If your child seems very unhappy about going to school, speak to his teacher; there may be things that can be done to help him settle in. A buddy system, such as having an older child help your child find his way around, might work. You could then invite that child to your home so they can get to know each other.

Inviting one or two children from your child's class to your home can also help build his social skills. It shouldn't take longer than six months for a child to feel more comfortable at school. After this time, you should speak to your child's teacher. Your child may need additional help.

Older children

Sometimes, an older or more confident child will come up with an excuse for not going to school. He might complain of a headache or of feeling sick when you think he's probably fine. If you think he's okay, try having him attend school. If you do let him have the day off from school, don't give him too much attention, so that he won't receive positive reinforcement for missing school.

If your child has previously been happy at school and suddenly doesn't want to go, it's possible that there's something worrying him. He may not like his teacher or he may be being bullied, which can occur at school. If your child seems

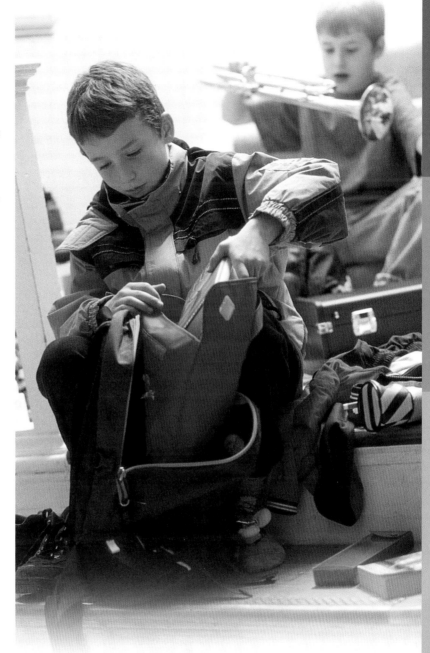

unhappy at school, cries on the way, and seems very reluctant to go, take it seriously. Bullying should never be ignored. Your child's school should have a policy to deal with bullying (*see p.151*).

Occasionally, if your child doesn't want to go to school, the problem can become very difficult. Talk to your child's teacher and agree on a

plan to help him. Rehearse his day, discussing each class subject. Remind him about reassuring things – for example, that he will be sitting next to a particular friend in math class. Positive statements about things he does well, such as "you're good in spelling," may help. Taking a favorite object or toy to school may also help, but check with the teacher first.

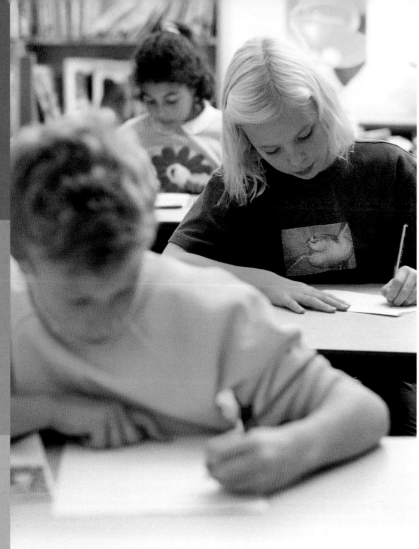

your child may be advised to skip a grade in school, this is not always appropriate. He may not be ready socially or emotionally to mix with older children. Allowing your child to take some advanced classes or giving him extra assignments while he remains in the same grade may be preferable.

Children who are exceptionally good at sports, music, or the creative arts could also be described as gifted. There may be school initiatives designed to promote the talents of gifted children; your child's school may have a policy on this. You can also do things to help at home. For example, if your child is good at music, take him to concerts and offer him lessons outside of school.

PROBLEMS WITH FRIENDS OR TEACHERS

Most children will come across at least one teacher and several classmates with whom they feel they don't get along during their school years, and if this happens your child should try to learn to deal with it quickly and effectively.

Make the experience into a learning one. Talk to him about how important it is to get along with different people and suggest some strategies for coping. Ideally, do not intervene directly; try to let him deal with the problem himself.

If you feel your child is being bullied, you should take this seriously (*see opposite*). If it seems to be more the case that the friendship is going through a negative phase, consider strategies that might help. For example, you could invite his friends over to your house, or get your child involved in after-school activities with them, or encourage him to make new friends.

Many children feel under great pressure to do well at school, and it is important to think carefully about how your expectations affect your child. You should ensure that he still has plenty of time in his day for enjoyable noncompetitive activities. If you can't get your child to go to school at all, ask your doctor for a referral to a mental health professional.

"…it is important to think carefully about how your expectations affect your child."

HELPING GIFTED CHILDREN

If your child excels academically, he'll need to feel challenged at school to help him make the most of his abilities. Teachers know that bright children can easily feel bored and frustrated if the pace of work is too slow for them, and this can lead to disruptive behavior. Although

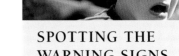

IF YOUR CHILD IS BULLIED

Unfortunately, bullying at school is a common problem. Most people think of bullying in terms of kicking, hitting, or other forms of violence. However, emotional bullying, which involves name-calling, sarcasm, spreading rumors, and/or persistent teasing or ignoring, is more usual and can be more difficult to deal with and prove. Persistent bullying of either kind can result in depression, low self-esteem, shyness, poor academic performance, isolation, or in extreme cases, even threatened or attempted suicide.

If you are worried that your child is being bullied, you must take the matter seriously. Try to establish the facts – ask him directly what is happening. Talk with his teacher and the principal. The school should have a policy for dealing with bullying. Keep a record of all incidents and submit a written copy to the principal.

If your child is being physically bullied, help him practice strategies such as calmly walking away or clearly and loudly stating "Stop doing that or I'm going to report you to the principal." If the bullying occurs at school, ask the teacher to separate the two adversaries so that they rarely cross paths. If it happens on the way to or from school, escort your child or have him go with a group of friends.

If your child is being emotionally bullied, teach him to avoid the children who are bothering him and encourage him to make friends with other children. Teach him to ignore name-calling or teasing, and explain that if he stops reacting to taunts, the bullies will soon lose interest.

IF YOUR CHILD IS A BULLY

If you discover that your child is bullying another child, try to stay calm. Talk to him and try to establish the facts, and talk to his teacher and the principal. Let your child know why bullying is wrong. Reassure him that you love him, but make it clear that you don't like his behavior. A reward system for good behavior might help. If he can't see that his actions are wrong or won't stop bullying, he may need referral to a specialist.

SPOTTING THE WARNING SIGNS OF BULLYING

Since your child may not tell you he is being bullied, look for these possible signs of bullying. If you suspect bullying, teach your child to immediately intervene and, if necessary, seek help from the teacher or principal.

Being frightened of walking to and from school or changing their usual route

Not wanting to go on the school bus

Begging you to drive them to school

Being unwilling to go to school

A sudden lack of interest in school

A drop in grades

Unexplained bruises and other physical injuries

Morning complaints of psychosomatic symptoms such as stomachaches or headaches

Depression or anxiety

Beginning to bully other children, including siblings

Becoming aggressive and unreasonable

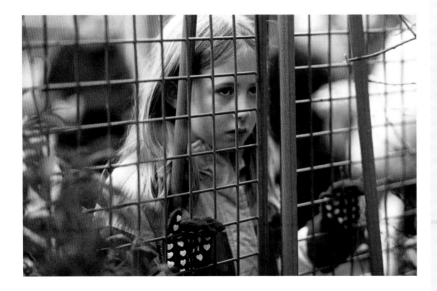

ADOLESCENT
DEVELOPMENT

P UBERTY INVOLVES PHYSICAL AND EMOTIONAL CHANGES as hormones guide your child from childhood to adulthood. All adolescents go through puberty, but there is a wide variation in when it occurs and the rate of development. Your child's emotional development will be slower than her physical development, so although she may begin to look like an adult, she will still need your guidance.

HORMONAL CHANGES

Both female and male hormones are present at low levels in children of both sexes from birth. However, the balance of these hormones changes dramatically at puberty as the levels of male sex hormones rise in boys and levels of female sex hormones rise in girls.

Up to a year before any physical changes appear, and as early as age 8 for girls and age 10 for boys, changes start taking place in the amount of certain hormones produced by the hypothalamus in the brain. These

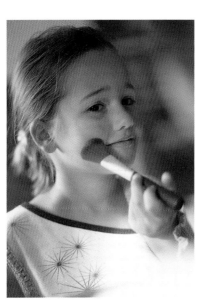

hormones cause the ovaries in a girl to develop follicles, which first produce the female sex hormone estrogen and later on, progesterone. In a boy, these hormones cause the testes to enlarge and begin producing the male hormone testosterone.

Estrogen and testosterone are the principal hormones that bring about the physical changes of puberty in girls and boys, although there is a contribution from the adrenal glands in stimulating the growth of pubic and underarm hair.

PHYSICAL CHANGES IN GIRLS

Girls usually start producing sex hormones between the ages of 8 and 11 years, with the average age of beginning puberty at around 10. The first and most obvious external sign that a girl is entering puberty is the development of breast buds. These may be asymmetrical in size at first and quite tender, which may require

some reassurance that this is normal.

This early breast development is usually accompanied by the adolescent growth spurt. There is often a feeling of awkwardness, since a girl's hands and feet may grow rapidly at first, with the legs and spine taking longer to catch up. There is also a change in body shape and fat distribution as girls gain fat in the area of their breasts and hips. This distribution of fat and the wider pelvis that girls have (which is needed in order to deliver a baby) account for the adult female figure being "curvier" than that of a man.

In addition to the obvious external changes, a girl's internal organs also increase in size and shape. Her uterus and vagina become larger and the lining of her vagina thickens and starts to produce clear secretions.

By the end of the pubertal process (which in both boys and girls may take up to five years from the first sign until adult height is reached),

"Your child's emotional development will be slower than her physical development, so although she may begin to look like an adult, she will still need your guidance."

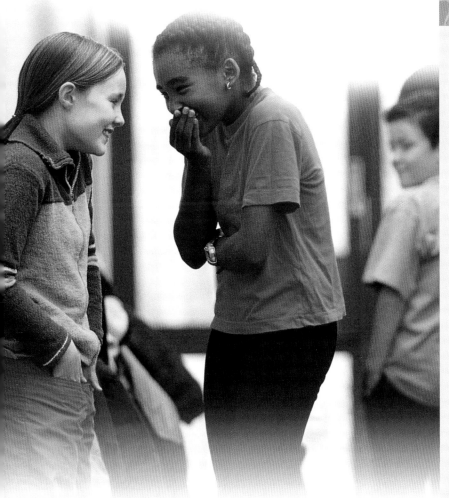

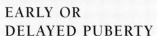

Early puberty in girls

You may want to visit your doctor if your daughter begins to develop breasts or pubic hair before age 8. While early puberty can run in families, it can also result from unusually early or excessive hormone production linked to a medical condition. Your daughter may need hormone measurements to determine if this is the case. She may also need a pelvic ultrasound scan, similar to those for pregnant women, to assess the size of her uterus and ovaries.

Delayed puberty in girls

Puberty is considered delayed if your daughter has no breast buds or pubic hair developing by the age of 14. You should also be concerned if her menstrual periods have not started within five years of the appearance of breast tissue. Again, delay can run in families. As is the case for early puberty, hormone levels may be measured with a blood test. In certain cases, puberty can be induced by giving extra hormones at the appropriate time.

Early puberty in boys

If your son has experienced an increase in the size of his testes and/or penis, or has developed any pubic hair, before age 9, visit your doctor. He may need hormone tests.

Delayed puberty in boys

You may also want to see your doctor if your son has not had any of the signs of pubertal development by the age of 14. He may simply be a late developer, especially if this runs in the family, but he could be producing insufficient hormones for a variety of reasons and may need medical tests.

a girl's height will increase by about 21 cm (9½ in), with only about 6 cm (2½ in) of this growth occurring after menstrual periods start.

Pubic hair is very different from the soft hair that may be present in young children. In girls it starts as coarse dark hair on the pubic mound and labia, subsequently increasing in both amount and area of distribution.

Pubic hair usually starts to appear after breast budding, but not always. In particular there may be an early "switch on" of the adrenal glands, which can occur around the age of 7 and is independent of true puberty. If this happens it is termed "premature adrenarche" and is most commonly seen in children who have a parent of African or Mediterranean descent.

In addition to pubic hair there may be some underarm hair and even some body odor. The appearance of "androgen" hair is often accompanied by other effects of androgen secretion, such as acne on the face and back, oiliness of the skin and scalp, and body odor. Your daughter may find she needs to wash her hair more frequently and also use a deodorant. Underarm hair develops at varying times but may be relatively late.

Menstruation

The onset of menstrual periods (menarche) usually occurs toward the end of puberty. Periods usually start when the breasts are well developed but not quite "adult" in size and shape (this takes up to four years) and as the adolescent growth spurt is coming to an end. On average, menarche occurs between the ages of 12 and 13 years, but may occur as early as 10 or as late as 15 years in normal girls.

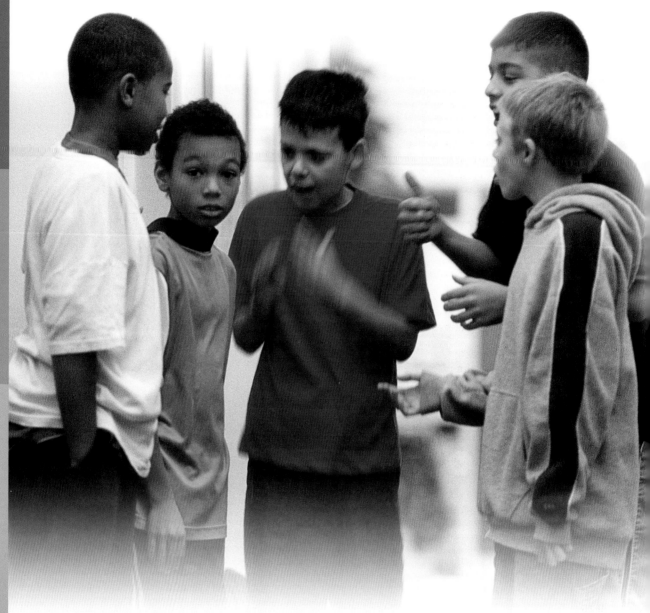

Menstrual periods during the first year often happen without the release of an egg (ovulation), so they may be irregular before settling into a cycle of between 28 and 35 days. Some girls do not establish a regular cycle during the first year or two. Address any concerns with your doctor at each annual checkup, or sooner if you suspect a problem (such as unusual cycles, very heavy bleeding or pain, or bleeding in between periods).

There is an impression that menarche occurs earlier than it did 30 or 40 years ago. The age of menarche, and probably the onset of puberty, has followed a trend to occur on average two to three months earlier per decade, probably reflecting improvements in nutrition and socioeconomic status, especially in the industrialized world. This trend is beginning to level off in most of western Europe and Canada.

However, the trend for an earlier age of menarche may be ongoing in parts of the developing world, where nutrition and living conditions are continuing to improve. It is certainly the case that genes play a strong role in the expected timing of puberty, with early or late menarche running in families, and girls from an African-American or Mediterranean background maturing earlier.

PHYSICAL CHANGES IN BOYS

Puberty in boys starts, on average, six months after it does in girls. The first sign of puberty – an enlargement of the testes – occurs at around 12 years of age, but can happen between the ages of 10½ and 14 in normal boys. Pubic hair development and growth of the penis usually begin within six months of the initial testicular increase, but the adolescent growth spurt in boys is a relatively late event, taking place on average at age 14 or so. This means that puberty in a boy may go unnoticed at first.

The testes continue to enlarge symmetrically as the rest of the physical changes occur, although one testis may be lower than the other. Inequality in the size of the testes or pain in either testis should be reported to your doctor. Pubic hair develops as coarse dark hairs around the base of the penis at first and then gradually spreads into the adult male distribution. Hair spreading up the lower abdomen or over the chest occurs relatively late, and in some boys not at all. As hair growth is happening the penis also begins to grow, at first just in length, but later in breadth also, with development of the glans, the sensitive tip of the penis. Underarm hair and oiliness of the skin and acne are later events, and the average age for the development of facial hair is around 15 years. Voice changes, which are partly due to growth in the voice box (larynx) and change in length and thickness of the vocal cords, usually start between the ages of 13 and 15 years.

A boy going through an "average puberty" may begin to experience nocturnal ejaculation, or "wet dreams," at around 13 or 14 years of age. This may worry him unless it has been explained to him before it starts. Nocturnal ejaculation is a reflection of normal semen production during puberty and will stop as the boy gets older.

As with girls, skeletal growth in boys is at first disproportionate. A boy's hands and feet grow more quickly than his arms and legs, which lengthen before his torso, creating an impression of gawkiness. This temporary unevenness also affects your son's face, since his chin, nose, lips, and ears may grow before his head attains its full adult size.

By the time puberty is completed, your son will have gained around 28 cm (11 in) in height. He will have become leaner, with more muscle than fat, and will, to a greater or lesser extent, have developed a more "male" body shape, with relatively broad shoulders and narrow hips. By this stage his facial hair will probably be growing more fully and he may need to shave occasionally.

As with girls, the surge of hormones and body changes may cause a boy to become moody, withdrawn, or aggressive. Because these behavioral changes are somewhat out of his control, try to ignore confrontational behavior and allow your teenager to develop into a mature adult while still preserving basic ground rules at home.

> "As with girls, the surge of hormones and body changes may cause a boy to become moody, withdrawn, or aggressive."

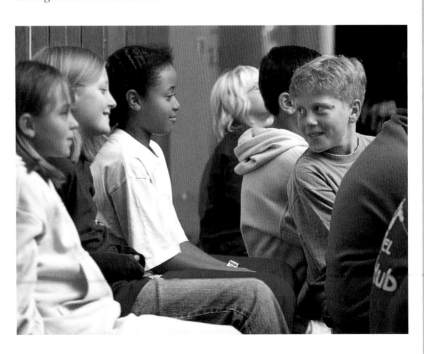

SEX EDUCATION

Talking to children about the facts of life isn't something that many parents find easy. How much information do you give your child? And when do you give it? The way you approach sex will depend on both you and your child. It's not something you can cover in one brief conversation. It's an ongoing process. Your child will need different information at different stages.

"...the best approach to sex education is to take the lead from your child"

WHEN IS THE RIGHT TIME TO START?

Many experts agree that the best approach is to take the lead from your child and wait until he asks you a question. "Where do babies come from?" is often the first. It's important that you be open and honest right from the start and

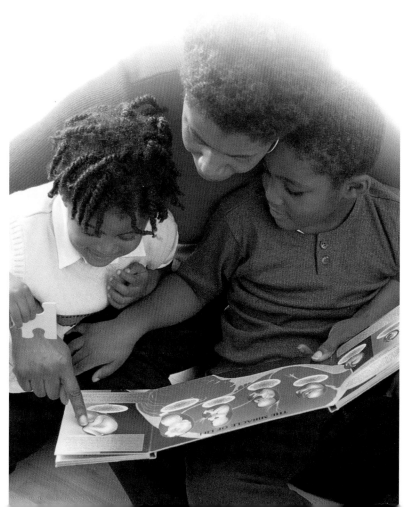

avoid stories about storks. They might seem easy explanations at the time, but as your child grows up and finds out what actually does happen, he will be less likely to trust you.

It's worth doing some preparation before your child is old enough to ask you questions. Think about how you might answer your child's questions when he asks them. Replies should be appropriate to his age and understanding. For instance, a child of 5 will probably be satisfied with hearing that a baby is made by a mommy and a daddy and grows in a special place in mommy's body. There's no need at this stage to go into a detailed biological explanation and you don't need to cover issues that he hasn't asked about. Doing so could just confuse him.

If your child asks you something that takes you by surprise and you're not sure how to reply, be honest. You could say something like: "That's an interesting question. I'm not sure what the answer is. Let me think about it a bit and we can talk later." This gives you time to think what to say, and for your child it leaves open the idea of talking about the subject again. It's worth investing in a book with simple diagrams that helps you show your child what you are explaining. There are many available for different age groups.

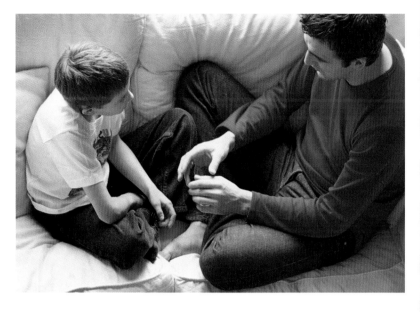

SEX EDUCATION IN SCHOOL

Sex education is now part of the curriculum in many schools, so most children will receive some information about it there. In grade school, children between 5 and 7 years may learn that animals, including humans, grow and reproduce. Between the ages of 7 and 11, students may learn more about life cycles and human reproduction. It's worth talking to your child's teacher to find out how the school tackles sex education specifically, and when it will happen. You can then be ready to talk to your child about what he has learned, make sure he has understood it properly, and give him the opportunity to ask any more questions. Parents also have the right to withdraw their children from sex education lessons if they feel they are inappropriate.

The content and tone of sex education lessons may be left to the discretion of schools or school districts and may vary from province to province and district to district. Many sex education programs in school will address recent concerns about a dramatic increase in the number of young people becoming pregnant at a young age or seeking help for sexually transmitted infections.

Sexuality and health

Children and adolescents need accurate, comprehensive sex education if they are to practice healthy sexual behavior as adults. Early or risky sexual activity may lead to unintended pregnancy and sexually transmitted infections (STIs). Teenage sexual activity and pregnancy remain high, and the incidence of STIs in teenagers is also high.

Your family doctor or local health center can play an important role. Unlike school-based instruction, discussion of sexuality with a doctor or public health nurse allows children and adolescents to ask questions or reveal personal information in a confidential setting.

ATTITUDES TOWARD NUDITY

Young children don't have any sense of privacy. They are often happiest when they don't have any clothes on and may be very interested in your body. Some parents are very relaxed about this and are happy to let their children see them without clothes. Others aren't. But if you are comfortable with it, it can be helpful for young children to see that you are relaxed and confident about your body. And it can help your child begin to realize how boys and girls and men and women are different.

Often, around the time of starting school, children tend to become more aware of their bodies and are less eager to take their clothes off. As your child's boundaries begin to emerge, be careful to respect them. Don't burst into the bathroom when your 8-year-old is in the bath, or into his room when the door is closed.

If you are concerned that your child doesn't show any inhibitions, you could gradually introduce the idea of personal privacy and boundaries. For example, you could close the door to your bedroom or bathroom and gently explain that there are some things that people prefer to keep private.

When children are young and happy to be seen naked it's easy to see anything obviously wrong. As your child grows older and becomes more inhibited, you should advise him that he needs to be aware of his body and talk to you if he notices anything different or unusual.

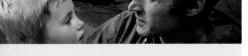

ANSWERING YOUR CHILD'S QUESTIONS

Answer your child honestly when he starts asking you questions about where babies come from. You don't need to give him details that he won't understand, but you can simply explain that he came from a special place in his mommy's body.

When your child is older, a good book with diagrams aimed at the appropriate age level is helpful in explaining how reproduction works.

Don't rely on sex education in schools to teach your child all he needs to know – your child may not understand issues about relationships and peer pressure.

Help your child understand that only a minority of teenagers are sexually active and that there are many important reasons to delay sexual intercourse.

Make sure at each stage of development that your child knows it's all right to approach you with any questions or problems about sex and relationships that he may have. Let him know that, whatever the question or issue, you are always there to listen to him.

Your doctor or public health nurse is also a good resource to help answer your child's questions.

Families and children may obtain education together or in a separate but coordinated manner.

While education about sex and relationships, pregnancy, HIV and AIDS, and other sexually transmitted infections may be provided in school, many sex education programs also center around teaching abstinence or discouraging early experimentation with sex.

PUTTING SEX EDUCATION IN CONTEXT

As children grow older, it is often easy for parents to assume that they will learn everything they need to

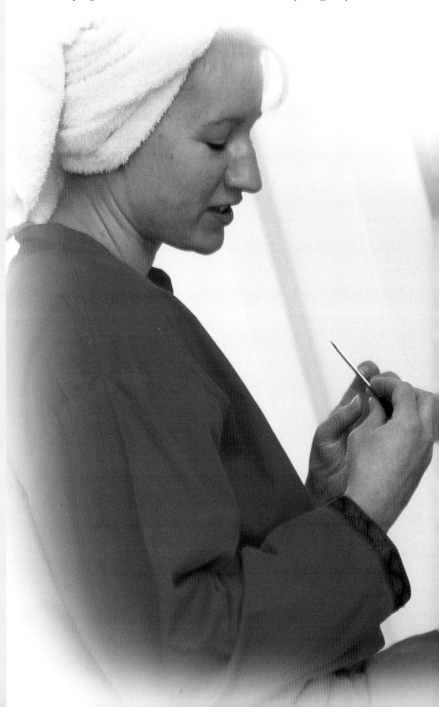

know about sex education in classes at school and to think that they understand more about sex, sexual development, and relationships than they really do.

Children are more sophisticated these days in terms of being aware of fashions and music, and they are used to seeing images of sexuality in the media – usually images of the bare-flesh variety rather than images depicting relationships.

Children may pick up on underlying, inaccurate messages from movies, videos, and music that all young people are sexually active. It is important for parents to be aware of and monitor their children's television and movie viewing, as well as their music choices, and discuss together any inaccuracies or stereotypes that are represented.

There is a huge amount of material on the Internet discussing sexual issues, and this is becoming an increasingly common source of information for young people. There can be some very helpful sites, but you may feel that some are too explicit for younger children. Be sure to monitor your child's usage of the Internet.

Most children say they would like to hear about sex and relationships from their parents as well as at school. For parents, it is useful to make sure your child has accurate information and above all to give guidance. With your help, your child can develop the confidence to make the right choices at the right times.

If your child enjoys reading magazines, a good starting place would be to pick out some of the information they contain and discuss it together. This would give you the opportunity to listen to any messages she may be picking up and to correct them if they're inaccurate. You can also give her the opportunity to ask you any questions.

Some children may be too embarrassed to talk openly about sex. Mentioning, almost casually, things that are relevant to sex education that you have read in the paper or seen on television together can give them the opportunity to ask questions or at least hear your views.

Talking to older children

Once the basic information on sex is imparted and children go through puberty, it can often become more difficult to talk about sex. Part of the reason for this may be that your child likes to appear as though he knows everything. Or, he may really think he knows all there is to know.

In reality, your child may know some facts about sex and reproduction but may not grasp their full implications. He also may not understand what the real issues are in relationships or how to resist pressure from peers or partners to be sexually active before he is ready. All of these things can be difficult for an adolescent to admit.

It may be helpful to reassure your child that at his age he's not expected to be able to deal with relationship issues or peer pressure alone. Being open may help your child feel more able to ask for your advice and more comfortable about receiving it.

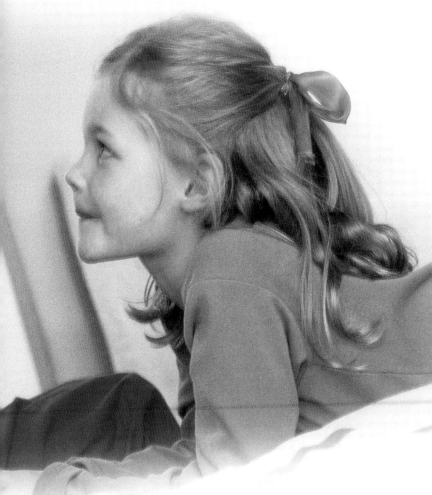

SUBSTANCE ABUSE
PREVENTION

THE USE OF TOBACCO, ALCOHOL, AND OTHER DRUGS is one of the biggest problems facing young people today. Drugs are more readily available than in the past, and the health effects of early drug use can be devastating. It may be difficult to shield young people from exposure to these substances, but early guidance from parents can discourage youth from experimenting and being harmed.

WHAT YOU CAN DO AS A PARENT

Although children are unlikely to drink alcohol, or use tobacco or other drugs during grade school, this is a crucial time to talk honestly and frequently about healthy choices and risky behaviors. Because children's bodies and brains are still developing, they are more sensitive to the dangerous effects of substance use. Drug use can lead to immediate problems such as depression or bronchitis; chronic problems such as brain damage, emphysema, cirrhosis (liver damage), heart disease, and cancer; and even death. Tobacco, alcohol, and drugs are addictive. There are no guarantees that your child won't use drugs, but you can influence her by providing guidance, setting clear rules about drugs, not using drugs yourself, and spending time with your child. Know the facts and correct your child's mistaken beliefs, such as "marijuana won't hurt you" or "everybody drinks."

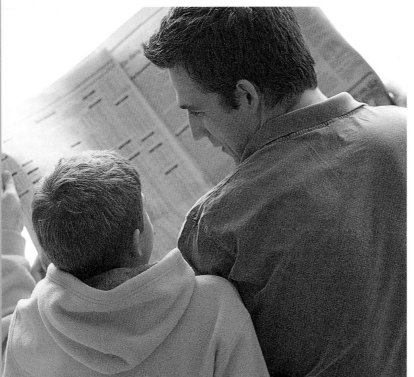

Teach children exactly how you expect them to respond if someone offers them drugs, such as firmly saying "No." Rehearse together other responses, such as stating reasons ("No thanks, I'm not into that."), suggesting other things to do, or leaving the situation.

Get your child involved in athletics, hobbies, school clubs, and other activities that reduce boredom and excess free time. Build self-confidence and encourage positive friendships and interests. Teach your child that doing something wrong is not a good way to try to feel accepted. Remind children that real friends do not urge others to use tobacco, alcohol, and other drugs, or reject them if they don't.

TOBACCO

It is important to remember that, although many Canadian teenagers smoke, the majority of teenagers choose not to smoke or use smokeless tobacco.

There is a significant impact on the health of a child who smokes. The adverse effects include being significantly more susceptible to colds, increased phlegm, wheezing, shortness of breath, and worsened asthma. Chewing tobacco can eventually lead to deadly mouth and throat cancers.

Young people are more likely to smoke if they live with a smoker, so you should set a good example. Passive smoking can lead to the same harmful effects on the body as active smoking, including more ear, throat, and lung ailments and greater risk for heart disease and cancer.

ALCOHOL

Alcohol acts as a nervous system depressant and is very addictive. The legal age for drinking alcohol in Canada varies from province to province, but is in the late teens. However, childhood drinking begins early, often between 11 and 13 years of age. While the most serious physical effects of excessive drinking typically take years to develop, binge drinking and high-risk behaviors while using alcohol are important causes of death and disease in teens. Alcohol is a major factor in the top four causes of teen death: traffic crashes, homicide, suicide, and drowning. Alcohol use can lead to experimentation with other drugs as well as to alcoholism, which may run in families. Parents can set a good example by discouraging illegal underage drinking and limiting their own alcohol use.

OTHER DRUGS

Although illicit drug use in adolescents has declined since it peaked in the 1970s, adolescents are now trying drugs at a younger age. In addition to illicit substances such as marijuana, LSD, ecstasy, and cocaine, household products such as aerosols or spray paint may be inhaled for their mind-altering effects. One of the keys to helping prevent children from experimenting with these substances is for parents, schools and communities to begin drug education prior to adolescence. Parental guidance may be the most effective of all methods for drug use prevention.

TOBACCO, ALCOHOL, AND THE MEDIA

A big influence on a child's decision to use tobacco or alcohol is the media. Young people today are surrounded by messages in the media that smoking cigarettes and drinking alcohol are normal, desirable, and harmless. Although tobacco products are not promoted in the Canadian media, many popular magazines available in Canada come from the US, where cigarette advertising is common. Alcohol advertisements are commonly associated with sporting events. Young people are the primary targets of many of these tobacco and alcohol ads.

Ads for these products appeal to young people by suggesting that drinking alcohol and smoking cigarettes will make them more popular, sexy, and successful.

Help children and teenagers understand the difference between the misleading messages in advertising and the truth about the dangers of using alcohol and tobacco products. Make sure the TV shows and movies your child watches do not glamorize the use of tobacco, alcohol, and other drugs.

HOW CAN I TELL IF MY CHILD IS USING DRUGS?

Despite your best efforts, your child or teen may still use drugs. Some warning signs of drug use are:

- Smell of alcohol, smoke, or other chemicals on your child's breath or clothing.
- Obvious intoxication, impairment, or unusual behavior.
- Change in dress, appearance, and grooming.
- Change in choice of friends.
- Frequent arguments, sudden mood changes, and unexplained violent actions.
- Change in eating and sleeping patterns.
- Skipping school and failing grades.
- Delinquent behavior and running away.
- Suicide attempts or depression.

If your child or teen is using drugs, he needs your help. Being able to recognize the signs of drug use is the first step. However, the problem could become too much for you to handle alone. Don't hesitate to seek professional help, such as your doctor, a counselor, support group, or treatment program.

"Because children's bodies and brains are still developing, they are more sensitive to the dangerous effects of substance use."

STAYING HEALTHY

W̲E ALL WANT TO KEEP OUR CHILDREN HEALTHY and may wonder what we can do to ensure that they stay as well as possible. As parents or caregivers, we are responsible for our children's well-being from day to day, and it is largely the things we do on a daily basis – such as providing balanced meals and making sure they get enough sleep – that keep them healthy and strong.

"...there are many simple ways that you can help your child to live healthily"

ENCOURAGING A HEALTHY LIFESTYLE

A great deal of emphasis is now placed on preventing illness and encouraging children to live as healthily as possible, and with good reason. As parents, you can help keep your child in the best possible physical health by providing a good, balanced diet, and ensuring he gets plenty of sleep and exercise. Mental health and emotional well-being are important too, so be sure to discuss any concerns with your child's doctor. A child who is raised in a loving, supportive family and grows up with a sense of self-worth and his own values and beliefs, will be getting a healthy start in life.

What you can do
There are many simple ways in which you can help your child live healthily. In addition to trying to prevent illness, take steps to ensure that your home is as safe as possible. Thousands of children need medical help every day due to unintentional injuries that happen at home. You can also keep your child protected in the sun. Above all, equip him with the information and confidence he needs to keep himself safe, and make sure that he knows what he should do in an emergency.

PREVENTING ILLNESS

Beginning in early childhood, encourage good personal hygiene by teaching your child to wash his hands before eating and after going to the bathroom as a way to prevent infections from spreading. Good dental practices can also prevent cavities, which are caused by bacteria and plaque on the teeth. Starting in infancy, immunizations are recommended to prevent infections. They are particularly important in the early months, when

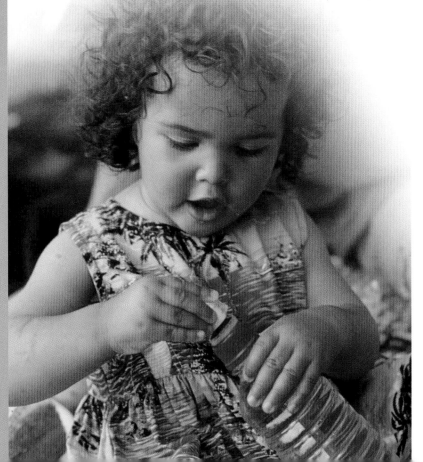

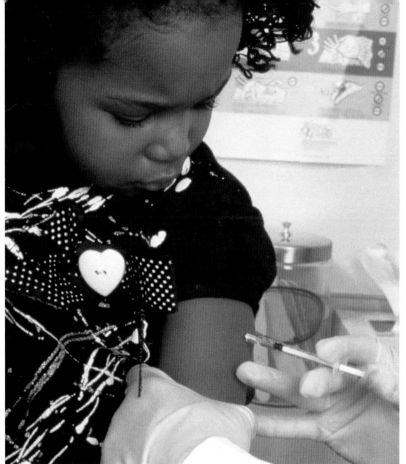

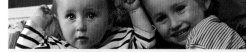

a baby's immune system is not fully developed and is most vulnerable.

Immunization

Immunizations help children build their own defenses against infections by forming antibodies (proteins that kill bacteria and viruses and protect against future infections). Prior to the development of immunizations (also called vaccines), many children died or were disabled by the effects of infectious diseases.

Making sure that your child is immunized appropriately will provide the best available defense against many dangerous childhood diseases. Recommended routine immunizations are usually given around birth and at 2, 4, 6, 12, 15, 18, and 24 months, and again before entering kindergarten, around 4 to 6 years. The immunizations will protect your child against hepatitis B, diphtheria, tetanus (lockjaw), pertussis (whooping cough), polio, HiB (*Haemophilus*

influenzae type B), measles, mumps, rubella (German measles), varicella (chickenpox), pneumococcus, and meningococcus. In some cases, children may also receive hepatitis A or influenza vaccines. Ongoing research continues to offer new and improved ways to protect children from serious diseases, so guidelines on immunization tend to change periodically. Consult your doctor about recommended vaccines.

Some of these vaccines may be combined, and many require more than one dose over a period of time. Studies and years of experience show that vaccines used for routine childhood immunizations can be safely given together. Side effects are no more common when multiple vaccines are given together than when each vaccine is given on separate occasions. Talk to your doctor if you are concerned about the number of vaccines your child is scheduled to receive.

Many of the infectious diseases discussed in this chapter do not occur or spread as much as they used to, thanks to better nutrition, less crowded living conditions, antibiotics, and, most importantly, vaccines. However, the bacteria and viruses that are responsible for these diseases still exist, so immunizations are still needed to protect children. Although immunizations have reduced most of these diseases to very low levels in Canada, some of these diseases are still common in other parts of the world. Travelers can bring these diseases into Canada. Although immunization rates here are higher than ever, some children are still not fully protected, so outbreaks can occur in areas of the country that are underimmunized. Immunizations help prevent these infections from spreading quickly.

Sometimes immunizations should be postponed or not given, such as if a child has an abnormal immune system, or currently has a high fever or serious illness. Minor illnesses such as colds and low-grade fevers should not prevent immunizations. Consult your doctor if you think your child may be too ill to receive his immunizations.

Occasionally, a child may have a minor reaction to immunizations. He may seem more irritable than usual or have a slight fever. There can be a local reaction, such as a small red lump around the injection site, which may swell to the size of a quarter. Report any larger swelling or area of redness, high fever, or other reactions to your doctor.

Immunizations and the diseases they prevent

All the recommended childhood vaccines have been scientifically proven to be safe, although there have been misperceptions about safety in the past. The Canadian Pediatric Society believes that immunizations are a safe and cost-effective way to prevent death, diseases, and disability, and advises parents to have their children immunized. The benefits of immunizations far outweigh the risks of these diseases, as well as any side effects of the vaccines. See below for information on specific diseases and vaccines.

DTaP (Diphtheria, tetanus, and pertussis)

Diphtheria causes sore throat, fever, and in some cases paralysis or heart failure. Before the immunization was developed, it was a major cause of death in children.

Tetanus (lockjaw) causes headaches and muscle spasms of the jaw, neck, arms, legs, and stomach. The bacteria that causes tetanus is found in dirt and is often spread through a puncture wound

or deep cut. Although it is a rare condition, this illness can be fatal.

Pertussis (whooping cough) causes severe coughing spells and affected infants may briefly stop breathing and often require hospitalization. It can also cause pneumonia, seizures, and brain damage. The "a" in DTaP stands for "acellular" and indicates that only part of the pertussis bacteria is used in the vaccine, which tends to have fewer side effects than the original DTP vaccine.

Hepatitis A

Hepatitis A affects the liver and causes fever, vomiting, and jaundice. It is spread through infected people or contaminated food or water. The vaccine is recommended for children in areas with high levels of hepatitis A and for people who are traveling to certain countries.

Hepatitis B

This virus also affects the liver and may cause jaundice, pain, vomiting, and diarrhea, or no symptoms at all. It is spread through contact with the blood, saliva, or other body fluids of an infected person. Hepatitis B is less common in children than in adults, but early immunization can provide lifelong protection.

HiB (Haemophilus influenzae type B)

This bacterium can cause meningitis (inflammation of the covering of the brain), pneumonia, and epiglottitis (inflammation and swelling in the throat). However, it has become very uncommon since the introduction of the HiB vaccine.

Influenza

The vaccine prevents the effects of certain strains of the influenza virus, including respiratory symptoms and

fever. It may be recommended for children with certain chronic diseases such as asthma, and may also be recommended for healthy children.

MMR (Measles, mumps, and rubella)

The measles virus causes fever, cold symptoms, and a rash, and in severe cases, pneumonia or encephalitis (an inflammation around the brain) leading to deafness, seizures, or mental retardation.

Mumps causes an inflammation of the glands under the jaw and of the pancreas and sometimes meningitis. Boys with mumps may develop swollen testes, which can lead to reduced fertility.

Rubella (German measles) causes fever and rash in children, but infected pregnant women can give birth to infants with birth defects.

The MMR vaccine is safe and effective. There has been concern that MMR may be associated with autism, but extensive scientific reports from the American Academy of Pediatrics, the Institute of Medicine, and the Centers for Disease Control and Prevention have concluded that there is no proven association between the vaccine and autism.

Pneumococcus

Pneumococcal bacteria can cause ear infections, pneumonia, bloodstream infections, and meningitis, and may cause death in the elderly or very young. Antibiotics may be effective treatment, but the bacteria is becoming resistant to them.

Polio

Polio is a virus that may cause mild cold symptoms but can also lead to paralysis or death. Polio has been eradicated in Canada, but is still common in a few areas of the world.

The inactivated polio vaccine (IPV) is used in Canada today.

Varicella (chickenpox)

Varicella is a virus that causes a rash of itchy blisters, fever, and sometimes skin infections, encephalitis (inflammation around the brain), and, rarely, death. Most people who receive the chickenpox vaccine will not get chickenpox. If someone who has been immunized does later get chickenpox, it is usually very mild.

Meningococcus

Meningococcal bacteria can cause meningitis and bloodstream infections. Although rare, the infection can be deadly, even with treatment.

CHILD SAFETY

Unintentional injuries can happen very quickly. Hundreds of children are taken to emergency rooms every day. Most have only minor injuries, but some are much more serious.

Many injuries can be prevented. Try to keep one step ahead of your child. Being aware of the risks your child faces at each age and stage of development will help you keep your home as safe as possible.

For children age 5 and under, unintentional injuries at home are the most common. Babies under the age of 1 are most often hurt through falls, even in their first months. A baby can wriggle off surfaces even before he learns to roll. Make sure your baby is never left unattended on any raised surface, even strapped into a car safety seat placed on a table. Install safety gates at the top and bottom of stairs before your baby learns to crawl and install catches that prevent windows from opening more than 10 cm (4 in).

It is also vital to keep your baby safe around water, even shallow

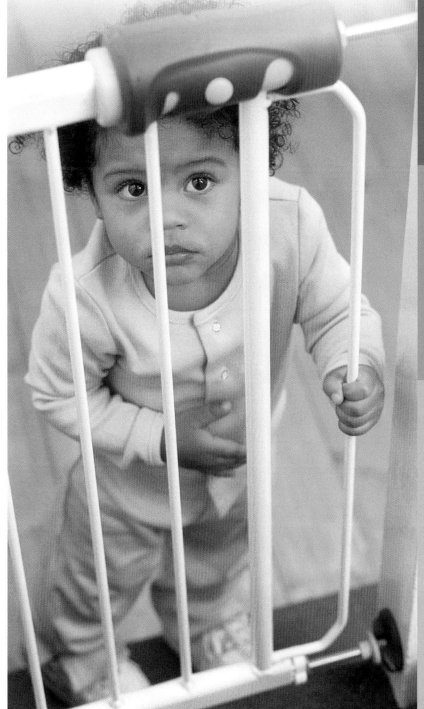

"Install safety gates at the top and bottom of stairs before your baby learns to crawl"

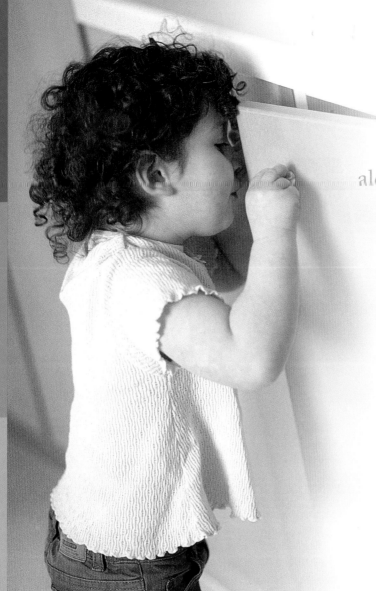

"Keep household cleaners, medicines, cosmetics, and alcohol in a locked cabinet."

child's reach. Use placemats rather than a tablecloth that your child could grab, and make sure she can't reach pot handles. Keep your hot water heater below 50°C (120°F).

Microwaved food and drinks can cause burns. Stir and test microwaved food before giving it to your child to even out any hot spots.

House fires are often caused by children playing with matches or lighters. Keep them out of sight and reach. Install smoke alarms and check them regularly, and always cover fireplaces with a guard.

Safety and older children
By the time your child starts school at about age 5, unintentional injuries outside the home are increasingly common. Make sure your child is always supervised when outside. Most children do not have the skills to handle traffic situations safely until at least 10 years of age. Also consider other factors in your decisions about independence and safety, such as location, traffic patterns, and your child's maturity and distractibility. Your child won't be ready to bicycle on the street yet, but you can let him bicycle in a safe place, such as a park. He should always wear a helmet.

For children ages 7–11, bicycling injuries become more common. Ensure your child takes responsibility for maintaining his bike and is aware of road safety. Find out about local bicycling proficiency courses. Ensure that your child always wears a helmet. It's also a good idea to wear reflective clothing.

water. Never leave a baby or small child alone in the bath, and make sure that children in wading pools are supervised at all times. Always fence or cover garden ponds if small children are playing in the yard.

Choking injuries are most common during your baby's first year. Babies love putting things in their mouths and can choke easily, even on liquids. Keep small objects out of reach and don't leave your baby alone with a bottle.

Young children, especially those between ages 1 and 3, are most commonly poisoned by household products such as cleaning supplies,

medications, and cosmetics. Keep household cleaners, especially those that look like candy, in their original containers, locked, and out of reach. Store medicines, alcohol, and cosmetics in a locked cabinet.

Preventing burns and scalds
Burns and scalds are also common. Each year thousands of children in Canada are injured by burns and scalds. If possible, keep your toddler out of the kitchen when you are cooking, and maybe even install a stair gate across the doorway.

Hot water is another hazard. Keep hot drinks and soups out of your

SAFETY IN THE SUN

Make sure your baby or child is fully protected in the sun. A baby's skin is much thinner than an adult's and is much more prone to sunburn. Damage may occur even before the skin turns red. Keep babies completely in the shade.

For toddlers and older children, applying sunscreen with a sun protection factor (SPF) of 30 or above with UVA and UVB protection is a must. You should apply it liberally 30 minutes before your child goes into the sun and again throughout the day, especially after swimming, even if it is waterproof. A hat with a wide brim or back flap is essential. Also, try to avoid being out in the middle of the day and early afternoon when the sun is strongest. Encourage your child to use sunglasses to protect his eyes, and give plenty of fluids to prevent dehydration.

Keep a close watch for symptoms of heat-related illness if your child is playing outside on a sunny day. These include headache, dizziness, and confusion; your child may also have hot, flushed, dry skin.

If you notice any of these symptoms in your child, get him to a cool place and take off his outer clothing, then seek immediate medical attention. If possible, cover him with a wet sheet. Alternatively, sponge his face and body with lukewarm water or fan him until he receives medical treatment.

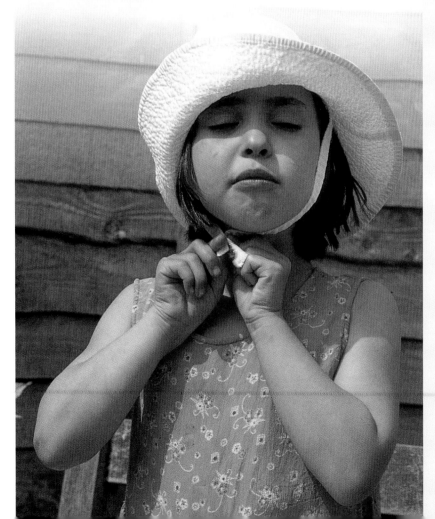

TEACHING YOUR CHILD ABOUT SAFETY

You can start talking to your child about safety very casually from the age of about 3 or 4 years.

Teach your child his full name and street address; some children may even be able to remember their telephone number. You should also discuss what your child might do if you became separated when you are out shopping. Suggest that your child stays where he is, and calls your name loudly a few times. If he can't see you, teach him that he should ask for help from a grown-up with children or a store worker who is behind the counter of the store.

Talk to your child about being safe at the playground. For example, make it a rule that your child should never walk in front of a swing or other moving play equipment, and encourage him to be extra careful on high equipment, such as jungle gyms. When you go swimming, talk to your child about pool safety, reminding him never to run in the pool area in case he slips, and never to dive into shallow water.

You could also raise his awareness about other safety issues, for example by pointing out the dangers of leaving toys on the stairs.

Explain what 911 is for and show your older child how to dial this number in an emergency.

Ask your child to tell you about any incident at all that makes him feel worried and to let you know if someone he doesn't know tries to talk to him or touch him.

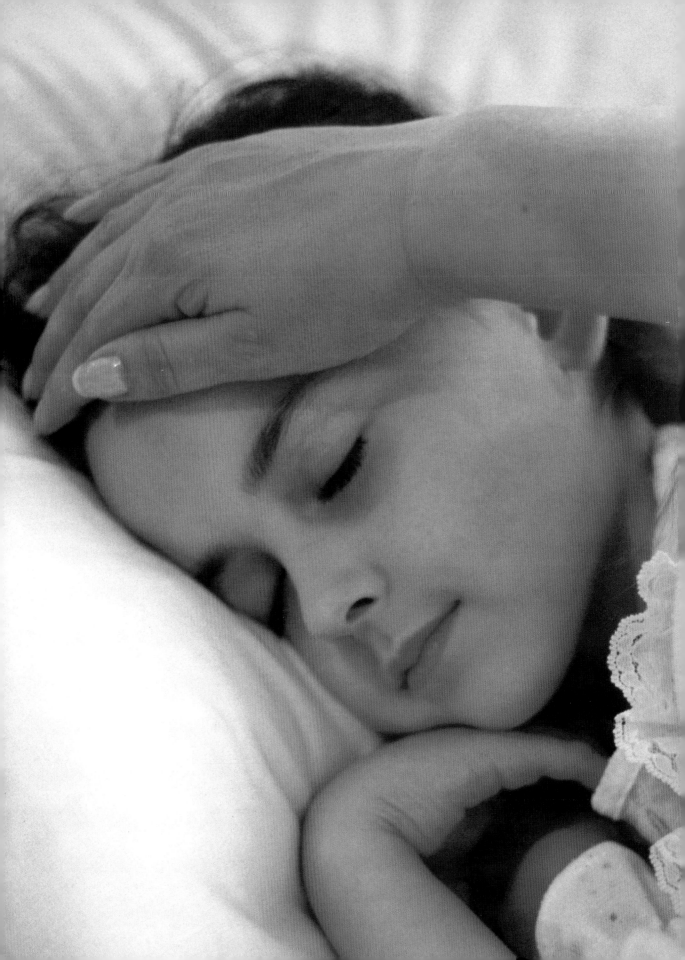

DIAGNOSIS CHARTS

CHAPTER THREE

One of the most worrying aspects of being a parent is when your child becomes ill, and it can be difficult to know if you can treat an illness at home or should seek medical help. The diagnosis charts in this chapter can help answer that question. Always consult your doctor if you are concerned about your child's health.

FEVER

A FEVER IS USUALLY A SIGN THAT THE BODY is fighting a bacterial or viral infection. Overheating may also be the cause. A temperature above 38°C (100.4°F) signifies a fever. Note other symptoms that may assist your doctor's diagnosis. See also RASH WITH FEVER (*p.186*) and FEVER IN BABIES (*p.58*).

SYMPTOM	POSSIBLE CAUSE
Does your child seem very sick and have a stiff neck, headache, abnormal drowsiness, or unusual irritability?	Meningitis (*p.294*).
Does your child have a cough, runny nose, and normal breathing?	A common cold (*p.221*) or influenza (*p.225*). Measles (*p.264*) is also a possibility.
Has your child been outside in the sun or in a hot room for several hours?	Your child may have become overheated.
Does your child have a sore throat or is he refusing solid food?	Tonsillitis (*see* Pharyngitis and tonsillitis, *p.223*).
Does your child have an earache or pull at either ear, or wake up screaming at night?	Inflammation of the middle ear (*p.240*).
Does your child have a cough, runny nose, and unusually noisy or rapid breathing?	Croup (*p.224*), asthma (*p.226*), bronchitis (*p.228*), or pneumonia (*p.227*).
Does your child vomit with or without diarrhea?	Gastroenteritis (*p.254*).
Does your child urinate more frequently than usual or have a painful or burning sensation when urinating?	Urinary tract infection (*p.275*).
Does your child have a swelling between the ear and the angle of the jaw on one or both sides?	Mumps (*p.268*).

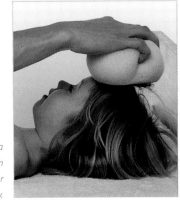

COOLING DOWN *Moisten a sponge with lukewarm water and place it on your child's forehead and body.*

ACTION NEEDED

Emergency! Seek immediate medical attention.

If she is no better in 48 hours, symptoms worsen, or other symptoms develop, consult your doctor.
Self-help Bringing down a temperature (*right*) and Relieving a cough (*p.197*).

If self-help measures don't lower the temperature (*right*), call your doctor immediately.

If he is no better after 24 hours, consult your doctor.
Self-help Bringing down a temperature (*right*) and Relieving a sore throat (*p.198*).

Get medical advice within 24 hours.
Self-help Bringing down a temperature (*right*) and Relieving an earache (*p.205*).

Call your doctor within 24 hours, or urgently if there are breathing problems.
Self-help Ease breathing in an asthma attack (*p.195*) and Bringing down a temperature (*right*).

See your doctor within 24 hours.
Self-help Giving extra fluids (*p.172*).

Get medical advice within 24 hours.
Self-help Bringing down a temperature (*right*).

See your doctor to confirm diagnosis.
Self-help Bringing down a temperature (*right*).

Bringing down a temperature

A rise in temperature is part of the body's normal reaction to infection. However, lowering the temperature will help your child feel better. A child whose temperature is allowed to rise may become very uncomfortable and may be at risk for a convulsion – called a febrile seizure. The following measures are simple things you can do to bring down and control your child's temperature:

- Monitor her temperature with a thermometer (*p.324*). Try a digital thermometer (*below*) or a tympanic thermometer, which measures the body's temperature through the ear canal.

- Consult your doctor regarding the appropriate dose of ibuprofen or acetaminophen. Ibuprofen use is approved for children 6 months or older, but it should not be given if your child is dehydrated or vomiting continuously. Do not use aspirin to treat your child's fever, as it may cause serious side effects.

- Remove excess clothing from her body – down to underwear or diaper if necessary.

- Remove any sheets or blankets if her illness confines her to bed.

- Keep the room ventilated and about 24°C (75°F).

- Make sure she drinks plenty of fluids – give small amounts regularly if she vomits easily.

- If her temperature reaches 40°C (104°F), sponge your child's skin and head with lukewarm water (*above left*). Alternatively, place her in a lukewarm bath.

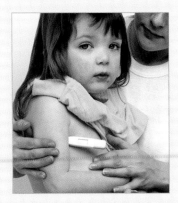

DIGITAL THERMOMETER
Place the digital thermometer in the child's armpit and gently hold the arm in place until you hear the "beep," usually about one minute. Remove the thermometer and simply read the digital display.

DIARRHEA

WHEN A CHILD PASSES FREQUENT runny stools, infection is usually the cause. Diarrhea usually lasts for 5–7 days at most. Make sure your child drinks plenty of fluid while it persists. If the diarrhea recurs or continues for more than a week, check with your doctor. See also DIARRHEA IN BABIES (*p.62*).

SYMPTOM	POSSIBLE CAUSE	ACTION NEEDED
If the diarrhea began within the last 3 days, is there abdominal pain, fever, or vomiting?	Gastroenteritis (*p.254*).	Call your doctor. **Self-help** Giving extra fluids (*below*).
Did the diarrhea start just before an exciting or stressful event or period of time?	A response to excitement or emotional stress. The diarrhea is likely to clear up quickly.	If the diarrhea persists or is distressing to your child, consult your doctor.
Has your child had constipation and diarrhea at the same time?	Overflow soiling as a result of chronic constipation (*p.255*).	Consult your doctor.
Have you been giving your child any medicine?	A side effect of the medicine she is taking.	Ask your doctor if the medicine may be the cause and if you should stop giving it.
Do your child's stools contain recognizable morsels of food?	Toddler diarrhea (*p.255*) if she is under 3.	Consult your doctor.
Are your child's stools uniformly runny?	Probably a reaction to food (*p.252*) or giardiasis (*p.262*).	Consult your doctor. **Self-help** Giving extra fluids (*below*).

DANGER SIGNS

Call your doctor immediately if your child has any of the following symptoms:

- Abdominal pain for a few hours
- Vomiting for several hours
- Refusing to drink for 6 hours
- Sunken eyes or abnormal drowsiness
- Passing no urine for over 6 hours in a day.

SELF-HELP

Giving extra fluids

The best way to give fluids is an oral rehydrating solution. These are widely available at pharmacies or ask your doctor for suggestions. Offer fluids every 2–3 hours while the diarrhea lasts. If your child is vomiting, give small sips every few minutes.

LOSS OF APPETITE

A CHILD MAY LOSE OR GAIN HIS APPETITE depending on how much energy he needs and whether he is in a period of growth. Provided he shows no other symptoms and his growth is normal for his age, you should not worry about any mild loss of appetite. For children under 1 year, see p.61.

SYMPTOM	POSSIBLE CAUSE	ACTION NEEDED
If your child lost his appetite less than a week ago, does he have a fever, sore throat, or rash?	Go to FEVER (*p.170*), SORE THROAT (*p.198*), or SPOTS AND RASHES (*p.184*).	Consult your doctor.
Did your child lose his appetite less than a week ago but has no other symptoms?	Snacking between meals or exercising less than usual. As long as your child seems well, there is no cause for concern.	If he feels ill, get medical advice within 24 hours. **Self-help** Healthy eating and Stimulating appetite (*below*).
Is your child failing to gain weight normally?	Poor growth or nutrition.	See your doctor.
Does your child have swollen glands in the neck?	Infectious mononucleosis (*p.270*).	See your doctor.
Does your child have pale stools and dark urine?	Viral hepatitis (*p.261*).	See your doctor.
Does your child urinate (or wet the bed) more frequently?	Urinary tract infection (*p.275*).	See your doctor within 24 hours.

SELF-HELP

Stimulating appetite

A child who is reluctant to eat or who has lost his appetite may need encouraging. Try the following tips:

- If the loss of appetite is caused by illness, do not force your child to eat. A sick child may only want liquids; ice cream and yogurt can soothe a painful throat and provide some nutrients.

- If your child is very young, make eating fun by preparing pizza faces or playing an eating game.

- Do not expect your child to eat as much as you do at mealtimes; five or six smaller meals or snacks each day may suit a child's immature digestive system and active metabolism.

- Tempt a picky eater with small portions of various foods.

VOMITING

VOMITING THAT RECURS IS OFTEN DUE TO AN INFECTION of the digestive tract, although an infection elsewhere in the body may also be responsible. A single episode of vomiting is not likely to be serious, however – it's probably due to overeating or excitement. See also VOMITING IN BABIES (*p.60*).

SYMPTOM	POSSIBLE CAUSE
Does your child have diarrhea?	Gastroenteritis (*p.254*).
Has your child had continuous abdominal pain for several hours?	Appendicitis (*p.253*).
Is your child's vomit greenish yellow?	Intestinal obstruction (*p.256*).
Does your child have two or more of the following: fever, pain on urinating, abdominal pain, or bed-wetting?	Urinary tract infection (*p.275*).
Does your child have pale stools and dark urine?	Hepatitis (*p.261*).
Is your child abnormally drowsy after recently suffering a blow to the head?	Head injury (*p.291*).
Is your child abnormally drowsy with a headache, stiff neck, or flat red or purple skin lesions that do not disappear when pressed?	Meningitis (*p.294*).
Did your child vomit after a bout of coughing?	A common cold (*p.221*) or pertussis (*p.269*).
Did your child vomit before or after an exciting or stressful event?	Children may vomit in reaction to an exciting event or to stress.
Did your child vomit during a trip or any type of motion activity?	Motion sickness.

Call your doctor immediately if your child has any of the following symptoms:

- Vomiting for several hours
- Abnormal drowsiness
- Refusing to drink for more than 6 hours
- Sunken eyes or dry tongue
- Not urinating for over 6 hours in a day.

Seek medical attention immediately if your child has any of the following symptoms:

- Greenish yellow vomit
- Abdominal pain for several hours
- Flat, red or purple spots on the skin that do not disappear when pressed.

ACTION NEEDED

Get medical advice within 24 hours.
Self-help Giving extra fluids (*p.172*).

Emergency! Seek immediate medical care. Do not give your child anything to eat or drink.

Emergency! Seek immediate medical care. While you wait, do not give your child anything to eat or drink.

See your doctor within 24 hours.
Self-help Bringing down a temperature (*p.170*).

Get medical advice within 24 hours.

Emergency! Seek immediate medical care. Do not give your child anything to eat or drink.

Emergency! Seek immediate medical care.

Consult your doctor within 24 hours.
Self-help Dealing with vomiting (*right*) and Relieving a cough (*p.197*).

If the vomiting persists, consult your doctor.

Stop the activity that is causing the problem. Consult your doctor about motion sickness remedies.

SELF-HELP

Dealing with vomiting

Try taking the following steps to bring relief to a child who is vomiting:

- Support the child's head while she is vomiting. Once she has stopped, sponge her forehead and face. Give her a sip of water so she can rinse out her mouth.

- Give your child plenty of reassurance because the experience may upset or frighten her.

- Encourage your child to drink small amounts of rehydrating solution (about 1 teaspoon every few minutes). This drink will help her replace the fluids which she has lost during vomiting (*see* Giving extra fluids, *p.172*).

- Let her lie down and rest for a while. Place a bowl beside her bed in case the vomiting recurs.

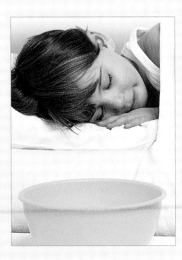

SICK BOWL *Place a bowl beside your child's bed so she doesn't have to worry about getting to the toilet.*

HEADACHE

A NY ACUTE INFECTION THAT TRIGGERS a fever may also cause a headache. Headaches may occur on their own or with various other illnesses and symptoms. Consult your doctor if a headache is persistent, recurrent, or severe, or if your child is having an unusual type of headache for the first time.

SYMPTOM	POSSIBLE CAUSE
Does your child occasionally suffer from headaches?	An occasional headache is rarely cause for concern.
Does your child get headaches after reading or after using a computer or watching television?	Eyesight problems (*see* Refractive errors, *p.245*) can sometimes cause headaches.
If your child seems generally well, might he be anxious about something?	Tension headaches (*see* Recurrent headaches, *p.291*) may be caused by anxiety.
If your child frequently suffers from headaches, does he get them every day?	Tension headaches, migraines, or other disorders (*see* Recurrent headaches, *p.291*).
Are the headaches accompanied or preceded by abdominal pain, nausea or vomiting, flashing lights, or other visual disturbances?	Migraine (*see* Recurrent headaches, *p.291*).
Has your child recently had a cold?	Sinusitis (*p.221*).
Does your child have a fever, vomiting, or other signs of illness?	Go to FEVER (*p.170*) or VOMITING (*p.174*).
Has your child recently had an injury to the head?	Concussion (*see* Head injury, *p.291*).
Does your child feel extremely sick, with two or more of these symptoms – drowsiness, stiff neck, fever, vomiting, refusal to drink, and flat red spots on the skin that do not fade under pressure?	Meningitis (*p.294*).

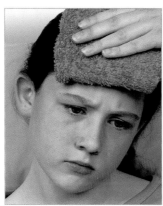

COLD COMPRESS *Fold a washcloth or a small towel and dip it in cold water. Wring it out and place it on your child's forehead or the back of his neck. Hold the compress there for two or three minutes and then repeat several times.*

ACTION NEEDED

Self-help Relieving a headache (*right*).

Consult your doctor or ophthalmologist.

If such headaches occur regularly and cause distress, consult your doctor.
Self-help Relieving a headache (*right*).

Consult your doctor.

For a first attack, a severe or prolonged headache, or for frequent attacks, consult your doctor.

Consult your doctor.

Urgent! Call your doctor immediately or seek medical attention.

Emergency! Seek immediate medical attention.

Relieving a headache

You can treat most of your child's headaches simply and effectively at home. However, some types of headaches are serious enough for you to consult your doctor immediately. These include headaches that last for more than about four hours; headaches that occur when your child seems very sick; headaches that accompany the development of other symptoms; or headaches that worry you. The following self-help measures might help relieve the pain of headaches:

- Give your child acetaminophen or ibuprofen in the recommended dose.

- Encourage your child to lie down in a cool, dark, peaceful room with his eyes closed. Falling asleep may relieve the headache.

- Hunger can sometimes cause a headache. If your child feels hungry, give him a drink of milk or an easily digestible snack, such as a plain cracker.

- Dehydration is a common cause of headache. Ask your child if he is thirsty or offer him a drink of water. Children who are in pain can vomit easily, so encourage him to sip the drink.

- A high-fiber snack – for example, a banana or whole-wheat bread or cereal – will raise the level of sugar in the bloodstream slowly. Encourage your child to eat one at the first signs of a headache. If your child suffers from headaches at school he could carry a "snack pack" with him.

- Teach him to breathe properly and to concentrate on relaxing the muscles in his shoulders and neck. If you suspect the headache is related to tension, consider giving him a relaxing massage. Gently massaging the muscles in his scalp, face, neck, and shoulders may be helpful.

- If you suspect a food intolerance is causing your child to have headaches, keep a journal of what food he eats and consult your doctor. If you think your child is sensitive to a particular food, remove it from his diet. Foods that can cause headaches in some people include sugary and carbohydrate-rich foods such as white bread, dried fruits, chocolate, peanut butter, hard cheeses, and certain food additives.

TOOTHACHE

I F YOUR CHILD IS SUFFERING FROM A TOOTHACHE, it is possible that one of her teeth is decaying. Take her to see the dentist as soon as you can if pain is affecting her teeth or gums, although you could try self-help measures in the meantime. While natural toothache remedies may help ease your child's discomfort, a toothache may be a sign of a problem that needs the attention of a dentist.

SYMPTOM	POSSIBLE CAUSE
Does your child have painful, red, swollen gums while new teeth are erupting?	Teething (*p.56*).
Does your child have bouts of severe throbbing pain or sharp pain lasting minutes and triggered by hot or cold food or drinks?	Your child may have a deep caries (*see* Tooth decay, *p.248*), a deep filling, or a tooth fracture which may have caused inflammation of the nerve tissue.
Does your child have continuous, dull pain in several back teeth?	The molars may be starting to emerge (or wisdom teeth in teenagers).
Does your child have continuous intense pain with or without fever?	Your child may be suffering from a dental abscess (*p.250*).
Does your child have tenderness around the upper teeth or jaw?	Your child may have sinusitis (*p.221*). This is an inflammation of the lining of the sinuses (air-filled cavities in the bones that surround the nose), which can cause pain in the upper back teeth.
If your child has had a filling recently, is she experiencing intermittent, unpredictable pain?	Your child may have a filling that is uneven or higher than the level of the tooth's biting surface which may cause pain when she bites down on it.
If your child has had a filling placed recently, does she experience pain only when she is biting or chewing on it?	A tooth that has been filled very recently is often slightly sensitive, particularly to cold temperatures. Sensitivity is especially likely if the child has had a deep filling.

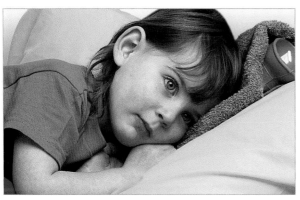

EASING TOOTHACHE *A warm or cold compress held against the affected side of her face may ease her toothache.*

ACTION NEEDED

Give your baby a hard object, such as a teething ring, to chew on. Over-the-counter remedies may also relieve the pain.
Self-help Relieving toothache (*right*).

Get dental help within 24 hours. Try the self-help suggestions while you wait (*right*).

Consult your dentist.

Urgent! Call your dentist immediately. Meanwhile, try the self-help suggestions (*right*).

Consult your doctor.

Consult your dentist. Until the child can see the dentist, give soft foods and liquids and ask her to chew on the other side of her mouth.

If sensitivity to heat develops, or if the pain intensifies or lasts for more than a few seconds, make an appointment with the dentist.

Preventing tooth decay

The following measures may help prevent tooth decay, which is a common cause of a toothache:

- Encourage your child to brush her teeth twice daily and floss at bedtime.

- Limit your child's intake of sticky, sweet foods and sugary beverages.

- Make sure your child gets enough fluoride. Children may begin to use a small amount of fluoridated toothpaste around age 2 or 3 years. Check whether your local water supply contains fluoride, and contact your dentist or doctor to see if your child needs a supplement.

Relieving toothache

The following measures may help relieve the pain of your child's toothache:

- Consult your doctor about an appropriate dose of ibuprofen or acetaminophen. Do not apply any of this medication directly to the tooth because a chemical burn may develop after prolonged contact.

- A young child may feel better if she is propped up against several pillows.

- A warm or cold compress, held against the affected side of the face, may help relieve the pain of a toothache.

- Encourage your child to rinse her mouth with warm salt water.

- Consult your doctor about over-the-counter numbing gels or other remedies. Numbing liquids should not be used in small infants, as they may affect their ability to swallow.

- Gently massage your teething infant's gums.

- A firm rubber teething ring may help. Avoid gel-filled rings, which sometimes burst.

- Never give your child an alcoholic beverage to ease a toothache.

FEELING SICK

I F YOUR CHILD FEELS SICK, take his temperature and look for symptoms such as a rash. Call your doctor immediately if your child is unresponsive or drowsy, has a temperature of 38°C (100.4°F) or more, has been vomiting for several hours, is breathing fast or noisily, or refuses to drink for 6 hours.

SYMPTOM	POSSIBLE CAUSE	ACTION NEEDED
Does your child have a fever – a temperature of 100.4°F (38°C) or above – and a rash?	Go to RASH WITH FEVER (p.186).	
Does your child have a fever without a rash?	If he is under a year, go to FEVER IN BABIES (p.58). If not, go to FEVER (p.170).	
Does your child have a rash?	Go to SPOTS AND RASHES (p.184)	
Does your child have a pain in his abdomen?	Go to ABDOMINAL PAIN (p.208)	
Does your child have diarrhea and vomiting?	Gastroenteritis (p.254).	Get medical advice within 24 hours. **Self-help** Preventing dehydration in babies (p.63) or Giving extra fluids (p.172).
Is your child refusing to eat and drink?	An infectious childhood disease, particularly if the child is listless or irritable, or is suffering from other symptoms.	If your child feels no better after 24 hours or develops other symptoms, consult your doctor.
Is your child refusing to eat?	Go to SORE THROAT (p.198).	
Has your child had contact with anyone with an infectious disease in the past 3 weeks?	An infectious childhood disease, as it incubates, might be the cause.	If your child feels no better after 24 hours, or develops other symptoms, consult your doctor.
Might your child be worried or anxious about something?	Problems at school can make a child feel sick (see Anxiety and fears, pp.131–132).	If the feeling lasts more than a day or if your child regularly refuses to go to school, consult your doctor.

ITCHING

ITCHING MAY BE DUE TO VARIOUS CAUSES, ranging from allergies to infestation by parasites, and may affect all of your child's body or just one part. Severe itching can be distressing and scratching can lead to infection, so consult your doctor about the underlying condition without delay.

SYMPTOM	POSSIBLE CAUSE	ACTION NEEDED
Does your child have a rash of itchy spots or patches of inflamed skin?	Go to SPOTS AND RASHES (p.184) or RASH WITH FEVER (p.186).	
Is the itching between the toes, or on the soles of her feet?	Athlete's foot (see FOOT PROBLEMS, p.192).	If the rash does not clear up within 2 weeks or if it affects your child's toenails, consult your doctor. **Self-help** Apply an antifungal powder, cream, or spray to every part of the rash.
Is the itching in the anal area?	Pinworms (p.262).	Consult your doctor.
Is the itching on the scalp?	Go to HAIR AND SCALP PROBLEMS (p.182).	
Is the itching in your daughter's genital area?	Go to GENITAL PROBLEMS IN GIRLS (p.215).	
If a large area of the body is itchy, has your child been wearing either wool or some kind of synthetic material next to the skin?	Sensitive skin or eczema (p.234).	Use a laundry soap made for people with delicate or sensitive skin. Ensure cotton is worn next to the skin.
Are there thin, gray lines on your child's fingerwebs, wrists, palms, or soles?	Scabies (p.232).	Consult your doctor.

HAIR & SCALP PROBLEMS

Hair and scalp problems in children are fairly common but are unlikely to be a cause for concern. Any problem with a child's scalp is likely to be due to an infection, a skin condition, or a parasite. Actual hair loss may be caused by constant pulling on the hair or tying the hair back tightly.

SYMPTOM	POSSIBLE CAUSE
Is your child's hair becoming thin, even though he is under 1 year old?	As the baby hair falls out, your infant's hair will become noticeably thinner until the new, stronger hair grows in. This process is normal and is not a cause for concern.
Is your child's hair becoming thin after a recent illness?	General thinning of the hair could be a result of a recent illness. The hair will probably return to its normal thickness over the next few months.
Is your child suffering from temporary hair loss?	Damage to the hair roots, caused by excessive pulling of the hair or wearing hair in a tight pony tail or braids.
Does your child habitually pull or twist his hair?	Habitual hair pulling may indicate an underlying psychological problem.
Is your child's hair becoming thin at the same time he is taking medicine?	The thinning of your child's hair could be a side effect of the medicine that he is taking.
Does your child have either a flaky scalp or an itchy scalp that gets better for a few days after a thorough shampoo?	Dandruff (*see* Seborrheic dermatitis, *p.230*).
Does your child have visible lice or an itchy scalp that doesn't improve after a thorough shampoo?	Head lice (*right and p.236*).
Does your child have bald patches where the exposed skin looks scaly and inflamed?	Ringworm (*p.236*).
Does your child have bald patches where the exposed skin looks normal?	A form of localized baldness, which often may have no apparent cause.

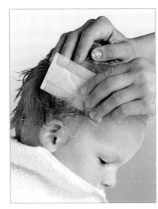

REMOVING HEAD LICE *Special shampoos and treatments for eradicating head lice are available over the counter or by prescription. Rinse hair over a sink rather than in the bath or shower to limit exposure to the treatment – the treatment may need to be repeated in 7 to 10 days. Some are more effective than others.*

ACTION NEEDED

Self-help Cover your baby's head to protect it from the sun and to keep it warm in cold weather.

If you are worried, consult your doctor.

Encourage your child to change her hairstyle or have a haircut.

If your child is losing a lot of hair or if he has other behavioral problems, consult your doctor.

Ask your doctor or pharmacist if the medicine may be causing your child's symptoms and whether you should stop giving it.

Self-help Wash your child's hair with an antidandruff shampoo. If the symptoms do not improve within 2 weeks, consult your doctor.

Self-help Wash your child's hair with an over-the-counter antilice shampoo. If your child is under 2 years old or has an allergy, consult your doctor before starting any treatment.

Consult your doctor.

Consult your doctor.

Treating dandruff and head lice

Dandruff
As an alternative to antidandruff shampoos, massage a small amount of olive oil into the scalp. Shampoo normally and brush the scales away.

Head lice
If your child has head lice, use an over-the-counter treatment or contact your doctor for recommended therapy. Lice treatments are usually applied to dry hair and left on for 10 minutes before being rinsed out. Your child may attend school the next day but should be retreated in 7 to 10 days if live lice are noticed again. Manual removal of nits (louse eggs) is not necessary after treatment, since the nits will not contain live lice. Because a child with lice has likely had the infection for a month or more by the time it is discovered and poses little risk to others, he or she should remain in school, but be discouraged from direct head contact with others.

Hair care

Try the following tips to improve the health of your child's hair naturally:

- Encourage your child to eat a healthy diet, including at least five portions of fruit and vegetables a day and oily fish twice a week. Any nutritional deficiency can exacerbate hair and scalp problems, so ask your doctor whether your child would benefit from a multivitamin and multimineral supplement.

- Encourage your child to wear a hat when he is outside in the sun.

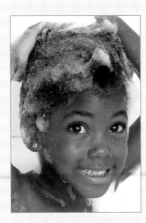

SHAMPOO *Wash your child's hair regularly with a mild shampoo, gently towel dry, and apply a conditioner. Avoid harsh chemicals such as the chlorine used in swimming pools and, if using a hairdryer, set it on medium or low heat to limit damage.*

SPOTS & RASHES

INFECTIONS AND ALLERGIC REACTIONS ARE RESPONSIBLE for most spots and rashes. If your child shows no other signs of being sick, the spots or rashes are probably not serious. But if her skin is very itchy or sore, or if she is showing signs of distress, call your doctor.

SYMPTOM	POSSIBLE CAUSE
Does the rash consist of slightly raised, bright red, blotchy patches?	Urticaria (*p.233*).
Urticaria (*see above*), and a swollen face or mouth or difficulty breathing or swallowing?	Anaphylactic shock (*p.189*).
Are you giving your child any medicine?	An allergic reaction to certain medicines.
If there's no itching, are there groups of small bumps, each with a central dimple?	Molluscum contagiosum (*p.235*), a mild viral infection that causes bumps on the skin.
Are there pus-filled areas or golden crusts, often on the face?	Impetigo (*p.235*).
Are there one or more firm, rough bumps?	Warts (*p.231*).
Is there a painful, red lump, possibly with a yellow top?	A boil (*right and p.233*).
Are there tiny, red, itchy spots or fluid-filled blisters?	Prickly heat, caused by unevaporated sweat.
Is the rash itchy, red, or scaly in patches mainly on the face and around the joints?	Eczema (atopic dermatitis) (*p.234*).
Are there round patches on the scalp, trunk, or limbs?	Ringworm (*p.236*).
Is the rash made up of small inflamed spots in one or more exposed areas?	Insect bites, possibly from mosquitoes or from cat or dog fleas.
Is there itching on skin that does not have the rash?	Scabies (*p.232*).
Are there small, oval, pink spots arranged in lines along the ribs or back?	Pityriasis rosea (*p.237*).

ACTION NEEDED

If the rash doesn't disappear in a few hours, or if your child has repeated attacks, consult your doctor.

Emergency! Seek medical attention immediately.

Urgent! Ask your doctor if the medicine could be the cause and if you should stop giving it.

Consult your doctor to confirm the diagnosis.

Get medical advice within 24 hours.

If troublesome, consult your doctor.

If painful, or if more form, consult your doctor.
Self-help Treating a boil (*right*).

Apply cool compresses.

If your child's rash is very itchy, extensive, or oozing, consult your doctor.

Consult your doctor.

Apply cool compresses to relieve the itching.

Consult your doctor.

Consult your doctor.
Self-help Relieving itching (*p.66*).

Treating a boil

A boil develops when a hair follicle becomes infected. After two or three days it will form a white or yellow head and will then either burst or heal on its own. Don't squeeze the boil and don't let your child scratch it. Boils often occur on the face or at pressure points where something rubs against the child's skin.

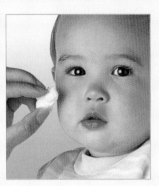

TACKLING A BOIL Wipe the boil with a cotton ball dipped in a salt solution (made from a teaspoon of salt in a cup of warm water) or an antiseptic solution such as rubbing alcohol. Cover with an adhesive bandage. Warm compresses may also help.

Lip licker's eczema

Too much licking of the lips or sucking of a thumb can cause a rash around the mouth. The saliva is irritating, making the lips turn dry and chapped while the skin around them becomes inflamed and scaly. Over-the-counter corticosteroid cream can help contain it, but the best way to deal with lip licker's eczema is to moisturize your child's lips with a lip balm and protect the skin with petroleum jelly.

As soon as the habit stops, the eczema heals. Don't make a big issue out of the habit because children usually grow out of it before too long. Just try to discourage it as soon as your child starts.

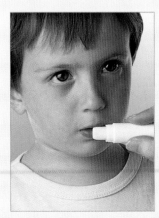

*MOISTURIZING THE LIPS
You may not be able to stop a child from excessively sucking his thumb or licking his lips, but you can cover his lips with a moisturizer in a lip balm. This will help reduce the irritating effects of the saliva.*

RASH WITH FEVER

A N INFECTIOUS DISEASE IS THE USUAL CAUSE of a rash combined with a fever (a temperature of 38°C (100.4°F) or over). Viruses are the culprits behind many of these infectious diseases and the body generally deals with them without the need for special medical treatment. Since some conditions may be very serious, always consult your doctor if your child has a rash with a fever.

SYMPTOM	POSSIBLE CAUSE
Did the rash appear after your child took some medicine?	Drug allergy.
Is your child's rash made up of flat red/purple spots that do not disappear when pressed?	Infection with meningococcus, a bacterium that causes meningitis (p.294) or another condition.
Is your child's rash bright red and confined to the cheeks, followed by a lacy red rash on the body?	Erythema infectiosum (p.266).
If your child's rash is raised and blotchy, or made up of fine spots that turn white when pressed, was it preceded by a runny nose, a cough, or red eyes?	Measles (p.264) or other viruses or conditions.
Is there a fine sandpaper-like pink rash that followed a sore throat?	Scarlet fever (p.267).
Is your child's rash made up of itchy bumps that blister and dry into scabs?	Chickenpox (p.265).
If the rash is made up of flat pink spots that start on the face or trunk, was your child's temperature 38°C (100.4°F) or above in the 3 or 4 days prior to the rash?	Roseola infantum (p.267).
Was your child's temperature 38°C (100.4°F) or a little below in the 3 or 4 days prior to the rash?	Rubella (p.264).

Call your doctor immediately if your child has any of the following symptoms during, or after apparent recovery from, any of the common childhood infectious diseases:

- Abnormal drowsiness or floppiness
- Seizures
- Temperature of 40°C (104°F) or above
- Abnormally fast breathing
- Noisy or difficult breathing
- Severe headache
- Refusing to drink for over 6 hours.

ACTION NEEDED

Urgent! Call your doctor immediately to find out whether the medicine may be causing the symptoms and whether you should stop giving it.

Emergency! Seek immediate medical attention.

If you are concerned, or if your child has sickle-cell anemia (*p.313*), consult your doctor. Avoid contact with pregnant women.

Get medical advice within 24 hours.
Self-help Bringing down a temperature (*p.59 and p.171*).

Get medical advice within 24 hours.
Self-help Bringing down a temperature (*p.59 and p.171*) and Relieving a sore throat (*p.198*).

Call your doctor.
Self-help Bringing down a temperature (*p.59 and p.171*).

Call your doctor.
Self-help Bringing down a temperature (*p.59 and p.171*).

Consult your doctor. Avoid contact with pregnant women.
Self-help Bringing down a temperature (*p.59 and p.171*).

Rashes of some common childhood diseases

The six photographs below can help you identify the rashes associated with some common infectious diseases in childhood (*see also* Infectious Diseases, *pp.263–272*). It is important to remember, however, that a rash may differ in its appearance depending on how severely a child is affected by the disease and on the complexion or color of the child's skin. Consequently, a firm diagnosis of a rash should always be made by a doctor. If you think your child's rash resembles the meningitis rash, seek medical care immediately.

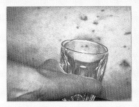

MENINGITIS
The spotty meningitis rash does not fade when pressed with a glass or your finger.

SCARLET FEVER
The tiny red spots of scarlet fever spread from behind the ears all over the body and last for about a week.

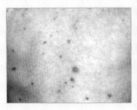

CHICKENPOX
Chickenpox spots appear after two or three weeks' incubation and contain fluid.

RUBELLA
The pink rubella spots start to appear behind the ears and spread to the forehead, chest and limbs.

MEASLES
The scattered pink spots of measles start at the hairline and spread down the body to the legs.

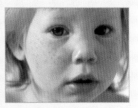

ROSEOLA INFANTUM
The tiny, distinct, pink spots of the roseola infantum rash usually develop on the head and the trunk of the body.

LUMPS & SWELLINGS

A LUMP OR SWELLING THAT APPEARS on, or just below, the surface of a child's skin may be due to a variety of causes. Lymph glands may swell in the fight against an infection in a nearby part of the body. Injuries, bites, and stings are other causes. If your child has a persistent or painful lump or swelling, consult your doctor.

SYMPTOM	POSSIBLE CAUSE
Does your child have a warm or painful red lump?	A boil (*p.185 and p.233*) or abscess.
Does your child have a slightly raised, bright red welt?	Your child may have been stung by an insect such as a bee or wasp.
Is the lump or swelling on the back of your child's neck?	A scalp infection (*p.236*) or a viral infection, such as a cold, causing lymph node enlargement.
Is the lump or swelling on the side of your child's neck, and accompanied by earache?	Inflammation of the middle ear (*p.240*), causing lymph node enlargement.
Is the lump or swelling on the side of your child's neck, and accompanied by a sore throat and a reluctance to eat and drink?	Pharyngitis or tonsillitis (*p.223*), causing lymph node enlargement.
Does your child have a tender swelling near an infected cut or abrasion?	The swelling is probably a nearby lymph gland, which has swollen as it helps to fight the infection.
Is the lump or swelling in the neck, armpit, and/or groin?	Infectious mononucleosis (*p.270*) or other condition, causing lymph node enlargement.
Is the lump or swelling between the ear and jaw?	Mumps (*p.268*).
Does your child have a large tender lump on the head after a blow to the head?	Swelling of skin or scalp (hematoma) or head injury (*p.291*).
Is your child's joint swollen?	Strain or sprain (*p.281*).
Is the swelling in your son's scrotum or penis?	Go to GENITAL PROBLEMS IN BOYS (*p.214*).
Is there a soft lump in the groin or navel area?	Inguinal or umbilical hernia (*see* Hernia, *p.260*).

Removing a stinger

Stings from a bee, wasp, or other insect are usually more painful than dangerous. The body's natural response to a sting is a mild swelling that is red and sore. If you can see the stinger, brush or scrape it off sideways with a credit card or your fingernail. Apply a cold compress to the affected area for at least 10 minutes to reduce the swelling and pain.

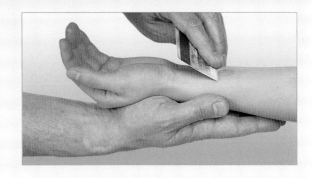

If a lump is very painful or if more than one lump forms, consult your doctor.

If your child has had an allergic reaction to a sting in the past, or shows symptoms of anaphylactic shock (right), seek medical care immediately.

Consult your doctor.

Get medical advice within 24 hours.
Self-help Relieving earache (p.205).

If your child feels no better after 24 hours, consult your doctor.
Self-help Relieving a sore throat (p.198).

If your child's swelling or pain persists for more than a week, consult your doctor.

Consult your doctor.

Consult your doctor.

Call your doctor. Seek medical care immediately if headache, vomiting, and drowsiness develop.

If pain is severe or there is no improvement after 24 hours, consult your doctor.

Get medical advice within 24 hours.

Anaphylactic shock

Sometimes, the sting of an insect – or a marine creature such as a jellyfish – produces a severe allergic reaction. The face and neck suddenly swell, the airways constrict, and breathing becomes very difficult. The body goes into anaphylactic shock, which requires urgent treatment. It can also occur after a child eats something, such as a peanut, to which she is especially sensitive. If your child goes into anaphylactic shock, take the following action:

• Dial 911 or call EMS immediately!

• Support your child in a way that makes it easiest for him to breathe. Reassure him while you wait for help.

• If he loses consciousness, check his condition. If he's breathing place him in the recovery position. If not, give him rescue breaths (see ABC, pp.326–328).

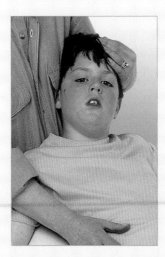

HELP WITH BREATHING *The most important help you can give in anaphylactic shock is to ensure that the child keeps breathing. Loosen the child's clothing at the neck and the waist to make breathing easier. Support the child in a semi-sitting position and provide reassurance.*

PAINFUL LIMBS

MINOR FALLS OR INJURIES CAUSE MANY CHILDREN to experience pain in an arm or a leg but such pain rarely requires medical attention. A child needs urgent treatment if he fractures a bone or dislocates a joint. If you are worried about an unexplained or persistent pain, consult your doctor.

SYMPTOM	POSSIBLE CAUSE	ACTION NEEDED
If your child fell or was injured recently, is movement painful or restricted, or does one of his limbs seem misshapen?	A broken bone or a dislocated joint (*see* Fractures and dislocations, *p.283*).	**Self-help** Broken bones (*p.334*).
Does your child have a fever, with a red or tender area over a bone?	Bone infection (*see* Bone and joint infection, *p.288*).	**Urgent!** Call your doctor immediately.
Is the pain centered around one or more joints or is it confined to the feet?	Go to PAINFUL JOINTS (*p.191*) or FOOT PROBLEMS (*p.192*).	
Is your child's limb swollen?	Bruised or strained muscles or sprained ligaments (*see* Strains and sprains, *p.281*).	If there's no improvement within 24 hours, consult your doctor. **Self-help** Treat the strain or sprain (*p.335*).
Has your child been experiencing bouts of pain in the lower leg that persist for a few minutes?	Cramp (*p.282*).	**Self-help** Gently massage or stretch the affected leg.
Does your child have a fever, with a headache, cough, or sore throat?	Influenza (*p.225*), which may cause body aches.	If there's no improvement within 48 hours, if breathing difficulties develop, or a rash appears, call your doctor immediately. **Self-help** Bringing down a temperature (*p.59 and p.171*).
Is your child experiencing none of the above symptoms yet still has a painful limb?	Bruised or strained muscles or sprained ligaments, possibly caused by an unnoticed injury (*see* Strains and sprains, *p.281*).	If your child is in severe pain, is reluctant to use the affected limb, or does not improve within 24 hours, consult your doctor.

PAINFUL JOINTS

Serious disorders of a joint are extremely rare in children. If there is any pain it is usually due to a minor sprain or strain of a muscle or ligament around a joint. If your child suffers from a persistent pain in a joint, or if there are any other symptoms, such as a fever, consult your doctor.

SYMPTOM	POSSIBLE CAUSE	ACTION NEEDED
If your child fell or was injured recently, is there restricted or painful movement in a joint, or is the joint misshapen?	A dislocated joint or a break in a bone near a joint (*see* Fractures and dislocations, *p.283*).	Contact your doctor's office or go to the nearest emergency room. **Self-help** Broken bones (*p.334*).
Is the joint red, hot, or swollen, and does your child have a fever or seem sick?	Infection of a joint (*see* Bone and joint infection, *p.288*). A short-lived arthritis or juvenile idiopathic arthritis (*p.288*) if more than one joint is involved.	**Urgent!** Call your doctor immediately.
Does your child have a painful knee?	A minor strain or sprain (*p.281*). Bone or joint infection (*p.288*) is possible. See also Limping (*p.281*).	If the pain is severe, is no better after 24 hours, or recurs, consult your doctor. **Self-help** Treat the strain or sprain (*p.335*).
Is your child's joint swollen?	Strained muscles or sprained ligaments near the joint (*see* Strains and sprains, *p.281*).	If the pain or swelling is severe or does not improve within 24 hours, call your doctor.
Does your child have a limp or a painful hip?	Developmental hip dysplasia (*p.286*) in a child just learning to walk. Perthes disease (*p.286*) or fracture in an older child. Bone or joint infection (*p.288*) or irritable hip (*p.285*) in a child of any age. See also Limping (*p.281*).	Get medical advice within 24 hours.
If more than one joint is involved, does your child have a purplish rash on her limbs?	Henoch-Schönlein purpura (*p.307*).	**Urgent!** Call your doctor immediately.

FOOT PROBLEMS

THE MOST COMMON FOOT PROBLEMS in childhood are caused by falls, conditions affecting the skin of one or both feet, and ill-fitting footwear. Few of these foot problems are serious. However, if your child suffers from a very painful or swollen foot, or if he finds walking difficult, consult your doctor.

SYMPTOM	POSSIBLE CAUSE
If your child's foot is painful after a recent fall or injury, can he walk on the affected foot?	A bone in your child's foot, toe, or ankle may have been fractured (*see* Fractures and dislocations, *p.283*).
Is walking painful but possible?	Bruised or strained muscles or strained ligaments (*see* Strains and sprains, *p.281*).
If a recent fall or injury is not the cause, and your child feels pain all the time, is there redness or swelling on his foot or toes?	Infection from a cut or a foreign body, such as a thorn or a splinter, may cause redness or swelling.
Is there an itchy, peeling rash?	Athlete's foot (*p.193*).
If your child feels pain only when weight is put on the foot, is there a flattened lump on the sole?	Plantar warts (*p.193 and* Warts, *p.231*).
Does your child feel pain only when wearing shoes?	Your child's shoes may not fit properly, or the lining may be worn.
If your child's feet appear to have bent or curly toes, are his socks and shoes too small?	Shoes or socks that are too small may cause your child's toes to curl.
If your child is 3 years or older, do his feet appear to be flat ?	Flat feet (*see* Minor skeletal problems, *p.284*).
If your child is younger than 3 years, do his feet appear to be flat ?	Undeveloped muscles and ligaments in the soles of the feet, which are not a cause for concern at this age (*see* Minor skeletal problems, *p.284*).

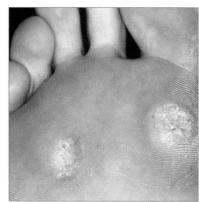

**REMOVING A
PLANTAR WART**
*Scrape the skin
of the plantar wart
and cover it with
a salicylic acid
bandage every day.*

ACTION NEEDED

Contact your doctor's office or take your child
to the nearest hospital emergency room. If you are
unable to move your child, dial 911 or call EMS.

If the pain or swelling is severe, consult your doctor.
Self-help Treat the strain or sprain (*p.335*).

Get medical advice within 24 hours.
Self-help Remove a foreign body with clean tweezers.
Cover with a sterile bandage and then elevate and
support the foot to reduce any swelling.

Self-help Apply an antifungal powder, cream, or
spray to the rash. Ensure your child's feet are dried
properly after bathing. If the rash doesn't clear up
within 2 weeks, or if your child's toenails are affected,
consult your doctor.

Self-help Treating plantar warts (*right*).

Replace tight or worn shoes with new shoes that are
long and wide enough. Try to buy from stores where
the employees are trained to fit children's shoes.

Replace your child's shoes and socks as soon as they
become tight.

If your child's feet are painful or you are worried
about them, consult your doctor.

If you feel your child's feet are not developing
properly, consult your doctor.

Treating plantar warts

**Plantar warts are hard, callused warts on the soles
of the feet. They are caused by a virus and are
flattened by the weight of the body. Plantar warts
can be painful – but usually the painful phase is
short-lived. Do not pick or scratch a wart because
it may spread.**

- Warts are highly infectious and are often acquired
  from walking barefoot in communal changing rooms,
  so encourage your child to wear flip-flops or sandals
  at a gym or swimming pool.

- Use a pumice stone to remove as much of the skin as
  possible and cover with a fresh salicylic acid bandage
  every day until the wart disappears.

- Your doctor can advise you on over-the-counter topical
  applications.

- Stubborn, painful warts may need treatment from a
  dermatologist.

Treating athlete's foot

**Athlete's foot is a fungal infection that thrives in the
warm, moist conditions between the toes.**

- Keep your child's feet clean and dry – use a hairdryer
  set on low if necessary. Use cotton socks and change
  them daily. Air your child's shoes after use.

- Sprinkle antifungal powder or spread antifungal cream
  between your child's toes twice a day.

- Contact your doctor if the infection lasts more than
  2 weeks.

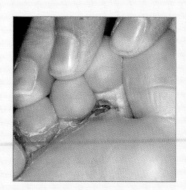

**ATHLETE'S FOOT
POWDER** *Keep your
child's feet clean
and dry and sprinkle
antifungal powder
in his socks and
shoes and between
his toes.*

BREATHING PROBLEMS

BREATHING PROBLEMS ARE OFTEN SERIOUS IN CHILDREN. Children may have difficulty inhaling or exhaling, or their breathing may be noisy or fast. Children with a minor respiratory infection may wheeze a little. Breathing problems accompanied by danger signs (*right*) require urgent attention.

SYMPTOM	POSSIBLE CAUSE
If your child's breathing problems started suddenly a few minutes ago, could she be choking on a small object?	Inhalation of a foreign body.
Does your child have a hoarse voice, noisy breathing, and a barking cough?	Croup (*p.224*).
Does your child suffer from repeated episodes of wheezing, shortness of breath, or coughing especially during the night?	Asthma (*p.226*).
Does your child show one or more of the danger signs (*above right*) and have a history of asthma?	Severe asthma (*p.226*) attack.
Is your child showing one or more of the danger signs (*above right*) without a history of asthma?	Bronchiolitis (*p.228*), pneumonia (*p.227*), severe croup (*p.224*), or asthma (*p.226*).
Has your child's breathing recently become faster or noisier accompanied by a fever and a cough?	Pneumonia (*p.227*), bronchiolitis (*p.228*), or croup (*p.224*).
Has your child's breathing been intermittently squeaky and noisy since birth?	Congenital laryngeal stridor (a harmless condition called laryngomalacia that your child will outgrow).

Dial 911 or call EMS immediately if your child:

- Has blue-tinged lips or tongue
- Is abnormally drowsy
- Can't talk or produce sounds normally.

Call your doctor immediately if:

- The areas between your child's ribs appear sunken when he breathes in.

ACTION NEEDED

Emergency! Dial 911 or call EMS.
Self-help Choking (*p.329*).

Urgent! Call your doctor immediately.

If your child seems very sick or if breathing difficulties develop, call your doctor immediately.
Self-help Ease breathing during an asthma attack (*right*).

Emergency! Dial 911 or call EMS.
Self-help Administer asthma medications as prescribed. See also Ease breathing during an asthma attack (*right*) and Giving rescue breaths (*pp.327–328*).

Emergency! Dial 911 or call EMS.
Self-help Giving rescue breaths (*pp.327–328*).

Urgent! Call your doctor immediately.
Self-help Ease breathing during an asthma attack (*right*) and Checking breathing rates (*above right*).

See your doctor.

Checking breathing rates

A child with an unusually rapid breathing rate may need medical attention. To check your child's rate, make sure she is resting and then count the number of breaths in one minute. As a child grows, the rate decreases. For a baby under two months the breathing rate is less than 60. For a baby between 2 and 11 months, it is less than 50. For a child between 1 and 5 years, the rate is less than 40. For a child over 5 years, it is less than 30.

Natural relief

Relaxation techniques
Techniques such as deep breathing may help your child relax and breathe calmly from the diaphragm. This will help her develop a sense of control when she has difficulties.

Better posture
Adopting a better posture may help your child relax her chest and improve breathing, so preventing difficulties from arising.

Ease breathing during an asthma attack

If your child is having an asthma attack, try the following while waiting for help:

- Help your child sit up (*below*).

- Give any prescribed asthma medicine right away.

- Keep her calm and limit distractions.

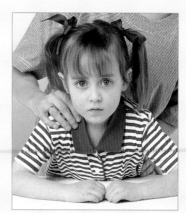

BREATHING POSITION
Help your child to adopt a good position to help her breathe. Encourage her to sit up and lean against a table or the back of a chair, using her arms and elbows as support.

COUGHING

I N OLDER CHILDREN, coughing is usually due to a minor respiratory infection, such as a cold. In very young babies, coughing is uncommon and may be a sign of a serious lung infection. Be alert to a sudden cough in any child who is otherwise well because the airway may be obstructed.

SYMPTOM	POSSIBLE CAUSE
If your child been coughing for less than 24 hours, was there a sudden onset?	Inhalation of a foreign body.
Is your child under a year old?	A common cold (*p.221*) or, less commonly, bronchiolitis (*p.228*) or pneumonia (*p.227*).
Has your child been coughing for less than 24 hours, with a stuffy or runny nose?	A common cold (*p.221*).
If your child has been coughing for 24 hours or more, is his nose persistently runny?	An allergy or a recurrent cold (*see* Common cold, *p.221*).
Does your child have a fever and a cough?	A common cold (*p.221*) or influenza (*p.225*).
Does your child cough mainly at night, whether or not he has a fever?	Asthma (*p.226*) or pertussis (*p.269*).
If your child coughs, does the cough come in bouts ending in a whoop, and is there vomiting?	Pertussis (*p.269*) or other infections.
If your child has been coughing for 2 weeks or more and doesn't have a runny nose, has he had pertussis or a viral infection recently?	Cough persisting after pertussis (*p.269*) or a viral infection.
Does your child have a fever, a cough, and a rash – or has he recently been exposed to measles?	Measles (*p.264*).
If your child has been coughing for 24 hours or more, is his nose persistently runny, does he snore and is his voice nasal?	Enlarged adenoids (*p.222*).

Dial 911 or call EMS immediately if your child:

- Has blue-tinged lips or tongue
- Is abnormallly drowsy
- Can't talk or produce sounds normally.

Call your doctor immediately if:

- The areas between your child's ribs appear sunken when he breathes in.

ACTION NEEDED

Urgent! Call your doctor immediately.
Self-help Choking (*p.329*).

If your child is very sick or if breathing difficulties develop, call your doctor immediately.
Self-help Relieving a cough (*right*).

If your child is distressed, consult your doctor.
Self-help Relieving a cough (*right*).

If your child seems generally sick or is upset by the cough, consult your doctor.
Self-help Relieving a cough (*right*).

If breathing difficulties develop, call your doctor. If a rash appears, get medical advice within 24 hours.
Self-help Relieving a cough (*right*) and Bringing down a temperature (*p.59 and p.171*).

Get medical advice within 24 hours.
Self-help Relieving a cough (*right*).

Get medical advice within 24 hours.
Self-help Relieving a cough (*right*).

If your child is distressed or feels sick, or if the cough persists for several weeks, consult your doctor.
Self-help Relieving a cough (*right*).

Get medical advice within 24 hours.
Self-help Bringing down a temperature (*p.59 and p.171*).

Consult your doctor.
Self-help If the ear infections are causing pain, see Relieving earache (*p.205*).

SELF-HELP

Relieving a cough

The following may help relieve your child's cough:

- Let the child drink soothing liquids, such as warm tea or water mixed with honey. But do not give honey to children under one year of age because it may cause botulism. Give plenty of other warm or cool drinks.

- Use a humidifier or vaporizer to moisten the air. Cool fresh air is a good home remedy for croup.

- A cold-water humidifier is just as effective as a hot-water vaporizer and is safer if accidentally knocked over. However, be sure to clean the device daily so that it does not become a breeding ground for harmful bacteria or fungi.

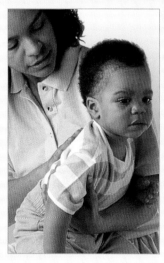

EASING A COUGH Try to keep your child calm during a coughing attack to help prevent breathing difficulty.

- Avoid excessive heating of your child's room because this will dry out the air and may increase coughing.

- Nighttime coughs can be disruptive to the whole household. It may help to elevate the head of your child's bed. If the cough is due to asthma, consult your doctor for appropriate treatment.

- Although cough medicines can be purchased without a prescription, they vary widely in their ingredients. Ask your doctor to recommend a brand and specify the correct dosage and frequency for your child. Only give these medicines with your doctor's approval.

SORE THROAT

Minor viral infections cause many of the sore throats that affect children. They usually clear up quickly without medical treatment. A very young child who is reluctant to eat or drink may have a sore throat. On occasion, a sore throat may be a symptom of a bacterial infection that requires antibiotics.

SYMPTOM	POSSIBLE CAUSE	ACTION NEEDED
Is your child sneezing with a runny nose and a cough?	A common cold (*p.221*) or allergic rhinitis (*p.224*), which can irritate the throat.	If symptoms last for more than a week, consult your doctor. **Self-help** Relieving a cough (*p.197*).
Does your child have a fever and either feel pain on swallowing or refuse to eat solids?	Pharyngitis or tonsillitis, (*p.223*).	If your child is no better after 24 hours, consult your doctor. **Self-help** Bringing down a temperature (*p.59* and *p.171*).
Does your child have a fever, vomiting, a rash, and a bright red tongue and throat?	Scarlet fever (*p.267*).	Call your doctor within 24 hours. **Self-help** Bringing down a temperature (*p.59* and *p.171*).
Does your child have no other symptoms except a sore throat?	Minor infection or irritation may cause the throat to be inflamed.	If her throat is still sore after 48 hours, consult your doctor.

SELF-HELP

Relieving a sore throat

The following tips may help relieve a sore throat:

- Offer your child cold, nonacidic drinks such as milk. A straw may make drinking easier. Also, ice cream and flavored gelatin may be soothing.

- Give your child acetaminophen or ibuprofen in the recommended dose.

- If she's over 8, let her gargle with warm, diluted saltwater.

- Throat lozenges or hard candy may be a choking hazard in young children.

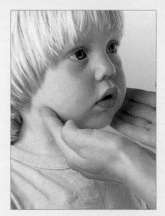

CHECKING THE GLANDS
Your child may complain of a difficulty swallowing as well as a sore throat. Ask your child to sit still while you run your fingertips below the jaw, from the ears to the chin, to feel the size of the glands. If they feel larger than a pea, they are swollen.

DROWSINESS

A MINOR ILLNESS, LACK OF SLEEP, or a serious disease, such as meningitis, can cause drowsiness. Dial 911 or call EMS immediately if your child is unconscious for more than a few minutes; is breathing irregularly, slowly, or quickly; is unresponsive or difficult to wake from sleep; or has blood or fluid leaking from the nose or ears.

SYMPTOM	POSSIBLE CAUSE	ACTION NEEDED
Has your child had a recent injury to the head?	Head injury (*p.291*).	**Emergency!** Seek immediate medical care. Meanwhile, do not give any food or drink.
Has your child swallowed something that may be poisonous?	Swallowed poisons may lead to a change in consciousness.	**Emergency!** Call the nearest Poison Control Center, or go to hospital immediately.
Does your child have a fever?	A high fever, resulting from any infection, may cause delirium, particularly if the temperature exceeds 102°F (39°C).	**Urgent!** Call your doctor immediately. **Self-help** Bringing down a temperature (*p.59 and p.171*).
Does your child have diarrhea with or without vomiting?	Dehydration resulting from gastroenteritis (*p.254*).	**Urgent!** Call your doctor immediately. **Self-help** Preventing dehydration in babies (*p.63*) or Giving extra fluids (*p.172*).
Does your child have a stiff neck, headache, vomiting, or flat spots that remain when pressed?	Meningitis (*p.294*).	**Emergency!** Seek immediate medical attention.
Is your child urinating often and very thirsty; or has he recently lost weight and been uncharacteristically tired?	Diabetes mellitus (*p.309*).	**Urgent!** Call your doctor immediately.
Does your child have red eyes, no appetite, mood swings, withdrawal, or aggression?	Substance abuse (*pp.160–161*).	Consult your doctor.
Have you been giving your child any medicine?	Certain medicines can cause confusion or have a sedative effect.	Ask your doctor whether you should stop giving the medicine.

DIZZINESS

FAINTING MAY BE ACCOMPANIED BY A FEELING OF DIZZINESS or lightheadedness. In fainting, a fall in blood pressure causes a brief loss of consciousness. In a seizure, the loss of consciousness that occurs is due to an abnormal electrical discharge in the brain.

SYMPTOM	POSSIBLE CAUSE
Has your child fallen to the ground unconscious, either with no other symptoms or looking pale and sweaty?	Fainting is a likely cause. Fainting is due to a fall in blood pressure, possibly caused by emotional stress, anxiety, not eating for some time, or being in an overcrowded or stuffy atmosphere for too long.
Your child falls to the ground unconscious – did her face or limbs twitch and did she urinate or bite her tongue?	Epilepsy (p.293).
Does your child feel her surroundings are spinning around?	Labyrinthitis (p.242) or motion sickness, which is due to a problem in the inner ear.
Does your child seems unaware of surroundings for a few moments?	An absence seizure (see Epilepsy, p.293).
If your child is being treated for diabetes mellitus, does she feel faint or unsteady?	Extremely low blood sugar level caused by diabetes mellitus (p.309) may cause your child to lose consciousness and, in some cases, to have a seizure.
If she is not being treated for diabetes mellitus, is she under 5 with a fever?	Febrile seizures (p.292).
Does your child feel faint or unsteady?	Low blood sugar level (hypoglycemia), caused by diabetes mellitus (p.309), or low blood pressure due to a quick change in posture.

DANGER SIGNS

Dial 911 or call EMS immediately if your child has lost consciousness and any of the following occur:

- Consciousness is not regained within a few minutes
- Breathing becomes slower
- Breathing is irregular or noisy.

SELF-HELP

Dealing with lightheadedness and fainting

If your child feels lightheaded, have her lie down with her legs up, and do the following:

- Loosen tight-fitting clothing and provide fresh air.
- Give calm reassurance.
- Offer a sugary drink or small snack to raise the sugar level in her blood. Do not offer food or drink if she is not fully conscious.
- If she loses consciousness, monitor her condition (pp.326–328). If she is breathing, place her in the recovery position (p.326). Dial 911 or call EMS if she doesn't regain consciousness within a few minutes.

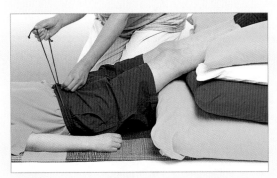

A FAINTING CHILD Prop the legs up to increase the blood supply to the brain, and loosen any tight-fitting clothing.

ACTION NEEDED

See your doctor immediately.
Self-help Dealing with faintness and fainting (right).

Urgent! Call your doctor immediately. Do not try to open her mouth.

Consult your doctor.

Consult your doctor.
Self-help Sit your child down quietly until she is fully recovered.

Emergency! Dial 911 or call EMS if she is having a seizure. If diabetes has already been diagnosed, give her a glucagon injection while you are waiting.
Self-help As soon as she feels faint, give her glucose tablets.

Urgent! Call your doctor immediately.
Self-help Bringing down a temperature (p.59 and p.171).

If your child often feels faint, consult your doctor.
Self-help As soon as your child feels faint, give glucose tablets or a glucose or sugary drink. See Dealing with lightheadedness and fainting (right).

Coping with a seizure

Children ages 6 months–5 years are susceptible to febrile seizures when their temperature rises abruptly at the start of a fever. This may appear serious but usually it is not. A child may sweat, have a hot forehead, and roll her eyes. Her fists may clench, as the back arches and the body stiffens and jerks. Help your child as the seizure runs its course and then go to the nearest hospital:

- Lay her down and arrange soft towels and pillows around her to prevent injury.
- Undress her and expose her to fresh, cool air.
- When she's cool the seizures will cease. Put her in the recovery position (p.326), under a light blanket.

EYE PROBLEMS

Most eye problems, such as itching, redness, watering, and discharge, are caused by infections or irritation and are rarely serious. If you cannot use self-help measures to help a child who has an eye injury or a foreign object in the eye, go to your doctor or the nearest emergency room.

SYMPTOM	POSSIBLE CAUSE	ACTION NEEDED
Do your child's eyes often produce tears when he is not crying?	Blocked tear duct if your child is under a year old.	Consult your doctor.
Does your child have itchy eyes?	Allergy, such as hay fever (*see* Allergic rhinitis, *p.224*).	Consult your doctor.
Can you see a foreign body, such as a speck of dirt, in your child's eye?	A foreign body often causes redness and watering.	If you cannot remove the foreign body or your child is in pain, call your doctor immediately. **Self-help** Removing a foreign body from the eye (*p.337*).
Is one or both of your child's eyes red or painful?	Eye irritation may be caused by smoke, chemicals, fumes, allergies, or infections. Iritis (*p.244*), a more serious condition, is also possible.	**Urgent!** Call your doctor immediately if your child is in pain. If there is no pain but redness continues for more than 24 hours, consult your doctor.
Does your child have a red eye accompanied by a sticky discharge?	Severe conjunctivitis (*p.244*).	Get medical advice within 24 hours.
Has your child developed a red lump on an eyelid?	Stye (*p.243*).	If the stye persists or becomes painful, see your doctor.
Does your child have red, itchy eyelids or white flakes on the lashes?	Blepharitis (*p.243*) or conjunctivitis (*p.244*).	Consult your doctor.
Does your child have any obvious damage to an eye?	Eye injury.	**Emergency!** Take your child to the nearest hospital emergency room.

VISION PROBLEMS

DEFECTS IN A CHILD'S VISION may be picked up in the eye tests routinely conducted at school or at the doctor's office. However, if you or your child's teacher notices that your child is having difficulty seeing, or has some other kind of vision problem, seek medical care promptly.

SYMPTOM	POSSIBLE CAUSE	ACTION NEEDED
Does your child have double or blurred vision and no other symptoms?	A refractive error (*p.245*) or strabismus (*p.245*).	Consult your doctor or ophthalmologist.
Does your child have difficulty seeing near or distant objects?	A refractive error (*p.245*).	Consult your doctor or ophthalmologist.
Do your child's eyes sometimes seem out of alignment?	Strabismus (*p.245*).	If your child is over 4 months old, consult your doctor.
Is the double or blurred vision associated with headaches?	Migraine (*see* Recurrent headaches, *p.291*).	Consult your doctor.
Does she regularly see flashing lights or floating spots, with a severe headache afterward?	Migraine (*see* Recurrent headaches, *p.291*).	If this is the first attack or if the attacks are frequent, see your doctor.
Is your child taking any medicine?	Some drugs may cause blurred vision.	Ask your doctor if the medicine may be the cause and if you should stop giving it.
Might your child have taken someone else's medicine or ingested poison?	Drugs, such as antidepressants, may cause blurred vision.	**Urgent!** Immediately call your doctor or the nearest Poison Control Center, or go to the nearest hospital.
Does the double/blurred vision follow a recent head injury?	Bleeding inside the skull (*see* Head injury, *p.291*).	**Emergency!** Dial 911 or call EMS.
Has your child lost all or part of her vision?	Injury to the eye or part of the brain is possible.	**Emergency!** Dial 911 or take your child to the nearest hospital.

EAR PROBLEMS

AR PROBLEMS SUCH AS EARACHE are usually caused by an infection. Middle ear infections are common in young children because the eustachian tubes connecting their ears with their nose and throat are immature and easily blocked, which predisposes them to infection. Disorders that affect a child's external ear canal cause such symptoms as itching, pain, and discharge.

SYMPTOM	POSSIBLE CAUSE
If your child's earache is not severe, might there be something in his ear?	A foreign body, such as an insect or bead, in the ear.
Can you see a red lump inside your child's ear canal?	A boil (p.233) in the outer ear canal.
If the earache is severe, does your child seem well with no red lump inside his ear?	Inflammation of the outer ear (p.240).
Does your child have an itchy ear?	Eczema (p.234) or inflammation of the outer ear (p.240).
If there is a discharge from the ear, does gently tugging on the earlobe make the pain worse?	Eczema (p.234) or inflammation of the outer ear (p.240).
Is there is a discharge from the ear but little or no reaction to tugging the earlobe?	Inflammation of the middle ear (p.240).
Does your child have hearing problems or an earache without any other symptoms?	Inflammation of the middle ear (p.240).
If the earache is severe, does your child have a fever or cold, or is he generally feeling sick?	Inflammation of the middle ear (p.240).
Did the pain in your child's ear start during or soon after a trip on an airplane?	Barotrauma (p.242).

Hearing problems

Hearing defects are often first noticed by the child's parents. In babies, the first sign of deafness is a failure to respond to sounds. In older children, the onset of hearing problems may cause schoolwork to deteriorate. The following are instances when your child may experience hearing problems. In each case, consult a doctor.

- Sneezing or a recent cold may cause the tubes connecting the ears and throat to become blocked. See Common cold (p.221) and Allergic rhinitis (p.224).

- Hearing problems can start during or shortly after a trip on an airplane, because of barotrauma (p.242).

- The problem may be due to otitis media with effusion (p.241), or middle ear inflammation (p.240) if it accompanies or follows earache.

- If the problem is not related to any other symptom then earwax may be blocking the external ear canal.

- Rarely, infectious diseases such as mumps, measles, and meningitis may have a long-term effect on hearing.

Get medical advice within 24 hours.
Self-help *see* Foreign objects in the ear, p.337.
If in doubt, seek medical advice.

Get medical advice within 24 hours.
Self-help Relieving earache (*right*).

See your doctor within 24 hours.
Self-help Relieving earache (*right*).

Get medical advice within 24 hours.
Self-help Relieving earache (*right*).

Get medical advice within 24 hours.
Self-help Relieving earache (*right*).

Get medical advice within 24 hours.
Self-help Relieving earache (*right*).

Get medical advice within 24 hours.
Self-help Relieving earache (*right*).

See your doctor within 24 hours.
Self-help Relieving earache (*right*) and Bringing down a temperature (p.59 and p.171).

Consult your doctor.
Self-help Relieving earache (*right*).

Relieving earache

You may be able to reduce the pain of your child's earache with the following:

- Give him the recommended dose of acetaminophen or ibuprofen.

- Wrap a warm water bottle in a towel for him to hold against his ear.

- Have your child sit up or prop up his head with pillows. It is possible that lying flat may make his earache worse.

- Consult your doctor before using ear drops or oil.

Preventing earaches

To prevent conditions that may lead to earaches, consider the following:

- Breastfeeding may decrease the risk of ear infections. Do not give a bottle or breastfeed while your child is lying flat.

- Immunize your child according to the recommended schedule.

- Avoid tobacco smoke, which may lead to ear infections and other health problems.

- If possible, avoid sick children and large group child care settings.

- Avoid giving pacifiers to children who are prone to ear infections.

MOUTH PROBLEMS

THE TONGUE, GUMS, LIPS, AND INSIDE LINING of the mouth are rarely affected by serious problems. A sore mouth may be upsetting for a child, largely because it hurts to eat and drink. An infant with mouth pain is probably teething – chewing on a hard or cold object can often bring relief.

SYMPTOM	POSSIBLE CAUSE
Does your child's mouth or tongue have painful areas with a creamy yellow or white discoloration that is not easily scraped off?	Oral thrush (*p.248*).
Does your child have painful discolored areas inside the mouth or on the tongue?	Mouth ulcers (*p.247*).
Does your child seem sick or have a fever at the same time as having painful, red areas with light yellow spots inside the mouth or on the tongue?	Gingivostomatitis (*p.247*).
Does your child have painful red areas with light yellow spots inside the mouth or on the tongue, as well as spots on the hands and feet?	Hand, foot, and mouth disease (*p.266*).
Does your child have tiny blisters on or around the lips?	Cold sores (*p.231*).
Does your child have redness around his mouth or cracks at the corners of her lips?	Lip licker's eczema (*p.185*).
Does your child have honey-colored crusts on or around the lips?	Impetigo (*p.235*).
Does your child have painful, red, and swollen gums?	Gingivitis (*p.249*).
Does your child have soreness affecting the tongue only?	Irritation of the tongue possibly caused by a rough tooth, contact with hot foods, or other trauma.

Relieving a sore mouth

Relieve your child's discomfort with the following:

- Rinse several times a day with ¼ teaspoon baking soda dissolved in 120 ml (4 fl.oz) of warm water.

- Give acetaminophen or ibuprofen as directed.

- Try soft foods, such as soup and ice cream. Avoid acidic drinks, such as citrus juices.

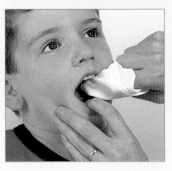

TREATING MOUTH ULCERS
Some mouth ulcers look like white "curds." Wrap a clean cloth around your index finger and wipe away the curds. Rinse the mouth out with a solution of baking soda.

Consult your doctor.

If the ulcers fail to heal in 7–10 days, see your doctor.

Self-help Relieving a sore mouth (*above*).

Consult your doctor.
Self-help Relieving a sore mouth (*above*) and Bringing down a temperature (*p.59 and p.171*).

Consult your doctor.
Self-help Relieving a sore mouth (*above*).

If the blisters are severe or persistent, consult your doctor.

Self-help Apply petroleum jelly to the affected area every few hours. Use a lip balm to moisturize and protect the lips themselves.

Get medical advice within 24 hours.

Consult your dentist.
Self-help Your child should continue to brush and floss her teeth with care. An antibacterial mouthwash may relieve inflammation. See Keeping your child's teeth healthy (Tooth decay, *p.248*).

Contact your doctor if you are concerned.

Combating cold sores

Small blisters on and around the lips may appear during an infection, after exposure to a cold wind or the sun, or as a result of stress. These cold sores are caused by the herpes simplex virus and go away on their own. You can relieve your child's discomfort and keep the sores under control.

- A cold drink may soothe the discomfort.

- An over-the-counter cream containing a pain reliever may help, especially if you apply it as soon as your child feels the tingling sensation that precedes the sores.

- Ask your doctor whether a prescribed antiviral medication may help.

Treating gingivitis

Children with red, swollen, and tender gums are probably not brushing or flossing their teeth properly – and when they do, the gums bleed. The best way to treat this gingivitis is to regularly brush both teeth and gums to remove the bacterial plaque that has accumulated. An antibacterial mouthwash may help relieve tenderness.

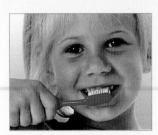

BRUSHING THE TEETH
Encourage her to brush her teeth and gums with a soft toothbrush and a little toothpaste after breakfast and before bedtime. Supervise her until she is 6 or 7 years old.

ABDOMINAL PAIN

ABDOMINAL PAIN IS NOT UNUSUAL in children and some children suffer pains that regularly recur. The cause is rarely serious and the pain usually soon goes away without any medical or self-help treatment. Occasionally, however, the pain may indicate an underlying disorder that requires prompt medical attention.

SYMPTOM	POSSIBLE CAUSE
Does defecation or vomiting relieve the pain, or is there diarrhea with or without vomiting?	Gastroenteritis (*p.254*).
Is your child's pain aggravated when the abdomen is gently pressed?	Appendicitis (*p.253*).
Has your child been in continuous pain for several hours?	Appendicitis (*p.253*).
Is your child vomiting and has he been in continuous pain for a few hours?	Appendicitis (*p.253*).
Is your child's vomit greenish yellow?	Intestinal obstruction (*p.256*).
Does your child have a painful swelling in the groin or scrotum?	Strangulated inguinal hernia (*see* Hernia, *p.260*) or testicular torsion (*see* Penis and testicle disorders, *p.277*).
Is there bloody mucus in your baby's stools?	Intussusception (*see* Intestinal obstruction, *p.256*).
Does your child have a sore throat, cough, or runny nose?	An upper respiratory tract infection, such as a common cold (*p.221*), causing lymph node swelling in the abdomen.
Does your child have two or more of the following: fever, pain on urinating, bed wetting (if toilet trained)?	Urinary tract infection (*p.275*).
Does your child often have recurrent bouts of abdominal pain without seeming sick?	Anxiety (*see pp.131–132*) or food intolerance (*see* Reactions to food, *p.252*) may be the explanation, but often there is no obvious cause.

Seek immediate medical care if your child has any of the following symptoms:

- Abdominal pain for several hours
- Pain or swelling in the groin or testes
- Greenish yellow vomit
- Red material in stools.

ACTION NEEDED

Get medical advice within 24 hours.
Self-help Preventing dehydration in babies (*p.63*).

If the pain continues for more than a few hours, call your doctor immediately.
Self-help Relieving abdominal pain (*right*).

Urgent! Call your doctor immediately. Do not give your child anything to eat or drink.

Urgent! Call your doctor immediately.
Self-help Relieving abdominal pain (*right*).

Emergency! Seek immediate medical care. Do not give your child anything to eat or drink.

Emergency! Seek immediate medical care. Do not give your child anything to eat or drink.

Emergency! Seek immediate medical care. Do not give your child anything to eat or drink.

If your child is distressed by his or symptoms, consult your doctor.
Self-help Relieving a cough (*p.197*), Relieving a sore throat (*p.198*), Relieving abdominal pain (*right*).

See your doctor within 24 hours.
Self-help If your child has a fever, see Bringing down a temperature (*p.59 and p.171*).

Consult your doctor.
Self-help Calm your child's anxiety. If you think food intolerance is the problem try to establish, and avoid, the triggers. See Relieving abdominal pain (*right*).

Relieving abdominal pain

The following tips may help you relieve your child's abdominal pain:

- Fill a water bottle with warm water and wrap it in a towel. Let your child hold it against his abdomen. Encourage him to lie down on a bed or sofa, or to sit in a chair.

- While your child is suffering from abdominal pain, do not give him anything to eat, and give only plain water to drink.

- If you suspect appendicitis or another serious disorder, your child might require surgery. Do not give him any food or drink until you have spoken to your doctor and know whether surgery is necessary.

Relieving anxiety

Talk with your child about the pain in his abdomen and see if you can establish whether it is linked to any concerns he may have.

- Children sometimes complain of pain when they are anxious – discussing their worries may ease the pain.

- If the pain is recurrent, and you suspect it is related to anxiety, consider giving him a relaxing massage (*p.321*).

- If your child has persistent anxiety or you have concerns, contact your doctor or seek the help of a mental health professional.

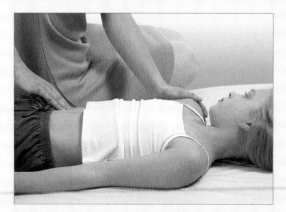

FEELING FOR ABDOMINAL PAIN *Press down firmly but not abruptly with the tips of your fingers to try to locate the pain.*

CONSTIPATION

CHILDREN CAN HAVE ERRATIC BOWEL MOVEMENTS. They may defecate four times a day or only once every four days; anything in between is normal. Changes in diet, a minor illness, or emotional stress may affect defecation in the short term. If the stools are hard, or painful to pass, your child is constipated.

SYMPTOM	POSSIBLE CAUSE
If your child has had a bowel movement in the last 24 hours, was the process painful and was there any blood?	Anal fissure (*see* Constipation, *p.255*).
If your child has had a bowel movement in the last 24 hours, were they hard and pelletlike?	Your child's diet may not contain enough fiber or sufficient fluid.
Does your child have abdominal pain?	Go to ABDOMINAL PAIN (*p.208*).
If your child usually moves her bowels daily, has she had a fever or been vomiting before becoming constipated?	Loss of fluid as a result of fever or vomiting can disrupt bowel movements, which will return to normal once your child has recovered.
Does your child usually move her bowels less than once every 4 days?	Constipation (*p.255*).
Is your child learning toilet training now or has she recently started?	Children who are anxious about toilet training may resist the urge to move their bowels.
If your child is constipated but has yet to start her toilet training or was trained a while ago, have you changed her diet recently?	Your child's diet may not contain enough fiber or sufficient fluid.

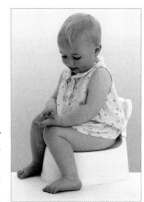

A REGULAR BOWEL HABIT
Encourage, but don't force, your child to sit on the potty or toilet at the same time each day.

ACTION NEEDED

Consult your doctor.
Self-help Preventing constipation (*right*).

Self-help Preventing constipation (*right*).

Self-help Encourage your child to drink plenty of fluids. See Bringing down a temperature (*p.59 and p.171*), Preventing dehydration in babies (*p.63*) or Giving extra fluids (*p.172*).

Consult your doctor.
Self-help Preventing constipation (*right*).

If your child does not pass any stools at all for longer than about 4 days, consult your doctor.
Self-help Perhaps you are anxious about how your child's toilet training is progressing and are making her nervous. Adopt a more relaxed attitude toward your child's toilet training.

Self-help Preventing constipation (*right*).

SELF-HELP

Preventing constipation

The following tips may help you relieve or prevent your child's constipation:

- Look at your child's diet to see if the meals she is eating contain a varied and nutritious mixture of foods. If necessary, increase the amount of fruit, vegetables, and other fiber-rich foods, such as wholegrain cereals.

- In addition to boosting her fiber intake, you will need to increase the amount of fluids that your child drinks, particularly water and some juices.

- Regular exercise is vital for a healthy digestive system. Encourage your child to be active every day.

- Don't force your child to sit on the potty or toilet for long periods "trying." Instead, have her try more often – such as after meals and before bedtime. Above all, don't make it a source of tension.

- Try to avoid unfamiliar bathrooms and hurried settings, which may create anxiety for your child.

- Never give your child a laxative unless specifically recommended or prescribed by your doctor. However, natural laxatives, such as prunes, may help relieve occasional constipation.

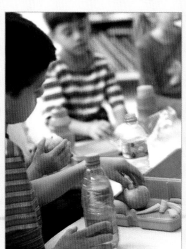

FIBER-RICH FOODS
Encourage your child to eat at least one fiber-rich food, such as wholegrain bread, vegetables, or fruit, at every meal.

ABNORMAL STOOLS

A CHANGE IN DIET IS ALMOST ALWAYS RESPONSIBLE when a child's bowel movements smell or look different. Changes in color, smell, consistency, and content do not usually last more than a few days and are of no concern. If you notice other symptoms, or if the abnormal stools persist, take your child to see the doctor.

SYMPTOM	POSSIBLE CAUSE	ACTION NEEDED
If his stools are yellow or green and runny, is he breastfed only?	Yellow or green, runny stools are normal in breastfed babies.	If he seems sick or has other symptoms, consult your doctor.
If your child is under a year old, are his stools red and jellylike?	Intussusception (*see* Intestinal obstruction, *p.256*).	**Emergency!** Seek immediate medical care. Do not give your child any food or drink.
If your child is one year old or more with very pale stools, has he just recovered from a bout of diarrhea or vomiting?	Gastroenteritis (*p.254*) may sometimes cause stools to be pale for several days.	If your child seems sick or if the stools do not return to their normal color in a few days, consult your doctor.
If your child's stools are pale, is his urine dark and are his skin and whites of the eyes yellowish?	Hepatitis (*p.261*), which may cause jaundice.	Get medical advice within 24 hours.
Are your child's stools very pale, floating, and foul-smelling?	Malabsorption (*p.258*), often caused by underlying disorders, such as reaction to food (*p.252*).	Consult your doctor.
Is there blood on your child's stools?	Gastroenteritis (*p.254*), anal fissure (*p.257*), or inflammatory bowel disease (*p.259*).	Get medical advice within 24 hours, or sooner if there is a large amount of blood.
Are your child's stools runny?	Go to DIARRHEA (*p.62 and p.172*).	
Is your child, whatever his age, taking any medicine?	Many medicines can affect the appearance of stools.	Ask your doctor if the medicine may be the cause and if you should stop giving it.

URINARY PROBLEMS

ROBLEMS WITH URINATING may be due to a minor infection or, more rarely, to a serious disorder, such as diabetes mellitus. If your child urinates more on some days than others, or if the urine color changes, this may not indicate a problem. If your child feels pain when urinating, consult your doctor.

SYMPTOM	POSSIBLE CAUSE	ACTION NEEDED
Does your child urinate frequently and feel sick or have a fever?	Urinary tract infection (*p.275*).	Call your doctor within 24 hours. **Self-help** Bringing down a temperature (*p.59 and p.171*).
Does your child feel pain when she urinates or have cloudy urine?	Urinary tract infection (*p.275*).	Call your doctor within 24 hours.
Is the color of your child's urine pink, red, or brown?	Glomerulonephritis (*p.276*) or urinary tract infection (*p.275*).	**Urgent!** Call your doctor immediately.
Does your child urinate often and in increased amounts, while also losing weight or being abnormally tired?	Diabetes mellitus (*p.309*).	Call your doctor within 24 hours.
Is her urine dark brown and clear, and her stools pale?	Hepatitis (*p.261*).	Call your doctor within 24 hours.
Is the color of your child's urine dark yellow, orange, or brown and clear, while her stools are normal?	Low fluid intake, vomiting, fever, or diarrhea concentrates the urine and thereby darkens it.	Give your child plenty to drink, especially if your child has had a fever or diarrhea (*p.172*).
Is the color of your child's urine green or blue?	Artificial coloring in food, drink, or medicine.	The coloring will soon pass out of your child's system naturally.
Is your child experiencing school difficulties, family problems, or a change of routine?	Anxiety (*pp.131–132*) or stress may result in your child using the toilet more often than usual.	If the problem does not clear up within a few days, call your doctor.
If your child urinates frequently, has she been taking any medicine recently?	Some drugs may cause frequent urination.	Ask your doctor if the medicine may be the cause and if you should stop giving it.

GENITAL PROBLEMS IN BOYS

BOYS OF ANY AGE CAN BE AFFECTED BY A PAIN or swelling in the penis or scrotum. They may also experience pain on urination or a discharge from the penis. Physical injuries to the genitals are most likely in boys of school age. If your son is suffering a severe or persistent genital pain, take him to see the doctor.

SYMPTOM	POSSIBLE CAUSE	ACTION NEEDED
Does your son have a painless swelling in the groin or scrotum?	Inguinal hernia (*see* Hernia, *p.260*) or hydrocele (*see* Penis and testis disorders, *p.277*).	Get medical advice within 24 hours.
If your son has a painful swelling in the groin or scrotum, has he just had an injury to his genitals?	Pain that does not subside following an injury may indicate damage to the testes.	**Urgent!** Call your doctor immediately.
If your son has a painful swelling in the groin or scrotum, has he had mumps in the past 2 weeks?	Orchitis (see Penis and testis disorders, *p.277*).	Get medical advice within 24 hours.
Does your son have a painful swelling in his groin or scrotum that is not the result of either an injury or a case of mumps?	Testicular torsion (*see* Penis and testis disorders, *p.277*) or strangulated inguinal hernia (*see* Hernia, *p.260*).	**Emergency!** Seek medical attention immediately. In the meantime, do not give your son anything to eat or drink.
Does your son have pain or a burning sensation on urinating?	Urinary tract infection (*p.275*).	Get medical advice within 24 hours.
Does your son have a swelling of the tip of his penis or a discharge from his foreskin?	Balanitis (*see* Penis and testis disorders, *p.277*).	Get medical advice within 24 hours.
Does your son have a grayish yellow discharge from his penis?	A foreign body in your son's urethra.	Consult your doctor.

GENITAL PROBLEMS IN GIRLS

ITCHING AND INFLAMMATION are the most common genital symptoms in girls. These may be painful or cause an abnormal vaginal discharge. Symptoms may be due to a fungal or bacterial infection. In some girls, irritation from scented soaps, bubble baths, or shampooing in the bathtub may cause the problem.

SYMPTOM	POSSIBLE CAUSE	ACTION NEEDED
If your daughter's genital area is itchy or sore, does she have a grayish yellow or greenish discharge from her vagina?	Infection of the vagina (*below and* Vulvovaginitis, *p.279*).	Get medical advice within 24 hours.
If your daughter's genital area is itchy or sore, does she have a thick white vaginal discharge?	Vaginal yeast and Vulvovaginitis, (*below and p.279*).	Get medical advice within 24 hours.
Is your daughter's genital area itchy or sore but without a discharge?	Poor hygiene, vulvovaginitis (*see below and p.279*), or pinworms (*p.262*).	Consult your doctor. **Self-help** Change her underwear daily, wash her vaginal area carefully, and avoid irritants.
If your daughter is over 10 years old, does she have a thin, white vaginal discharge?	Increased production of sex hormones at puberty.	If irritation accompanies the discharge, see your doctor.

SELF-HELP

Preventing vulvovaginitis

Teach girls basic hygiene for preventing vulvovaginitis and urinary tract infection. Your daughter should always wipe from front to back after going to the bathroom in order to avoid contaminating the bladder and vaginal opening with traces of stools. A few tablespoons of baking soda added to bathwater may relieve discomfort from vulvovaginitis.

You should encourage your daughter to wear cotton underpants. She should also avoid wearing tight-fitting pants and wearing leotards or wet swimsuits for a prolonged period of time. Some girls can avoid vulvovaginitis by taking showers rather than baths. If your daughter prefers baths, save soaps and shampoos until the end, and then be sure to rinse well with clean water.

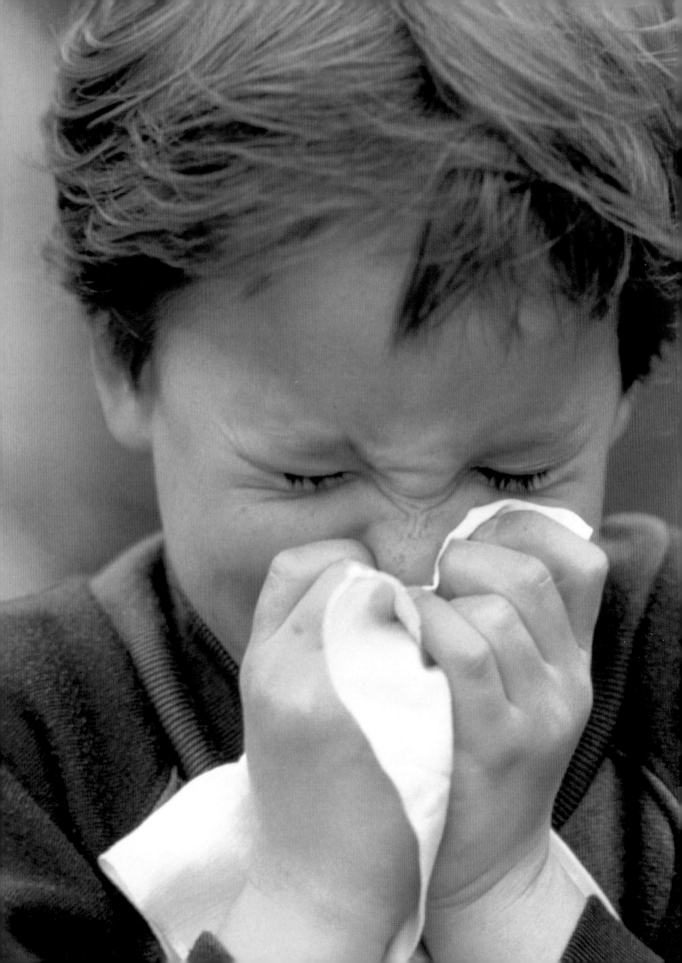

DISEASES
& DISORDERS

VISITING
THE DOCTOR
OR THE HOSPITAL

A LL CHILDREN GET SICK at some point. Most illnesses in children are minor,
but some serious conditions will require a trip to the hospital or emergency
room. Start building a good relationship with your doctor while your child
is healthy so that communication will be easier if she gets sick. Preparing for visits
to the doctor or the hospital can ease the way to a healthy recovery.

HAVING A GOOD RELATIONSHIP WITH YOUR CHILD'S DOCTOR

Don't wait until your child is sick
or needs a checkup to choose a
doctor. Find one as soon as you can,
whether you are having a new baby
or moving. Family doctors and
pediatricians are trained to prevent
and manage health problems in
infants, children, teens, and young
adults. A pediatrician is a specialist

in children's health. You can contact
a nearby hospital or provincial
medical association for a list of
doctors in your area.

Once you have a doctor, think
about getting the most out of your
visits. Bring to the appointment a list
of questions and record of facts, such
as what symptoms were noticed,
when an illness started, and how
eating, sleeping, or behavior may
have changed.

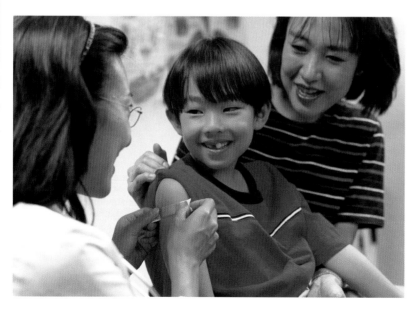

During the visit, make notes of
key points and ask your doctor
to explain anything you do not
understand. If you can, take a partner,
relative, or friend along with you to
your child's appointment. Having
another person to discuss it with
afterward may help you remember
what's been said.

If medication is prescribed, get
the full instructions on when and
how to administer it and ask about
any possible side effects. For further
information, talk to the pharmacist
when you fill the prescription.

You should always feel free to
contact your doctor's office, either
during office hours for routine
questions or at any time for an
emergency. Call right away if you
are worried about your child. Some
offices have special phone times for
nonurgent matters, while others
offer advice during and after office
hours. Find out in advance how
your doctor likes to handle routine
questions – by phone, via email, or
during appointments. If your doctor
will be calling you back, turn off any
call block features on your telephone
and keep phone lines open. Have a

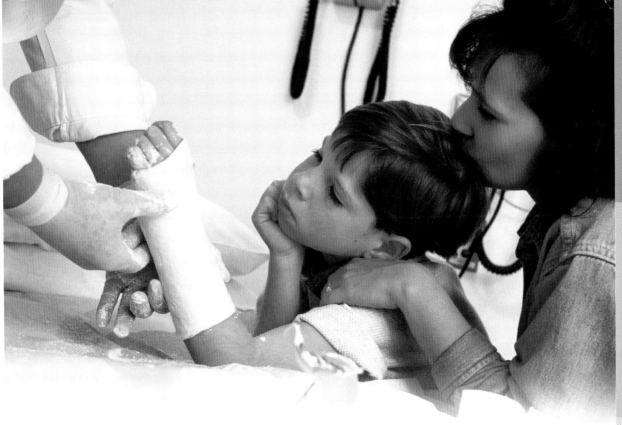

pen and paper ready to write down any instructions or questions. Be prepared to provide pertinent information such as your child's weight, temperature, symptoms, past medical problems, allergies, current medications, and your pharmacy's phone number.

PREPARING YOUR CHILD FOR A HOSPITAL STAY

If your child has a medical test or operation coming up, you can plan for it. Children who are prepared before a hospital stay tend to be less anxious, cope more effectively with medical problems, need less medication, and adapt more quickly to being back at home than children who have not been informed of what to expect. Think about how you present the subject. Children are very influenced by the reactions of their parents and if you have negative feelings about

hospitals, your child may pick this up and feel worried. It's often better to spread information out over a couple of days rather than give it all at once to help your child absorb it. Also, consider timing – if your child is younger or more anxious, leave less time between talking about the visit and the visit itself.

Find out as much as you can. Most hospitals have welcome booklets and many run preadmission tours that give you and your child the chance to look around, ask questions, and meet staff. Children may worry about an anesthetic and waking up afterward. If your child is concerned, ask to meet an anesthesiologist and visit the recovery room.

Be open and honest with your child as you describe, in terms he will understand, what will happen. Props may help younger children. Talk it through using a favorite doll or stuffed animal or play with a toy

doctor's bag so your child can see a stethoscope or blood pressure cuff. There are a lot of good books for different ages on preparing for a hospital visit, so it's worth a trip to a library or bookstore.

EMERGENCY TREATMENT

Since emergency situations are unplanned, preparing is more difficult. Every day in Canada, hundreds of children seek emergency treatment. Stay with your child to give him reassurance and comfort. As you meet members of the medical team, find out what will happen next so you can give your child a running commentary in terms he will understand.

When you get home, encourage your child to "play out" the situation, perhaps with a toy in the role of patient. Drawing and painting may help a child express feelings. With an older child, discuss the visit and see if you can detect any concerns.

RESPIRATORY PROBLEMS

YOUNG CHILDREN ARE PARTICULARLY LIKELY to catch colds and other disorders because they have not yet fully built up their immune systems. Allergic disorders, such as asthma and allergic rhinitis (hay fever), are the other main respiratory problems affecting children and asthma is becoming increasingly common. The best protection against respiratory problems is prevention: avoidance of tobacco smoke, good hand-washing, fresh air, a healthy diet, and plenty of exercise can boost your child's immune system and help him resist infection.

ANATOMY OF THE RESPIRATORY SYSTEM

▶ *HOW THE RESPIRATORY SYSTEM WORKS*

The respiratory system is made up of the lungs, air passages such as the nose and windpipe, and breathing muscles, including the diaphragm. The airways branch many times into small bronchioles that end in tiny air sacs, where the blood collects oxygen in exchange for carbon dioxide.

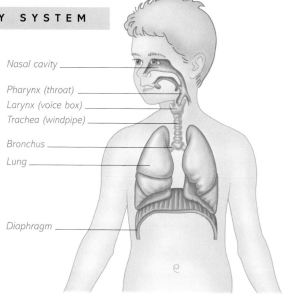

Nasal cavity

Pharynx (throat)

Larynx (voice box)

Trachea (windpipe)

Bronchus

Lung

Diaphragm

COMMON COLD

A viral infection of the nose and throat, the common cold is one of the most frequent illnesses in children. Most have at least six colds a year, more if they attend child care or preschool. Some otherwise healthy children have more than 10 colds a year.

Causes

The common cold can be caused by a range of different viruses. Immunity as a result of infection with one virus does not protect children against others, so they may get one cold followed by a different one.

Children attending school are particularly likely to catch colds because they are exposed to a wide variety of viruses to which they have not yet built up immunity. Cold viruses are spread in droplets that are sneezed or coughed out and then inhaled by others. The viruses may also be spread through direct contact with an infected person or object.

Medical treatment

Take your child to the doctor if her cough or fever has not improved after 5 days, other symptoms last longer than 10 days, or new symptoms develop.

Take your baby to see the doctor within 24 hours if she refuses feedings, has a fever over 39°C (102°F), or is very sick. A baby under 2 months should be seen right away if she has any of these symptoms.

How to help your child

Most colds will clear up on their own within a week. In the meantime, the following tips may help you make your child more comfortable.

Keep her room warm (but not too hot) and increase the moisture in the atmosphere with a humidifier or vaporizer. Give your child plenty of liquids to drink. A baby with a cold should be fed small amounts more frequently than usual. Giving ibuprofen or acetaminophen, at an appropriate dose for your child's age and weight, may relieve a fever and any accompanying aches.

Possible complications

A cold can spread down into the lungs, causing bronchiolitis (*see* p.228), bronchitis (*see* p.228), or pneumonia (*see* p.227). In some cases, these illnesses are complicated by another, secondary infection caused by bacteria.

The viral infection may also spread up the eustachian tubes and affect the ears, causing inflammation of the middle ear (*see* p.240), or the sinuses, causing sinusitis (*see below*). In children who have asthma (*see* p.226), a cold may be enough to trigger an attack.

⬛ SYMPTOMS

Symptoms start 1–3 days after infection.
- Tickly or scratchy feeling in the throat.
- Runny nose.
- Sneezing.
- Stuffy nose, which may make feeding difficult for a baby.
- Cough and sore throat.
- Watery eyes.
- Aching body.
- Possibly a fever.

SINUSITIS

This condition is an inflammation of the lining of the sinuses (air-filled cavities in the bones that surround the nose). The first indication of sinusitis may be symptoms of a common cold, such as a runny nose and coughing, that persist longer than usual.

Causes

Sinusitis is most often caused by bacterial infection following a cold when mucus produced in the sinuses traps bacteria.

Cilia, the tiny hairlike structures that project from the lining of the sinuses, normally move the mucus along until it drains through narrow passages into the nose and throat. However, if a viral infection such as a cold causes inflammation of the tissues, these passages may become blocked. Mucus then collects in the sinuses, blocking them and allowing bacteria to multiply.

⬛ SYMPTOMS

- Runny nose and a persistent nasal discharge.
- Feeling of fullness, or an ache or pain in the cheeks and sometimes the forehead.
- Cough.
- Headache.
- Possible severe pain in the upper back teeth.
- Loss of the sense of smell.
- Bad breath.
- Sometimes, fever.

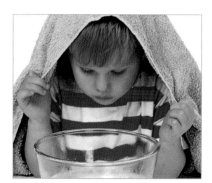

STEAM INHALATION *One way to relieve the congestion is to make a towel tent over your child's head. Ask your child to inhale the steam from a bowl of hot water.*

Medical treatment

Take your child to the doctor if nasal discharge lasts longer than 7 to 10 days. The doctor will examine him and, if sinusitis seems likely, may prescribe antibiotics and/or decongestants. With treatment, the symptoms of sinusitis usually clear up within a week.

How to help your child

If the sinusitis is painful, give your child ibuprofen or acetaminophen in the dose recommended by your doctor. Encourage him to drink plenty of fluids. Steam inhalation can relieve a stuffy nose rapidly. One way is to use a towel tent. Make sure he does not scald his face: place the bowl on a table, put the towel over his head. Tell him not to lean too close to the water. Do not leave him unsupervised. Do this a few times a day. Consult your doctor before adding any medication or oils to the water.

Alternatively, take your child into the bathroom, turn on the hot water to humidify the air, and encourage him to inhale. Keep the air in the house moist and let him walk in open air.

ENLARGED ADENOIDS

The adenoids are made of lymphatic tissue, which is rich in the white blood cells that help fight infection. In some children, they become enlarged following repeated infections and may hamper breathing or obstruct drainage of the middle ears.

Medical treatment

A child with mild symptoms does not usually need any treatment because the adenoids shrink naturally with age. But if your child has severe snoring or speech problems, or often has ear infections, take her to the doctor.

The doctor may refer your child to an ear, nose, and throat specialist, who may assess the size of the adenoids from an X-ray or by using a special scope to look at them.

Surgical removal of the adenoids, called an adenoidectomy, may be recommended. This is done at the hospital under a general anesthetic. The process allows the child to breathe more easily through her nose and stop snoring.

How to help your child

To relieve a dry mouth caused by persistent breathing through the mouth, moisten the air in your child's room with a humidifier or vaporizer. Encourage your child to sleep on her side or on her front to make snoring less likely.

Outlook

In children whose adenoids have not been surgically removed, the symptoms usually start to improve around the age of 7 – this is when the adenoids begin to shrink naturally. By the time your child has reached adolescence, the adenoids will probably have disappeared completely.

LOCATION OF ADENOIDS

The adenoids are pads of lymphatic tissue located at the back of the nasal cavity, beside the entrance to the eustachian tubes and above the tonsils.

SYMPTOMS

- Snoring.
- Waking frequently due to breathing problems, causing fatigue.
- Breathing through the mouth.
- Nasal voice.

Blocked eustachian tubes may cause ear infections (see Inflammation of the middle ear, p.240), which may lead to Otitis media with effusion (see p.241) and decreased hearing.

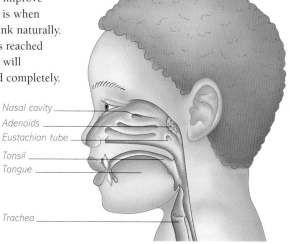

Nasal cavity

Adenoids

Eustachian tube

Tonsil

Tongue

Trachea

PHARYNGITIS AND TONSILLITIS

Often part of a common cold, pharyngitis is an inflammation of the throat and is the most common cause of a sore throat. Tonsillitis (inflammation of the tonsils) often occurs with pharyngitis in children.

Causes
Both conditions may be caused by either viruses or bacteria. Pharyngitis and tonsillitis have similar symptoms, although those of tonsillitis are usually more severe.

Medical treatment
If symptoms persist for more than 24 hours or get worse, call your doctor. She will examine your child and, if a bacterial infection is likely, may prescribe antibiotics. To confirm the diagnosis, the throat may be swabbed for analysis. Rare cases of an abscess on the tonsils may need surgical drainage.

How to help your child
Give ibuprofen or acetaminophen and fluids. She is most contagious just before the sore throat starts.

Outlook
Occasionally, surgical removal of the tonsils is recommended for children who have several bouts of tonsillitis a year due to confirmed streptococcal infections.

SWOLLEN TONSILS *In tonsillitis, the tonsils are swollen, fiery red, and sometimes flecked with yellow or white pus. Rarely, they get so enlarged they block the airway.*

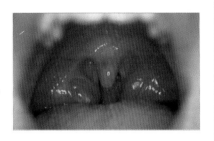

SYMPTOMS

- Sore, inflamed throat.
- Fever.
- Discomfort during swallowing (young children may refuse to eat).
- Enlarged, tender glands in the neck.
- Earache.
- In tonsillitis, red, swollen tonsils.

Symptoms usually disappear in 3 days. Rarely, an abscess may form around a tonsil, causing a high fever and increased difficulty swallowing.

EPIGLOTTITIS

Epiglottitis is inflammation of the epiglottis, the flap of cartilage at the entrance of the trachea that closes when a child swallows. It mainly affects children between 2 and 6 years old. It can be fatal, but immunization has lowered its incidence dramatically.

Causes
Epiglottitis is caused by the bacterium *Haemophilus influenzae*, which makes the epiglottis swell so much that the passage of air is obstructed.

Immediate action
If your child has difficulty swallowing and breathing, there is a risk that her airway may be completely obstructed. You should dial 911 or call EMS immediately or take her to a hospital emergency room. Keep your child calm. Don't try to look down your child's throat to see if something is blocking it, because she may start to cry. Crying will increase the production of secretions, which may totally block the narrowed airway.

Medical treatment
After examination, your child will be given antibiotics. In some cases, an anesthetic may be needed so a tube can be inserted through the nose and into the trachea. Children who are treated promptly make a complete recovery, usually within a week.

SYMPTOMS

- Difficulty and pain on swallowing.
- Drooling because the child cannot swallow her saliva.
- Fever.
- Noisy breathing that becomes quieter as the illness worsens.
- Increasing difficulty in breathing.
- Bluish discoloration of the tongue and sometimes the skin.
- Sits leaning forward to breathe better.

PREVENTION

Immunization against *Haemophilus influenzae* will very significantly reduce the risk of your child contracting epiglottitis.

CROUP

Croup is an inflammation and narrowing of the main airway to the lungs, usually caused by a viral infection. It is most common in children age 6 months–3 years. Although it is a mild illness, it can cause severe breathing difficulties needing emergency treatment. Croup starts like a cold with a runny nose and sneezing. Other symptoms develop a day or two later.

SYMPTOMS

- Noisy breathing.
- Persistent, barking cough.
- Hoarse voice.
- Breathing difficult or abnormally fast.
- Bluish tongue or lips; sometimes the skin is also bluish.

Croup tends to get worse at night and may last for a few days.

Immediate action
If your child is suffering from an attack of croup, with a barking cough that may be accompanied by stridor (noisy breathing) and shortness of breath, you should call your doctor immediately.

If you notice that your child's symptoms have gotten any worse, or if more severe symptoms develop, particularly a bluish tongue or lips, you should seek medical attention immediately.

Medical treatment
After checking how bad the attack is and considering other causes for your child's symptoms, the doctor may treat mild croup with steroids, either by

mouth or by an injection. Self-help measures (*see below*) may relieve the symptoms.

Children with a severe attack of croup may be admitted to a hospital. They may be given oxygen and medicated inhalations to ease breathing. If the airways are severely obstructed, a tube may be inserted through the nose or mouth into the trachea to help the child breathe. A child with severe croup usually takes a few days to recover.

How to help your child
At home, you should keep the air in your child's room moist, using a humidifier or vaporizer. To ease an acute attack, take her into the

bathroom and turn on the hot water to humidify the air rapidly and encourage your child to breathe.

Outlook
Most children do not suffer from a second attack of croup. However, some appear to be susceptible to the illness. For example, children with asthma (*see p.226*) in particular may be prone to further attacks, and for these children, doctors may recommend treatment with drugs for preventing asthma. Doctors may also prescribe corticosteroids, which can be taken at the first signs of an attack of croup.

ALLERGIC RHINITIS

This is an inflammation of the lining of the nose due to an allergic reaction. There are two forms: the seasonal variety, known as hay fever, affecting people during various seasons, while the perennial variety affects individuals throughout the year. Allergic rhinitis often runs in families and is most common in children with other allergies. Symptoms of both forms are similar.

SYMPTOMS

- Itchy eyes, nose, and throat.
- Stuffy, runny nose.
- Sneezing.
- Red, sore, watery eyes.
- Occasionally, dry skin.

Causes
Allergic rhinitis develops when a child inhales an allergen (a substance that causes an allergic reaction) and her immune system produces antibodies and white blood cells as if the allergen

were a bacterium or virus. The most common allergens are the pollen of grasses, trees, and weeds. Perennial allergic rhinitis is most often caused by dust mites, animal dander (flakes of animal skin), or mold spores.

Medical treatment
You should take your child to the doctor if she has severe or persistent symptoms that are not improved by self-help measures. The doctor may prescribe a nasal spray or oral

medication to alleviate the symptoms. In many children, the rhinitis becomes less severe as they grow older and eventually disappears.

How to help your child

If you know what causes the problem, try to reduce or eliminate exposure to it. A child who has hay fever should stay indoors as much as possible during the pollen season. Keep the windows closed, especially on hot, dry, breezy days, when pollen counts may be high.

If your child is allergic to animal dander, keep animals away from her.

If dust mites are causing the problem, keep house dust to a minimum. You can dust all surfaces with a damp cloth and treat carpets with an insecticide to kill the mites. You may want to enclose your child's mattress in a plastic cover and avoid down comforters and pillows.

If your child has an allergy to mold spores, you should make sure her bedroom is well ventilated and free of mold and dust. Oral antihistamines that are available over the counter may help if your child's hay fever is severe or if she cannot avoid going outside.

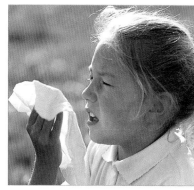

ALLERGIC RHINITIS *The delicate membranes of the eyes often suffer in an attack of allergic rhinitis. The eyes become red, itchy, and watery.*

INFLUENZA

A viral infection of the upper respiratory tract, influenza (flu) can affect children of all ages. The influenza virus is spread by coughing and sneezing, and by direct contact. There are small outbreaks of influenza every year.

Medical treatment

If your child is under 2 years of age or at a high risk of complications and has developed flu symptoms, call your doctor immediately. Also call a doctor immediately if any of the following symptoms develop:
a temperature above 39°C (102°F); abnormally fast breathing; drowsiness; or an unwillingness to eat.

If there is a secondary bacterial infection, the doctor may prescribe antibiotics. If the symptoms are severe, or if your child is at high risk of complications – for example, because of a chronic disorder – she may be admitted to a hospital.

How to help your child

The first 2–5 days of the illness are usually the worst. Most cases of flu clear up within about 10 days. Keep your child in bed in a warm, well-

ventilated, humidified room until her temperature returns to normal. Give her the appropriate dose of ibuprofen or acetaminophen for the aches and fever and plenty of warm fluids.

Possible complications

The flu virus may spread down to the lungs, causing pneumonia (*see p.227*) or bronchitis (*see p.228*). These are often complicated by secondary bacterial infection. This infection may also affect the sinuses (*see* Sinusitis, *p.221*) or ears (*see* Inflammation of the middle ear, *p.240*).

Disorders that put children at high risk for influenza include chronic heart, lung, or kidney disease; diabetes mellitus (*see p.309*); cystic fibrosis (*see p.315*); or a depressed immune system. Febrile seizures (*see p.292*) are a possible complication in babies and young children.

ASTHMA

Asthma causes periodic episodes of wheezing and shortness of breath. It is the most common chronic lung disease among children and is increasing. Most children who develop asthma have had their first attack by the age of 4 or 5. Untreated, asthma may slow a child's growth and reduce her capacity to exercise. In young children, the first sign is often a recurring cough, especially with a cold or after exercise. The first sign of asthma sometimes is coughing that occurs only at night.

SYMPTOMS

- Wheezing.
- Shortness of breath.
- Tightness in the chest.

During severe attacks of asthma, the symptoms may include:
- Difficult and noisy breathing.
- Difficulty speaking.
- Drowsiness.
- Disturbed sleep.
- Blue lips or tongue.
- Refusal to eat or drink.

Causes

Some asthmatic children have other allergic conditions, such as allergic rhinitis (*see p.224*) or eczema (*see p.234*). There may be a family history of asthma and other allergic disorders. Individual attacks are usually triggered by a viral infection or an allergen, such as dust mites or, more rarely, a particular food. Exercising, especially in cold air, may bring on an asthma attack. Emotional triggers such as anxiety, stress, sadness, excitement, and others may cause or worsen attacks. Other asthma triggers include tobacco smoke, acid reflux, mold, fragrances, and other chemicals.

Asthma symptoms are caused by narrowing of the airways in the lungs: the trachea, bronchi, and bronchioles. This occurs because the walls of these airways become inflamed and swollen, the muscle walls contract, and more mucus is produced.

Medical treatment

If you think your child has asthma, take him to the doctor within 24 hours. If the symptoms are severe, immediately dial 911 or call EMS or take your child to the nearest hospital emergency room. The doctor will ask about any possible exposure to triggering factors.

To check the severity of your child's condition, the doctor may use a peak-flow meter, which measures the capacity to exhale air. A chest X ray may be carried out to check for any associated infection.

If your child's asthma is mild, the doctor will prescribe a bronchodilator drug – this is a drug that dilates, or widens, the bronchi and bronchioles. The bronchodilator is inhaled to ease the child's breathing during asthma attacks.

If the asthma is more severe, the doctor may also prescribe other drugs for quick relief. Some children require corticosteroids or regular treatment with an inhaled, long-acting bronchodilator drug to prevent future asthmatic attacks.

A spacer (*see left*) should be used to inhale the drugs given by inhaler. Some children may need to use a nebulizer which disperses the drug as a fine mist at higher concentrations.

How to help your child

For a child ages 6 years or over, the doctor may suggest using a peak-flow meter to monitor the child's asthma and to warn you of an impending attack. You should keep an asthma

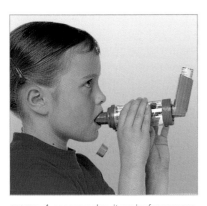

SPACER *A spacer makes it easier for younger children to inhale the drug, which is usually delivered as a spray. The spacer holds the drug before it is inhaled. Always supervise a child who is using an inhaler.*

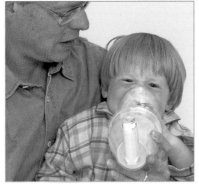

MASK *A spacer with a mask may be used for younger children. The mask fits snugly against the face, covering the nose and mouth to deliver the medication properly.*

diary to keep a record of symptoms and chart the peak-flow meter readings from day to day. This record will help the doctor adapt your child's treatment as the asthma changes, develops, or subsides.

You should always keep a bronchodilator handy in case your child has an attack. If your child has a severe attack of asthma, and the normal inhaler does not work, she should take a repeat dose. If the repeat dose also fails to ease the condition, you will need to call your doctor or seek medical care immediately.

Outlook
At least half of the children who develop asthma will stop having attacks by the time they reach adulthood. Effective treatment can help control symptoms of asthma, keep children from missing school, and allow them to take part in normal physical activity.

PNEUMONIA

Pneumonia is an inflammation of the lungs, usually caused by a viral or bacterial infection. It is most often a complication of an upper respiratory tract infection, such as a common cold, or of an infectious disease, such as chickenpox. Children with cystic fibrosis (see p.315) are particularly prone to pneumonia. Pneumonia may start with symptoms of a common cold, such as sneezing and a runny nose.

Immediate action
Call your doctor immediately if your child is breathing fast while resting; if a cough and fever last for more than a few days; or if your child seems far more ill than usual with an ordinary cold. Dial 911 or call EMS if your child is drowsy, refuses to eat or drink, or has blue lips and tongue.

Medical treatment
The doctor will listen to your child's chest through a stethoscope and may send a throat swab or blood sample for tests to identify an infection. She may prescribe antibiotics.

Pneumonia can usually be treated at home, but if your child's condition is severe, a hospital stay may be required. A chest X-ray can confirm the diagnosis of pneumonia. Your child may receive oxygen; rarely,

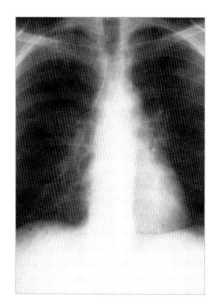

CHEST X-RAY Pneumonia causes some air sacs in the lungs to fill with fluid. A dense, white area on an X-ray can confirm the diagnosis.

mechanical ventilation will be required. Your child should be able to go home after a few days. She may continue to have a cough for a few weeks after she has otherwise recovered. Pneumonia should not result in any permanent damage to the lungs.

How to help your child
Make sure she has plenty of warm fluids to drink. Ibuprofen or acetaminophen can reduce her fever and relieve a headache. Most children recover within a week. After discharge from the hospital, your child should not do any vigorous exercise for about a week. Going outside will not harm your child.

BRONCHITIS

Bronchitis is an inflammation of the bronchi (the larger airways of the lungs). The condition is usually a complication of a viral infection such as a common cold or influenza, but is sometimes caused by a bacterial infection.

- Runny nose.
- Persistent cough. Usually dry at first, but may later produce yellowish green phlegm if there is a bacterial infection.
- Wheezing and shortness of breath.
- Sometimes, a fever.

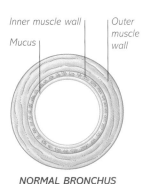

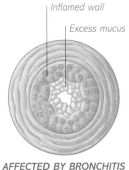

Inner muscle wall

Outer muscle wall

Mucus

Inflamed wall

Excess mucus

NORMAL BRONCHUS

AFFECTED BY BRONCHITIS

THE EFFECTS ON THE AIRWAYS
In bronchitis, the walls of the bronchi become inflamed, and the glands that line the walls produce excess mucus (see cross-sections, left). The central air channel is narrowed, making breathing difficult.

How to help your child

Keep your child's room moist. Steam inhalations may help decongest her airways. Give warm drinks to relieve the cough and acetaminophen or ibuprofen to reduce a fever. Most children recover fully within a week. If she does not improve after 24 hours, call your doctor – but call immediately if breathing becomes abnormally fast or the fever rises above 39°C (102°F). Seek immediate medical care if she is drowsy or becomes dehydrated.

Medical treatment

If your child is displaying symptoms of bronchitis, she will be examined by your doctor to see if she has a more serious condition, such as pneumonia or bronchiolitis. The doctor may prescribe antibiotics if a bacterial infection is suspected and your child may need a bronchodilator drug to relieve the wheezing.

BRONCHIOLITIS

This viral infection inflames the bronchioles (the smallest airways of the lungs). It may start like a common cold, usually occurs in epidemics during winter, and mainly affects children under 3 years. It can be more severe in babies born prematurely.

- Increased nasal mucus and congestion.
- Dry, rasping cough.
- Wheezing and/or rapid, difficult breathing. In some infants, long pauses (more than 10 seconds) occur between each breath.
- Reluctance to feed.
- Bluish lips and tongue.
- Abnormal drowsiness.

Immediate action

If your child is under 1 year and is coughing and/or wheezing, call your doctor immediately. Dial 911 or call EMS if breathing is difficult, if the lips and tongue are blue, or if your child becomes drowsy.

Medical treatment

For mild bronchiolitis, the doctor may prescribe a bronchodilator drug and advise you to treat your child at home. Give her plenty of fluids and frequent small meals. The recommended dose of acetaminophen or ibuprofen can help bring down a fever. Mild cases usually improve within about a week.

A child who needs to be treated in the hospital may be given oxygen. She may need to be fed by a tube inserted through the nose or, sometimes, intravenously. In severe cases, mechanical ventilation may be required. The child will be allowed to go home when she is able to breathe and feed normally again, usually within 7 days. The cough, however, may persist for up to 6 weeks.

Outlook

Bronchiolitis may recur, usually with a different virus. Some children may cough and wheeze with subsequent colds, especially if there is a family history of asthma or allergies. As children get older, they are at lower risk for developing bronchiolitis.

SKIN DISORDERS

TINY YELLOW-WHITE SPOTS OFTEN APPEAR on the faces of newborn children and young babies, but they soon vanish. In the first couple of days, many newborn babies develop a red blotchy rash, called erythema toxicum, on the face, chest, and back. This, too, soon goes away. For the next few years, until their skin becomes less sensitive, children are prone to skin disorders. For example, a skin reaction may be caused by an illness such as chickenpox or by irritation from detergents or other substances. Infections (*see also* Infectious Diseases, *pp.263–272*) and allergies can also cause skin reactions. Most of the skin problems that affect children aren't too serious and usually clear up rapidly. This section may help you find out what is causing the disorder – the diagnosis charts between pages 180 and 187 could also help you. If you are in any doubt, check with your doctor.

SEBORRHEIC DERMATITIS

This common inflammation of the skin may affect the scalp, face, and body. Its cause is unknown but it may initially appear in the first few months of life. The symptoms vary in severity over a number of months, but generally clear up by the age of 2.

Medical treatment

Check with your doctor if the rash is extensive, looks infected, or fails to improve in a few weeks; the scalp is inflamed; or other symptoms develop. He may prescribe a mild corticosteroid cream or a non-steroid cream.

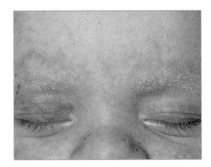

RASH ON A BABY'S FACE *Seborrheic dermatitis can affect the skin on any part of the head, including the scalp, as in cradle cap, and even the eyelids.*

How to help your child

As soon as the symptoms appear, clean the affected areas of your child's skin with an emulsifying ointment, not soap. Then apply a mild corticosteroid cream. Try to keep your child from scratching the affected skin because this can lead to a bacterial infection, such as impetigo (*see p.235*), causing the rash to become raw and ooze.

Cradle cap often disappears on its own within a few weeks or months. You can remove thick scales by gently massaging baby oil or olive oil into your baby's scalp and leaving it overnight. The next day, comb your baby's hair to dislodge the softened scales and then wash them away.

Over-the-counter shampoos with selenium sulfide may control cradle cap. Regular use of a special shampoo or combing your baby's hair daily may

SYMPTOMS

Infants
- A scaly, blotchy rash, usually in the skin creases of the neck, armpits, or diaper area.
- Sometimes slight itchiness.
- Thick yellowish scales on the scalp (cradle cap) and sometimes scaly areas on the forehead, behind the ears, and in the eyebrows.

Puberty
- A scaly, blotchy rash occurs on the face; behind the ears; on the neck, chest, and back; and in the armpits and groin.
- Sometimes, itchiness.
- Dandruff, if the scalp is affected. Greasy flakes of skin can be seen in the hair, usually at the hairline.

stop the scaly patches from forming. Use over-the-counter antidandruff shampoos to control dandruff.

Some children with seborrheic dermatitis may develop eczema. This condition may recur during puberty.

CONTACT DERMATITIS

This dermatitis is an inflammation of the skin caused by contact with irritating substances such as nickel in jewelry, rubber, fabric dyes, adhesive bandages, plants, bubble baths, medicinal creams, detergents, and cosmetics.

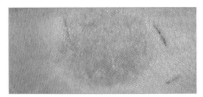

CONTACT DERMATITIS *The symptoms may take several days to appear after contact; how long they persist depends on the irritant.*

Medical treatment

A rash caused by something such as jewelry may be confined to one part of the body. If products such as bubble bath or scented soap are the cause, the rash may be more widespread.

If you know the cause, remove it or restrict your child's contact with it. An over-the-counter corticosteroid

SYMPTOMS

- An inflamed, scaly rash.
- Intense itchiness.
- Sometimes, blistering and oozing (often caused by contact with plants).

cream or calamine lotion may help relieve the symptoms. If you cannot identify the cause, see your doctor. He may arrange for some tests – small amounts of a range of suspected irritants are applied to your child's skin to see if there's a reaction.

COLD SORES

Cold sores are small blisters that develop singly or in clusters on and around a child's lips. Smaller and more regular in shape than impetigo sores, they may be brought on by fever, acute infection, anxiety or emotional stress, or exposure to sun or cold winds.

Causes

Cold sores are caused by a strain of the herpes simplex virus. After the first infection, which may go unnoticed, the virus lies dormant in nerve cells until it is reactivated.

How to help your child

The blisters burst within a few days to form a crust, and heal on their own within 2 weeks. Few children need treatment, but if the sores cause discomfort, a cold drink or popsicle may bring relief.

If your child gets cold sores often, or if they are severe and upsetting, consult your doctor. A prescription cream, ointment, or oral medication containing an antiviral drug may

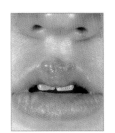

COLD SORE CLUSTER *Cold sores often appear in clusters on or around the lips. The blisters are clear at first; they turn cloudy and form crusts.*

reduce the severity and duration of an attack. These are most effective when used as soon as your child feels the initial tingling sensation around the mouth, before blisters appear. Over-the-counter preparations may also help ease discomfort.

If you can identify the trigger, you may be able to prevent the sores. For example, if they tend to develop after

□ **SYMPTOMS**

- A tingling feeling around the mouth, which starts 4–12 hours before any blisters appear.
- Small blisters, which may be itchy or sore and surrounded by a slightly inflamed area.

exposure to the sun, apply a sunscreen or sunblock to your child's lips before he goes outside.

To reduce the chance of spreading the virus, both to other people and to other parts of your child's body, explain that he should not touch the blisters or suck his fingers, and should wash his hands frequently.

Outlook

With no cure for cold sores, your child may have recurrences throughout life, but outbreaks usually become less frequent with time.

WARTS

Warts are harmless growths on the skin, usually on the hands and feet, caused by a virus. They are contagious, but some people are more susceptible than others. Most disappear naturally within a few months, while some last for years if they are not treated.

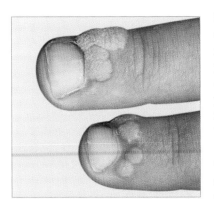

Medical treatment

Consult your doctor if home treatment is unsuccessful or if a wart causes your child either discomfort or embarrassment. The doctor may refer your child to a dermatologist, who may remove the warts by freezing, a technique known as cryotherapy.

COMMON WART *These hard, rough growths on the surface of the skin may be frozen off by a physician.*

□ **TYPES**

There are several types of wart, any of which may occur singly or in clusters. The ones that most often affect children are:

- Common warts. These are firm, raised growths, usually with a hard, rough surface. They generally occur on the hands, feet, knees, and face.
- Plane (flat) warts. These are smooth growths level with the skin or slightly raised. They occur on the hands or face and may cause slight itchiness.
- Plantar warts. These hard, horny warts occur on the sole of the foot. They appear flat and are often painful because the child's weight has pushed them into the skin.

Plantar warts (*see p.193*) may be scraped off in a technique known as curettage.

How to help your child

It is important that you tell your child not to touch the warts because picking or scratching may cause them to spread to another part of the body. If you do want to do something about the warts, you can treat warts on the hands and feet at home. However, you should never attempt to remove a wart that is located on your child's mouth or face.

The simplest way of treating your child's common or plane wart is to cover the wart with a salicylic acid bandage. The bandage should be changed every day. If the wart does not respond to this treatment within about 3 weeks, you can try applying a wart medication available over the counter; be sure to follow the instructions carefully. You can protect the unaffected skin around the wart by covering it with a layer of petroleum jelly before you apply the medication.

If your child has a plantar wart, you can rub the the surface of the wart with a pumice stone to remove as much of the thick overlying skin as possible. Cut a piece of salicylic acid bandage to the exact size of the wart and tape it in place over the wart. You should replace the bandage every day until the wart disappears, which may take up to 3 months. You should consult your doctor if you are considering this or other remedies for treating a wart.

Outlook

Eventually, most warts will disappear on their own without any treatment. However, warts do sometimes recur for no apparent reason, even after you have treated them. You may need to apply several treatments to such persistent warts in order to eliminate them entirely.

SCABIES

Scabies is caused by infestation of the skin by parasitic mites. Anyone can catch scabies – it has nothing to do with a lack of personal hygiene. Both extremely itchy and very contagious, scabies is passed from person to person by close bodily contact, and, to a lesser extent, through the sharing of infected sheets and blankets, clothes, and towels.

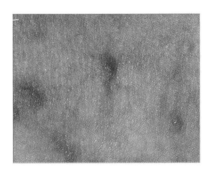

SCABIES MITE BURROW *Thin, gray lines on the skin are the burrows made by female mites. Burrows may be obscured by sores and scabs caused by scratching.*

Causes

Scabies is caused by the mite *Sarcoptes scabiei*, also known as the itch mite. The female mites burrow into the skin to lay their eggs. This causes the intense itching. The eggs hatch in 3 or 4 days and reach adulthood in about two weeks, when they mate again on the skin and the cycle begins once more. The symptoms of scabies may take up to 6 weeks to appear after infection occurs.

Medical treatment

If your child is scratching intensely or shows any other signs of scabies, take him to the doctor within 24 hours. Scabies will not clear up without treatment and scratching may cause impetigo (*see p.235*). The doctor will prescribe a medication that kills scabies mites. After a bath, apply this lotion to your child's body from the

> **SYMPTOMS**
>
> • Intense itchiness, especially at night.
> • Thin, gray lines (the mites' burrows) between the fingers, on the wrists, in the armpits, between the buttocks, or around the genitals. In infants, the palms and soles may be affected.
> • Sores, blisters, and scabs, resulting from scratching.
> • Inflamed bumps on the body.

neck down including the soles of the feet. Wash it off after 8 to 14 hours. Treat all members of your household at the same time, even if they have no obvious signs. After treatment, wash and dry all clothing and bed linen using the hottest setting.

The mites will usually die within 3 days of treatment, but the itching may continue for up to 2–3 weeks. The doctor may prescribe a medication to relieve the itchiness. Tell any people you and your child have been in contact with, so that they can be examined, and treated if necessary.

BOILS

A painful, pus-filled swelling in the skin, a boil develops when bacteria infect a hair follicle. Most burst, releasing their pus, although occasionally pus drains away into the surrounding area. Boils generally clear up in two weeks.

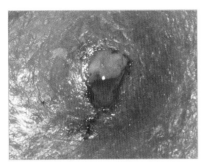

APPEARANCE OF A BOIL *The lump covered by white flakes of dead skin is a boil. Pus has escaped to form a greenish scab at its center. The surrounding skin is red because the infection has spread outside the follicle.*

Medical treatment
If your child has a boil that lasts longer than 2 weeks or is very large or painful, you should take her to see your doctor. The doctor may prescribe oral antibiotics to clear up the infection and may make a small cut in the boil to release pus.

If your child continues to get boils, the doctor may prescribe an antibiotic cream for you to apply to areas such as the inside of the nose. The doctor may also suggest that you have your child wash with antibacterial soap.

> **SYMPTOMS**
>
> - A small, red lump that becomes larger as it fills with pus.
> - Pain and tenderness around the boil.
> - A white or yellow "head" of pus at the center of the boil.

How to help your child
To help a boil drain more quickly, apply a warm compress to it several times a day. When the boil does drain, you should carefully wipe away the pus with a cotton ball soaked in an antiseptic solution and cover the affected skin with a bandage. Don't poke or squeeze the boil to make it burst or you may spread the infection. Tell your child not to poke it either. (*See* Treating a boil, *p.185.*)

URTICARIA

An intensely itchy, raised rash, urticaria is also known as hives. There are two forms: acute urticaria, which lasts between 30 minutes and several days, and chronic urticaria, which may persist for up to several months. Both may recur.

Causes
In many cases, the cause of urticaria is not known. Sometimes urticaria may be caused by an allergic reaction, possibly to a food (such as fish), an insect sting, a drug (such as penicillin), or a plant. The rash may affect a small area or it may be widespread.

Very rarely, urticaria is part of anaphylactic shock (*see p.189*). You should seek medical treatment immediately if your child has swelling of the face or mouth, noisy or difficult breathing, difficulty swallowing, and abnormal drowsiness.

Medical treatment
If your child often has attacks of urticaria, try to identify the cause so you can help your child avoid it, if at all possible. An oral antihistamine may relieve the symptoms during an attack – your doctor may advise you to continue this treatment for up to several weeks after the rash disappears.

If antihistamines do not help the attacks, you should notify the doctor, who may prescribe an oral corticosteroid or obtain tests to establish the cause. As your child gets older, attacks of urticaria will probably become less frequent.

> **SYMPTOMS**
>
> - Smooth, raised pale welt surrounded by an inflamed area of skin.
> - Extreme itchiness.

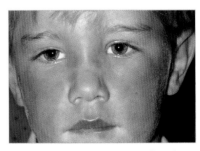

URTICARIAL RASH *The patches of affected skin in urticaria vary in size and shape. The patches are raised and pale and have red edges, which distinguish them from the surrounding normal skin.*

ECZEMA (ATOPIC DERMATITIS)

About 1 child in 20 develops eczema. The itchy rash usually appears for the first time before a child is 18 months old, and may come and go over a number of years. The cause is unknown, but most affected children have a close relative with eczema or an allergic disorder, such as asthma or hay fever. Intolerance to certain foods may also be responsible.

Medical treatment

If your child has not had the rash before, take him to the doctor. If your child has already been diagnosed with eczema, and the rash does not respond to treatment or gets worse, call your doctor in case the rash has become infected.

The doctor may prescribe a mild corticosteroid cream or ointment to reduce the inflammation and itching during flare-ups. It is particularly important to use corticosteroid creams as directed and to stop when the skin has recovered. If the itching is keeping your child awake at night, he may be given an antihistamine. Emollient creams to moisten the skin are important and should be used liberally. Alternatives to soap may also be prescribed. If the eczema is severe or widespread, the doctor may suggest that your child stop eating certain foods, although this is usually not helpful or necessary.

How to help your child

Use creams or ointments as directed by your doctor and try the following tips to keep your child's skin from becoming too dry.

When you bathe your child, use a mild cleanser such as a moisturizing cream or fragrance-free soap. You may want to add a bath oil that is specially formulated for eczema, but do not use scented bubble bath or soap.

Keep your child's skin soft and well moisturized by regularly applying an emollient, such as a moisturizing cream or ointment, particularly to warm, wet skin after a bath. Use the emollient several times a day on the affected areas.

In some children, eczema is worse in cold weather, while in others hot weather prompts a flare-up. Wearing cotton clothing next to the skin can help reduce irritation.

Keep your child away from anyone who has cold sores. Don't give him peanuts, or let him use creams or bath oils containing peanut oil.

Possible complications

If your child scratches the rash, the skin may become infected, resulting in oozing blisters. Your doctor may then prescribe an antibiotic.

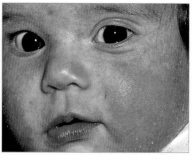

APPEARANCE OF ECZEMA *The rash seen here has the typical appearance of eczema in children under the age of 4 years: the skin is inflamed and may ooze slightly. The cheeks are one of the prime sites for the rash to develop.*

▣ SYMPTOMS

Children under 4 years
- Itchy, inflamed skin, which may ooze slightly.
- Worst on scalp, cheeks, forearms, fronts of the legs, and trunk, although the rash may appear anywhere on the child's body.

Children aged 4–10 years
- Itchy, dry, and scaly patches, as well as cracked skin.
- Worst on face, neck, insides of the elbows, wrists, backs of the knees, and ankles.
- Skin in affected areas may become thickened over time.

Eczema herpeticum is a rare, but more serious, complication. It can develop if a child with eczema is infected by the herpes simplex virus (*see* Cold sores, *p.231*). This disorder causes a widespread rash of blisters and open sores, sometimes accompanied by a high fever of 40–41°C (104–106°F). The child's lymph nodes may be enlarged. If your child has eczema herpeticum, she may have to go to a hospital and may be given the antiviral drug acyclovir orally or intravenously.

Outlook

In young children, the rash often disappears before they reach 4 years and may never come back. In other children, the rash may reappear (or appear for the first time) between the ages of 4 and 10 years. As your child grows older, the rash will probably be less extensive and it will probably disappear by adolescence. However, up to 50 percent of children who are affected by eczema develop other allergic conditions as well, such as asthma.

MOLLUSCUM CONTAGIOSUM

This mild viral infection, which causes small, shiny bumps on the skin, is common in children between 2 and 5 years of age. It is easily spread, either by direct contact or indirectly – for example, by touching the skin of an infected person.

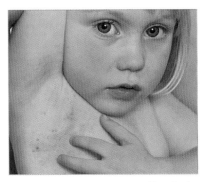

MOLLUSCUM CONTAGIOSUM PIMPLES *The pimples usually appear on a child's skin in groups, although they may occur singly.*

SYMPTOMS

The bumps appear 2–7 weeks after infection, usually on the trunk, face, hands, and (rarely) palms or soles. The bumps are:
- Dome-shaped with a central dimple.
- Pearly white or flesh-colored.

Medical treatment

The characteristic appearance of the bumps can be confirmed by your doctor. They will disappear without treatment and usually leave no scars, but this can take a few weeks to a few years. Most children have about 25 lesions. Open lesions let the virus spread to other parts of the body.

If your child is receiving treatment that affects her immune system – for example, for leukemia – the bumps can be more widespread and last longer. If your child has lowered immunity or many disfiguring bumps on a visible area, such as the face, your doctor may refer her to a dermatologist to remove the growths.

After applying an anesthetic cream to the area, the dermatologist may pierce the pimples with an instrument dipped in podophyllin paint. Alternatively, he may remove the lesions by scraping or by freezing.

IMPETIGO

A highly contagious bacterial skin infection, impetigo mainly affects young children, including babies. It may appear anywhere on the body, but is most common around the mouth and nose area in children, and the diaper area in babies.

Causes

Bacteria enter and infect the skin when it is broken by a cut, an insect bite, or a skin condition such as eczema (*see opposite*) or scabies (*see p.232*).

Medical treatment

Take your child to the doctor within 24 hours if you suspect impetigo. The doctor may prescribe an antibiotic ointment to be put on the sores, or an oral antibiotic, if the infection is widespread.

How to help your child

Before applying the ointment, gently dab the crusts with gauze soaked in warm water and then dry the area to remove them. With treatment, impetigo usually gets better within about 5 days.

Tell your child not to touch the sores to stop the infection from spreading. Keep his bedding, towels, and washcloth separate, and keep him away from other children until the infection has cleared up. Encourage him to shower or bathe daily. Keep his nails short and clean so that infection is less likely to be introduced through scratching. If your child has a cold or a runny nose, apply a little petroleum jelly to the nose and upper lip to keep constant wiping from breaking the skin.

SYMPTOMS

- First, the skin reddens and crops of small blisters appear.
- The blisters then burst, leaving raw, moist sores that gradually enlarge.
- Honey-colored crusts form as the surface of the sores dries.

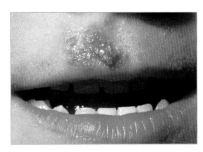

IMPETIGO *Impetigo sores are not painful, although they may be slightly itchy. Without treatment, the condition may last for weeks, or even months.*

HEAD LICE

Small, flat, wingless insects, head lice live on the scalp and feed on blood. Children catch them easily through direct contact with classmates or by sharing hats or combs. They are not associated with poor hygiene.

Checking for head lice
If you think your child has lice, check his hair. The eggs (nits) are more easily seen than the small and almost transparent adults. After the insects hatch, the empty nit shells can be seen as small white bumps near the bases of the hairs. If you wet your child's hair and comb it with a fine-toothed comb over a white piece of paper, you may see the lice crawling. If your child does have head lice, check the rest of the family and tell his school.

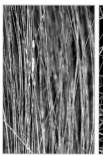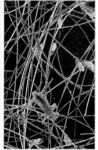

HEAD LICE AND EGGS *The tiny, white ovals are louse eggs. They are firmly attached to the hair shafts. Several head lice are also visible clinging to hairs.*

How to help your child
You can treat head lice without a doctor's advice, but if your child is less than 2 years old or has allergies, talk to your doctor before using lice preparations.

To eradicate the head lice, wash his hair with a special shampoo or lotion from the drugstore (*see p.183*). Some can be applied once; others must be applied repeatedly over several days.

Because head lice are highly contagious, all family members and contacts should be examined and possibly treated to get rid of the lice completely and to prevent your child from becoming reinfested. Wash and dry clothing, linens, and other items that have come into contact with your child's head.

Preventing head lice
To reduce your child's chances of catching lice, discourage him from sharing hats, combs, and brushes with family members or friends. If there is an outbreak at your child's school, examine your child or see your doctor if you are concerned.

RINGWORM

Ringworm (or tinea) is a fungal infection that affects the scalp or the skin of the body or face. Children can catch it directly from other people, an animal, or soil. They can also acquire it indirectly from hats, combs, clothing, or household items, such as carpets.

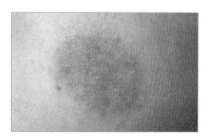

RINGWORM *The fungi can infect any part of the body but they particularly thrive in the damp and warm areas.*

Medical treatment
Take your child to the doctor if you suspect ringworm. For infections on the body or face, the doctor may recommend an antifungal lotion or cream. If the infection on your child's body or face is very widespread, or if her scalp is affected, your doctor may prescribe an oral antifungal medicine.

To help prevent your child from developing ringworm, keep her away from infected people or animals, and discourage the sharing of personal items, such as combs.

ACNE

Acne consists of bumps, whiteheads, or blackheads on the face, chest, back, and/or arms. It is most common in adolescents and tends to appear at the onset of puberty. It often runs in families and is usually more common and severe in boys than in girls.

Causes
At puberty, the skin produces more oily sebum. Acne lesions develop when excess sebum and, sometimes, dead skin cells form a plug that blocks a hair follicle. Trapped bacteria multiply, causing the skin around the follicle to become inflamed. Oily substances on the skin, such as cosmetics or hair oil, may make the problem worse.

How to help your child
In order to prevent the bacteria from spreading, your child should not pick, squeeze, or scrub the lesions. You should encourage him to wash his face twice daily with soap and water, and then apply an over-the-counter acne product to the affected areas. These preparations are available in different strengths – your child should try the mildest first and follow the instructions precisely. As a self-help measure, you may find that exposure to sunlight helps clear up the acne.

If this treatment does not improve the acne after 2–3 months, you should take your child to your doctor or dermatologist, who may prescribe oral antibiotics. Each course may last a few months or longer. The doctor may prescribe a retinoid drug. Dryness, peeling, or itching of the skin being treated are possible side effects of the drug treatment.

◻ SYMPTOMS

- Pimples (small, raised red spots).
- Blackheads (tiny black spots).
- Whiteheads (tender, inflamed lumps with a white center).
- Cysts (fluid-filled swellings).
- Purplish marks left by healed spots, which gradually fade.

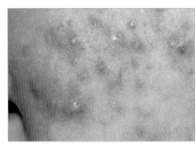

ACNE AFFECTING THE FACE *These lesions are typical of acne. The slightly indented purplish marks on the skin are the result of areas that have healed.*

PITYRIASIS ROSEA

A rash of flat, scaly spots, pityriasis rosea generally affects the trunk, arms, and legs and is most common in adolescents. Although no specific virus has been isolated, it is believed to be caused by a viral infection.

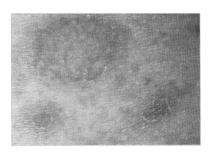

PITYRIASIS ROSEA *The rash first appears on the trunk, running along the lines of the ribs. It may then spread up toward the neck and down along the arms and legs.*

Medical treatment
Although it is not a serious rash and usually gets better without treatment, take your child to the doctor within a few days to make sure there is not a more serious skin disease. A corticosteroid cream may soothe any itching, but if it is severe, the doctor may prescribe an oral antihistamine.

Pityriasis rosea generally takes between 3 and 8 weeks to clear up. Once your child has had the rash, she is unlikely to develop it again.

◻ SYMPTOMS

- An initial spot (the herald patch) is oval or round, flat, and scaly.
- Flat, oval, copper-colored or dark pink spots, which appear 3–10 days after the herald patch. After a week, each lesion develops a scaly edge.
- Occasionally, itchiness.

How to help your child
The rash usually fades below the elbows and knees and seldom appears on the face. Whenever possible, keep the skin cool and moisturize the areas of skin affected by the rash. You may find that sunlight helps clear up the rash more rapidly.

PSORIASIS

This chronic skin condition rarely affects children under the age of 10. The rash may itch and can be uncomfortable. Its appearance may upset your child. It tends to vary in severity and often gets worse during illness or emotional stress.

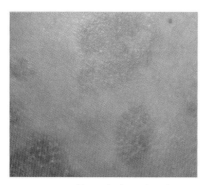

PSORIASIS RASH *The rash shown here is characteristic of psoriasis. The affected area of skin is a sharply defined red patch which is raised and covered by silvery-white scales of dead skin. A large patch such as this may appear on areas of a child's body, such as the elbows or knees.*

Medical treatment

Psoriasis cannot be cured and is likely to recur, but individual attacks can be controlled with prompt treatment. If the rash is severe, widespread, or upsetting to your child, consult your doctor, who may refer him to a dermatologist for assessment.

For psoriasis limited to a few small areas, such as the scalp, knees, or elbows, the doctor may prescribe medication containing a corticosteroid, coal tar, or salicylic acid. There are many treatments for psoriasis. The doctor or dermatologist may prescribe particular treatments alone or in combination with others. Ultraviolet light and a topical

medication called calcipotriene may also be used.

How to help your child

If your child has mild psoriasis, you may be able to control the condition by keeping the skin well moisturized with an emollient cream. Exposing affected areas to the sun sometimes helps clear up the rash, but do not let your child get sunburned.

TINEA VERSICOLOR

An overgrowth of a yeast normally present on the skin, possibly triggered by exposure to sunlight or a hot, humid environment, causes the discolored patches of this skin condition. It is rare in children before they reach puberty.

Medical treatment

Take your child to the doctor if he shows the symptoms of tinea versicolor. Although it is not harmful or contagious, the condition may persist indefinitely if not treated.

The doctor will prescribe an antifungal cream or lotion which should be applied to the affected areas. This treatment reduces the yeast to its normal levels in about a week, but should be continued for at least 3 weeks in order to reduce the chances

of the condition recurring. You should encourage your child to expose the affected areas of his skin to the air as much as possible since this can also help discourage regrowth of the yeast. However, it may be weeks or even months before the skin color evens out.

TINEA VERSICOLOR *On dark or tanned skin, areas affected by tinea versicolor appear as round, flat, pale patches with clearly defined borders.*

EAR & EYE DISORDERS

EAR AND EYE INFECTIONS may be caused by viruses or bacteria and are common in young children. By the time they reach the age of 7 or 8, most children have become immune to the more common viruses, and infections become less frequent. Ear and eye infections can cause severe illness and symptoms should be addressed promptly. Persistent ear infections may lead to hearing difficulties, which can delay speech and learning. Vision problems need to be identified and treated promptly so a child's sight can develop normally.

ANATOMY OF THE EYE AND EAR

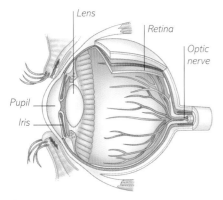

▲ **HOW THE EYE WORKS**

Sight is the most complex sense. Light rays enter through the pupil and register on the retina, where they are converted to nerve impulses that are sent to the brain.

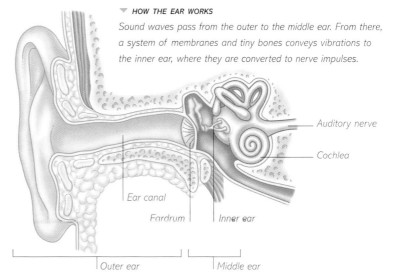

▼ **HOW THE EAR WORKS**

Sound waves pass from the outer to the middle ear. From there, a system of membranes and tiny bones conveys vibrations to the inner ear, where they are converted to nerve impulses.

INFLAMMATION OF THE OUTER EAR

This can be caused by bacteria or by seborrheic dermatitis and eczema. Infection is more likely if the ear canal is exposed to contaminated water, or if it is scratched or irritated by a foreign body or by long-standing wax blockage.

Medical treatment

Take your child to the doctor within 24 hours if she has an earache, a discharge from the outer ear canal, or difficulty hearing. The doctor will probably look into her ear with an otoscope. If there is a discharge of pus, a sample may be sent for tests. If the doctor finds a foreign body or plug of wax, she may remove it, and then clean and dry the canal. This may be done using an anesthetic. Antibiotic ear drops may be prescribed.

If either seborrheic dermatitis or eczema is the cause, the doctor may prescribe corticosteroid ear drops for your child to relieve any itching and tenderness. With treatment, inflammation of the outer ear will usually clear up within 7–10 days.

How to help your child

The appropriate dose of acetaminophen or ibuprofen may relieve the pain and a water bottle

SYMPTOMS

- Itching, usually followed by pain.
- Discharge from the canal, which may be thick and white or yellowish.
- Partial hearing loss, if wax or discharge is blocking the canal.
- Oozing, crusting blisters.
- Tenderness when the outer, fleshy part of the ear is touched or moved.

(filled with warm, not hot, water) or a warm cloth against the ear may also bring relief.

If ear drops are prescribed for your child, ask her to lie down with the affected ear upward. Hold her head still while you give the drops and for about a minute afterward.

Do not let her swim or get the ear wet until the inflammation has cleared up. Cover the ear with a shower cap during a bath or shower and sponge her hair clean instead of washing it.

AN INFECTED EAR CANAL
If there is a discharge from the ear canal, you can gently wipe some of it away. The doctor may also send a sample for tests to determine the cause.

INFLAMMATION OF THE MIDDLE EAR

Also called otitis media, this is often a painful complication of an upper respiratory tract infection, such as a common cold, or a throat infection, such as pharyngitis or tonsillitis. It is a common cause of earache in children up to 8 years old.

Causes

The middle ear is connected to the back of the throat by the eustachian tube. In young children this tube is immature and does not always function well.

When a viral or bacterial infection spreads to the eustachian tube, the sensitive tissues lining the middle ear become inflamed and produce fluid, and sometimes pus. These secretions are unable to drain away because the tube is blocked by the inflammation or by enlarged adenoids (*see p.222*). The secretions accumulate, causing pain as they press against the eardrum, which may subsequently rupture.

Medical treatment

Take your child to the doctor within 24 hours if you suspect a middle ear inflammation. If she is very young or the pain is severe, you should call the doctor immediately. The doctor

SYMPTOMS

- Earache.
- Fever and vomiting.
- Waking at night, crying.
- Tugging at or rubbing ears.
- Decreased hearing and irritability.
- A discharge from the ear.

will examine the ear with an otoscope to try to find the cause of the problem.

The doctor may take a sample of any discharge and send it for tests to identify the infection. She may prescribe a course of antibiotics or ear drops, which should treat the infection and any drainage and consequently bring down your child's temperature and relieve the pain.

If the earache and fever show no sign of improving after about three days, the doctor may prescribe a different antibiotic or recommend other interventions. Antibiotics may be effective if the infection is caused by a bacterium, not a virus.

The fluid sometimes remains in the middle ear for as long as three months after the infection, which may mean that your child continues to experience some decreased hearing.

How to help your child

You should give your child acetaminophen or ibuprofen in the recommended dose to combat the

inflammation and ease the pain until you see the doctor. A water bottle wrapped in a towel may also be soothing – fill the bottle with warm, not hot, water. Encourage your child to rest with the affected side of her head turned downward in order to allow any discharge to drain out. If the eardrum has ruptured, it should heal within about a week.

Your doctor may test your child's hearing three months after the illness. If your child's hearing is still impaired, otitis media with effusion may be the cause (*see below*).

Outlook

As your child grows, the eustachian tubes in both ears mature so that air can get into the middle ear. As a result,

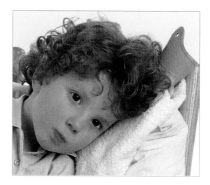

EASING EARACHE *Lying flat may make the earache worse. Prop your child up with pillows while she rests the painful ear on a warm water bottle.*

her middle ears gradually become less vulnerable to infection. Your child is unlikely to have bouts of otitis media after she is about 8 years of age.

OTITIS MEDIA WITH EFFUSION

This condition develops when the middle ear becomes filled with a thick, gluelike mucus. The child's hearing is usually affected because sounds cannot be transmitted to the organs of the inner ear. Some children are more prone to the condition than others.

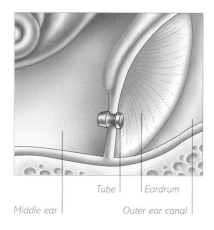

| Tube | Eardrum |
| Middle ear | Outer ear canal |

TYMPANOSTOMY TUBE *A small tube is inserted into the eardrum to let air circulate and dry out the middle ear. The tube falls out about two months to two years later and the eardrum heals.*

Causes

When air cannot enter the middle ear, the mucus can accumulate, particularly if the eustachian tube is blocked.

Medical treatment

You should see your doctor if you suspect that your child has otitis media with effusion. The doctor will check your child's ears with an otoscope, and may send her to an ear, nose, and throat (ENT) specialist. This specialist will test your child's hearing and may also measure the movements of the eardrum.

Fluid in the middle ear can persist after an ear infection or may develop following ventilation problems. If the buildup of fluid in your child's ear

SYMPTOMS

- Child may complain of partial hearing loss and hearing may be worse at some times than at others.
- Child may seem inattentive and slow at speaking and/or learning. Pain is seldom a symptom, so your child may be affected for some time before the condition is detected.

does not resolve, a tiny tube (called a tympanostomy, ventilation, or pressure-equalization tube) may be placed through the eardrum to ventilate the middle ear.

Outlook

As your child grows, the eustachian tubes function better and usually prevent fluid accumulation in the middle ear. Otitis media with effusion is less common in children over about 8 years old.

LABYRINTHITIS

The inner ear, also called the labyrinth, contains fluid-filled chambers that are concerned with balance and hearing. Labyrinthitis, or inflammation of the labyrinth, can be a complication of a viral infection and causes dizziness and nausea.

Causes

This rare but distressing condition results when a bacterium or virus that has caused a respiratory tract infection then infects the fluid inside the sensitive inner ear. Children lose their balance and hearing and become unsteady on their feet, and may feel nauseous and as if they are moving.

Medical treatment

If you are worried about your child's unsteadiness and think she might be suffering from labyrinthitis, seek medical care immediately.

The doctor will examine your child and will ask about any recent infectious illnesses. An ear, nose, and throat (ENT) specialist will evaluate your child's hearing and balance function. She may prescribe bed rest for about a week as well as a special type of antihistamine syrup to relieve the vomiting and dizziness. Other treatments, such as antibiotics, may be required.

SYMPTOMS

- Vertigo, making your child feel that everything is spinning around uncontrollably.
- Unsteadiness and falling down. She may need to lean on something to support herself.
- Nausea and vomiting.
- Ringing in the ear or hearing loss.

Outlook

Labyrinthitis usually lasts days to several weeks, then gradually improves. It can cause permanent impairment, but children can often compensate well for balance problems that may result.

BAROTRAUMA

This is a temporary blockage of the eustachian tube (the passage that connects the middle ear and the throat), in which one or both of a child's eardrums bulges in or out. It is usually caused by abrupt changes in atmospheric pressure.

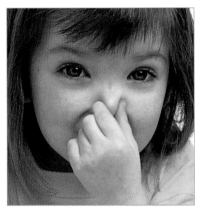

THE VALSALVA MANEUVER *When the aircraft begins its descent, encourage your child to pinch her nose while keeping her mouth closed, and gently blow down her nose until her ears go "pop."*

Causes

Air travel is the usual cause of barotrauma. Airflow through the eustachian tube normally keeps the air pressure inside and outside the middle ear the same. When an aircraft climbs, the air pressure in the cabin falls, and so does the pressure inside the middle ear. When the aircraft descends, pressure outside the middle ear increases, causing the eustachian tube to shut and pushing the eardrum inward. An upper respiratory tract infection, such as a common cold (*see* p.221), hay fever (*see* Allergic rhinitis, p.224), or an ear infection (*see* Inflammation of the middle ear, p.240) makes barotrauma more likely.

SYMPTOMS

- Pain as the eardrum bulges or retracts.
- Partial hearing loss.
- Ringing in the ears.
The symptoms of barotrauma usually disappear within a few hours and do not usually cause any lasting damage.

How to help your child

When an aircraft is landing, age-appropriate action such as sucking on a hard candy, yawning, swallowing, chewing gum, or using the Valsalva maneuver (*see left*) may open the eustachian tube, allowing air to flow into the middle ear. An appropriate dose of ibuprofen or acetaminophen may relieve any pain. Feeding during the aircraft's descent may prevent barotrauma in babies. These measures are particularly important if a child has a cold, hay fever, or an ear infection.

BLEPHARITIS

Blepharitis is an inflammation of the eyelid edges and is often associated with dandruff. It is common in children who have seborrheic dermatitis (greasy, flaky skin patches) and can also be caused by viral or bacterial infections.

Causes
There are two kinds of blepharitis – infectious and seborrheic. The first is caused by bacteria or, more rarely, a virus, and may be accompanied by conjunctivitis (*see p.244*). The second is usually caused by an accumulation of dandruff in the eyelashes. Blepharitis may sometimes be caused by an allergy to eye makeup such as mascara.

Medical treatment
Take your child to your doctor if you suspect blepharitis. The doctor will show you how to wipe off any crusting scales from the eyelid margins using a cotton ball or clean, soft cloth

moistened with warm water. The doctor may swab some scales from the eyelids if she suspects an infection and send the sample for tests. If confirmed, the doctor may prescribe an antibiotic ointment or cream, which you can apply at home after you have removed all the scales.

Infectious blepharitis usually clears up within 2 weeks, but you may be advised to apply the ointment or cream for a further 2 weeks or more to prevent a recurrence.

Seborrheic blepharitis tends to be persistent. Once you have removed the scales of dandruff, try to keep it under control to help prevent flare-ups.

SYMPTOMS

- Burning, redness, and itching of the edges of the eyelid.
- Scales at the roots of the lashes. The scales in the seborrheic form of blepharitis are yellow and oily.
- Sometimes, eyelashes that grow in the wrong direction or fall out.

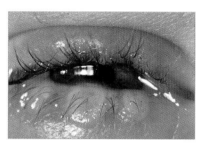

INFECTIOUS BLEPHARITIS *The eyelids are red, swollen, and crusted with scales. The white of the eye is red, indicating that conjunctivitis is also present.*

STYES

A stye is a pus-filled swelling that forms at the base of an eyelash. Styes are common in children. Like other eyelid disorders such as blepharitis, they can be uncomfortable and painful but are not serious.

Causes
When an oil-producing (sebaceous) gland beside an eyelash is blocked and inflamed, a painless swelling develops. If it becomes infected, a stye forms around the bottom of the eyelash. A stye may develop as a complication of blepharitis (*see above*).

Medical treatment
If your child develops persistent or recurrent styes, take her to the doctor, who may give her an antibiotic ointment. Applying the ointment to a

stye as prescribed can prevent it from recurring. A stye usually gets better in a few days.

How to help your child
Don't try to squeeze the stye to get rid of the pus. To relieve the discomfort, get your child to press a warm cloth to the infected area 2–4 times a day. This helps the pus to discharge, which hastens healing. To avoid spreading the infection, make sure your child washes her hands frequently and doesn't share a towel or washcloth.

SYMPTOMS

- A yellow head of pus on the eyelid around the base of an eyelash.
- Swollen and inflamed eyelid skin surrounding the head of pus.
- Pain or tenderness to the touch.

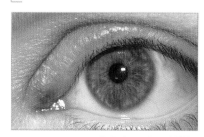

A STYE ON AN EYELID *A stye develops on an eyelid when a blocked sebaceous gland at the base of an eyelash becomes infected, inflamed, and painful.*

CONJUNCTIVITIS

This is an inflammation of the thin, transparent membrane (conjunctiva) that covers the whites of the eyes and lines the eyelids. One or both eyes may be affected. Conjunctivitis may be caused by an infection or by irritation from chemicals or allergens.

Causes

The usual cause in older children is viral infection. In a newborn baby it may be the result of infection by bacteria in the birth canal. In rare cases, infection is transmitted by a mother with gonorrhea, genital herpes, or a chlamydial infection. A baby infected during delivery should fully recover with prompt treatment. It may also be a symptom of hay fever.

Medical treatment

Conjunctivitis in a baby may be treated at the hospital soon after birth. See your doctor immediately if symptoms develop later. In older children, viral conjunctivitis is not serious, but contact a doctor to rule out a more serious disorder. It is contagious but usually clears up without treatment within a week.

For bacterial infections the doctor may prescribe an antibiotic ointment or eye drops that usually clear up the problem in a week. Severe infections may need intravenous or oral antibiotics; they may take several weeks to get better. Anti-inflammatory eye drops may relieve the discomfort of allergic conjunctivitis.

How to help your child

Gently dab the sticky pus from the eyelashes as often as necessary with a moist, clean cloth or cotton ball. To prevent the spread of infection, wash your hands thoroughly after touching the infected eyes, and do not let your child share washcloths or towels.

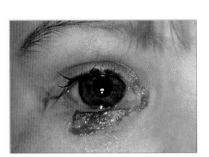

APPEARANCE OF BACTERIAL CONJUNCTIVITIS
The white of the eye is bloodshot and the eyelashes are gummy with yellow pus. Pus has also collected in the corner of the eye.

SYMPTOMS

- Redness of the white of the eye and the inside of the eyelid.
- Itchiness and irritation in the eye.
- In bacterial conjunctivitis, yellow, sticky pus in the corner of the eye and on the eyelashes. The eye is hard to open in the morning.
- In allergic conjunctivitis, swollen eyelids and a clear discharge from the eye that is not sticky, plus itchiness.

IRITIS

This is an inflammation of the iris, the colored muscular ring that surrounds the pupil. It often results from an eye injury and may affect one or both eyes. Serious attacks are rare except in children with juvenile idiopathic arthritis.

Medical treatment

Call your doctor immediately if you think your child may have iritis. She may prescribe eye drops or an ointment containing a corticosteroid to reduce the inflammation.

If it is treated promptly, iritis often clears up within 1–2 weeks, without any long-term ill effects or concerns about the child's vision. However, if the iritis is left untreated, or if it is persistent or keeps recurring, then a child's vision can be at risk of permanent damage.

How to help your child

Holding a clean, moist cloth to the affected eye may help relieve the symptoms. Sunglasses may also help reduce sensitivity.

SYMPTOMS

- Pain, which may be dull or severe, in the affected eye.
- Acute sensitivity to light.
- Redness of the white of the eye, particularly of the part around the edge of the iris.
- Blurred vision.
- An irregularly shaped pupil, which (if only one eye is affected by iritis) is smaller than the pupil of the unaffected eye.
- Watering of the affected eye.

STRABISMUS

Strabismus is an abnormality in the alignment of the eyes. Many young babies occasionally cross their eyes up to the age of 2–4 months, but crossing after the age of 4 months or a persistent crossing at any age is abnormal.

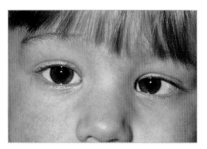

CONVERGENT STRABISMUS *This child's left eye is crossing. The right eye looks ahead, while the left eye is pointing inward.*

which the eyes adjust for near focus too strongly, forcing one eye inward.

Strabismus may be due to unequal refraction, which causes the two eyes to produce conflicting images. The weaker eye is poorly focused and its image is suppressed. To prevent the double vision produced by strabismus, the brain ignores the image from the weaker eye; because the eye is not used, its vision may eventually become permanently impaired.

Causes

A baby may develop strabismus because the mechanism coordinating the eyes is not fully developed. In older children, strabismus may be due to severe farsightedness (*see below*), in

Medical treatment

If your child develops strabismus after the age of 4 months or has persistent strabismus, consult your doctor. It is important to deal with this as soon as possible while her

vision is developing. The doctor may send your child to an ophthalmologist who will evaluate her vision and may prescribe glasses if she has a refractive error (*see below*).

Treatment may also involve covering the normal eye with a patch, forcing your child to use the affected eye. In some cases, the position of the deviating eye may be corrected by an operation. If treatment is provided in early childhood, a child's vision should develop normally.

■ SYMPTOMS

- The child's eye turns too far in or out (convergent or divergent strabismus), or up or down (vertical strabismus), when she looks directly at an object.
- Poor vision in the affected eye.
- Double or blurred vision, which the child may try to remedy by closing or covering the affected eye.

REFRACTIVE ERRORS

Nearsightedness, farsightedness, and astigmatism are focusing problems that cause blurred vision and are often inherited. Astigmatism and farsightedness may be present from birth. Nearsightedness usually develops a few years before adolescence.

Medical treatment

If you think that your child has a focusing problem, take her to your doctor, who will probably refer her to an ophthalmologist. Her sharpness of vision will be tested and she may be examined with retinoscopy. This technique involves observing the movement of a light shone into the eye and reflected from the retina at the back of the eye. The measurements obtained from the retinoscopy will

help the ophthalmologist determine whether your child needs glasses and, if so, which kind.

Outlook

In most cases, refractive errors do not become any worse once body growth is complete. But because the focusing power of the lens decreases with age, farsightedness that did not produce any symptoms in a child may become apparent during middle age.

■ SYMPTOMS

If your child has a refractive error, she may be unaware that anything is wrong. You may notice when your child:

- Complains that objects appear blurry.
- Sits too close to the television.
- Cannot see what is going on at the front of the classroom or cannot read materials clearly.

Because children often don't complain of visual difficulties, visual acuity screening should be performed starting around age 3. Early detection and treatment of visual problems is important to avoid lifelong visual impairments.

MOUTH PROBLEMS

Most of the body is protected by tough skin, but the mouth is not and therefore is more vulnerable: the tongue and lining of the mouth are damaged easily by chewing coarse food or abrasive objects, and are exposed to a wide variety of potentially damaging infections as well as excessively hot or cold food and drink. A child's primary teeth are replaced by permanent (secondary) teeth, which begin to emerge around the age of 6 years. Both sets must be cared for properly to avoid tooth decay and gum problems, such as gingivitis.

ANATOMY OF THE TEETH AND TONGUE

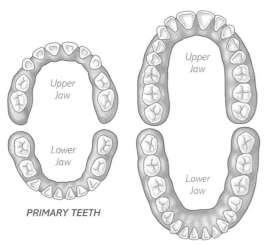

PRIMARY TEETH

SECONDARY TEETH

Upper Jaw

Lower Jaw

◁ **DEVELOPMENT OF THE TEETH** *At birth, the primary teeth are already developing in the jaws. The first of these erupt around 6 months. By the age of 3 years, the entire set of 20 primary teeth has come through. Meanwhile, the secondary set of 32 teeth is developing in the jaws and will appear between the ages of 6 and 16 years. As these teeth erupt, the primary teeth are displaced and consequently fall out. The third molars (wisdom teeth) usually break through at 16 or older, although sometimes they never appear.*

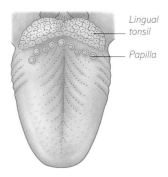

Lingual tonsil

Papilla

▲ **UPPER SURFACE OF THE TONGUE** *Taste buds are located mainly within the papillae on the surface of the tongue. Different types of these papillae, arranged over the surface of the tongue, can detect the four main tastes – sweet, salty, bitter, and sour.*

MOUTH ULCERS

Ulcers, or "cankers," are open sores on the lining of the mouth or on the tongue. They usually develop for no obvious reason and tend to recur. Ulcers may make the mouth very painful, but they are not serious and usually heal on their own. Children who get repeated ulcers usually grow out of the problem. They may also be due to minor injury or, rarely, to an underlying disorder.

Medical treatment

If your child is in pain, or if the ulcers fail to heal within 10 days, or appear often, take him to your doctor. If an ulcer returns to the same place, a sharp tooth may be the cause.

If several mouth ulcers appear and your child has never had ulcers before, they may be due to a first

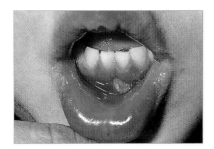

A MOUTH ULCER *This ulcer at the base of the gums has a gray, hollowed-out center, with a raised, paler rim. The area around the ulcer is inflamed.*

attack of oral herpes simplex (*see* Gingivostomatitis, *below*).

If your doctor thinks the ulcers are caused by an underlying disease, your child might need tests to find out if anything else is wrong.

How to help your child

Most ulcers heal without treatment within 4–10 days. Ulcers less than 2 mm (½ in) in diameter heal quickly; larger ulcers may take longer. Rinsing your child's mouth with a solution of baking soda – mix ¼ teaspoon of baking soda in 120 ml (4 fl.oz) of warm water – may help relieve pain or tenderness. An over-the-counter anesthetic ointment or gel can soothe ulcers and the appropriate dose of acetaminophen or ibuprofen can relieve the pain.

Another home remedy uses a mixture of over-the-counter liquid

antacid and diphenhydramine elixir in equal amounts. Doctors and dentists sometimes advise parents to swab a small amount of the mixture onto the mouth sores. Older children may be able to swish around the mouth and then spit out a teaspoon of the liquid every few hours for pain relief. Consult your doctor before trying this treatment.

Acidic, spicy, hot, or salty food or drinks may irritate the ulcers. If chewing is very painful, give your child soft foods or liquids. Drinking through a straw may help prevent liquid from bathing the ulcers.

SYMPTOMS

- A single ulcer or a cluster of ulcers inside the cheeks or lips or on the margin of the tongue. Each ulcer has a gray center with a pale white or yellow rim and a red border.
- Pain and tenderness in the mouth, which may make your child reluctant to eat or to brush his teeth.
- Before the ulcers appear, there may be a sore or burning sensation on the lining of the mouth, the insides of the lips, or the tongue.

GINGIVOSTOMATITIS

Gingivostomatitis is most common in children between the ages of 6 months and 4 years and causes very painful ulcers to appear in the mouth. It results from a first infection by the herpes simplex virus, which also causes cold sores.

Medical treatment

Consult your doctor if you think your child may have gingivostomatitis. The doctor may prescribe a pain reliever or other medication. A child who is very

ill or has been refusing fluids may need to be admitted to the hospital so that antiviral medication and rehydrating fluids can be given intravenously.

SYMPTOMS

- Fever and a sore mouth are usually the first signs and the following symptoms then develop.
- Painful, shallow ulcers on the gums, tongue, and palate.
- Red, swollen gums that are prone to bleeding easily.
- Swelling of lymph nodes in the neck.

ORAL THRUSH

This yeast infection is most common in babies under 12 months. It is caused when the yeast *Candida albicans*, which lives naturally in the mouth, grows quickly after the oral bacteria that keep it in control are altered by something such as a course of antibiotics.

Medical treatment

If you think your baby may have oral thrush, check with your doctor within a few days. The doctor will examine him and may take scrapings from the inside lining of his mouth for analysis.

You may be given antifungal drops to apply to the inside of his mouth. He may also develop yeast in the diaper area and this will need to be treated at the same time. To help prevent reinfection, be extra careful when cleaning feeding bottles and nipples. For mothers who are breastfeeding, an antifungal cream to treat the nipples may be recommended.

ORAL THRUSH *Raised, white spots appear in the mouth and on the gums and soft palate. They form a bumpy coating, which cannot be wiped away, on the tongue.*

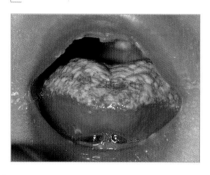

☐ SYMPTOMS

- A sore mouth, making your baby reluctant to feed.
- Creamy yellow or white spots on the tongue and the lining of the mouth.

TOOTH DECAY

Tooth decay is the most common childhood disease, but has greatly decreased, mainly because of fluoride in drinking water and in toothpastes. However, tooth decay continues to occur in many children, so good oral hygiene is extremely important.

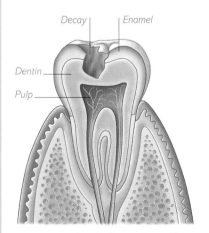

TOOTH DECAY *A cavity forms when acids produced by the bacterial breakdown of food erode the tooth's hard outer surface of enamel. The softer layer of dentin beneath is exposed, and as it too is eroded, the cavity gradually enlarges.*

Causes

Tooth decay is caused by the bacteria that live in plaque, a sticky coating of saliva and food debris that forms on the surface of the teeth. The bacteria use components of food and drinks (mainly sugars) for energy and, in breaking them down, produce acids. These acids, which are held in close contact with the teeth by plaque, cause calcium and phosphate to be lost from the tooth's enamel (demineralization).

If this continues unchecked, the enamel and eventually the dentin beneath is destroyed. If the problem is left untreated at this stage, the pulp at the center of the tooth may become infected, resulting in permanent damage to the nerves and blood vessels that it contains.

☐ SYMPTOMS

Early tooth decay does not usually cause any symptoms. The main symptoms of established decay are:

- Sensitivity of the tooth to hot, cold, and/or sweet foods or liquids.
- In very advanced decay, the tooth may be brown with visible pits or holes in the enamel surface, and may also be very painful.

Dental treatment

You should take your child to a dentist regularly so tooth decay can be detected at an early stage. If you notice that any symptoms of tooth decay have developed between regular checkups, make an appointment for your child to see your dentist within a few days.

At your child's routine dental examination, the dentist will look at the teeth for signs of tooth decay. X-rays may also be taken to detect areas of decay that are hidden in the crevices of the teeth's biting surfaces.

If the dentist finds any signs of very early decay or an area of demineralization, he may simply clean the teeth and scrape them to remove the plaque. This treatment allows the surface of the teeth to come into contact with saliva, which has a natural ability to remineralize tooth enamel. The dentist may also apply a fluoride gel.

To deal with more advanced tooth decay, the dentist may drill the tooth to remove the decayed portion and then insert a filling. If the nerve of the tooth has been irreversibly damaged or destroyed by bacterial infection, it may need to be removed. If the dentist finds that the decay is very advanced, the entire tooth may need to be taken out.

How to help your child
One of the most important steps you can take to prevent tooth decay is to limit the amount of sweet foods and drinks that your child consumes. Do not let him indulge in sweets too

often. Try to discourage him from having sugary snacks and drinks between meals.

Make sure your child keeps acidic food and drinks, including fruit juice and all sodas (both diet and regular), to a minimum. Ideally, your child should have fruit juice and soda only with a meal, and should drink water most of the time.

Do not give a baby sweetened drinks in a bottle because the liquid will bathe the teeth in sugar and may lead to tooth decay. Ask your doctor or dentist whether your water supply is fluoridated and if fluoride treatment or supplements would be advisable for your child.

Teach your child to brush his teeth twice a day with a fluoride toothpaste – the best times are either following meals or after breakfast and especially last thing at night. You should brush your child's teeth for him or supervise him closely until he reaches the age of 7 years. Before then, children do not have the dexterity to brush their own teeth properly. Children should also floss daily.

Dental sealants protect the chewing surfaces of the teeth. You should ask your dentist if your child would benefit from dental sealants.

Starting in the early toddler years, you should schedule a regular dental checkup for your child.

PREVENTION
- Keep your child's diet as low in sugar as you can.
- Teach your child the principles of good oral hygiene.
- Take your child to the dentist regularly.
- Make sure your child gets plenty of the minerals required for forming tooth enamel. They include calcium (found in milk), fluoride (added to most toothpastes), phosphorus (found in meat, fish, and eggs), and magnesium (found in spinach, bananas, and wholegrain bread).
- Don't allow babies to fall asleep while drinking a bottle containing anything but water.
- Don't sweeten pacifiers with sugar or honey.

GINGIVITIS

This inflammation of the gums may develop if a child does not clean his teeth and gums thoroughly. It is caused by the irritant effect of bacteria in plaque, a sticky layer of food debris and saliva that collects on and around the teeth, and at the gum margins.

SYMPTOMS
- Red, swollen, and tender gums.
- Gums bleed easily when they are brushed.

How to help your child
Take your child to the dentist if you think he has gingivitis. For mild gingivitis, the dentist may simply encourage your child to care for his teeth properly (see above for advice on oral hygiene). If the gingivitis is more advanced, the dentist may also recommend that your child rinse his mouth with an antibacterial

mouthwash to relieve inflammation and tenderness.

When your child's gums are less tender, the dentist may scale (scrape) the teeth to remove plaque and calculus (hardened plaque). Although gingivitis is a minor problem if left untreated, it may go on to cause a more serious infection, and teeth may be lost as a result.

Outlook
If you and your child care for his teeth properly and regularly, his gums should get better in a few months. Good oral hygiene, combined with regular visits to the dentist for checkups and scaling, can help prevent your child from getting gingivitis again.

DENTAL ABSCESS

A collection of pus around the root of a tooth, a dental abscess develops when the pulp at the tooth's sensitive core is invaded and destroyed by bacteria. Bacteria enter the pulp cavity if the tooth has been badly damaged or has become severely decayed.

Dental treatment
You should take your child to see a dentist within a few hours of any of the symptoms appearing. The dentist will drill into the tooth to release the pus and relieve the pressure. The dead and dying pulp is removed, and the resulting cavity is washed, dried, and filled – a procedure known as a root canal. The dentist may extract the tooth if it is severely affected. A course of antibiotics may be prescribed to clear up any remaining infection. Following a root canal, the tooth usually functions as well as a healthy tooth. If a tooth has been removed, the other teeth often move into the space.

How to help your child
To relieve the pain until seeing the dentist, give your child the appropriate dose of acetaminophen or ibuprofen. A warm or cold compress held against the affected side of the face may also provide relief.

You can protect your child from abscesses in the future by teaching him the basics of good oral hygiene, such as brushing his teeth two to three times a day and flossing at bedtime (*see* Tooth decay, *p.248*). You can also help your child by encouraging sensible eating habits (such as avoiding sweet foods and drinks), and taking him for regular dental checkups to maintain healthy teeth and to recognize and treat dental cavities promptly.

> ### ☐ SYMPTOMS
>
> - A persistent and throbbing toothache.
> - Severe pain in the tooth when biting or chewing, or when consuming hot foods or liquids.
> - Tenderness, redness, and swelling of the gum around the affected tooth.
> - Occasionally, a discharge of foul-tasting pus through an opening in the gum, after which the pain tends to subside.
> - Looseness of the affected tooth.
>
> *If the infection spreads into surrounding tissue, the face and lymph glands in the neck may swell. Eventually, the child might develop symptoms of general infection, such as fever and headache.*

MALOCCLUSION

Malocclusion is a poor fit between the upper and lower teeth when they bite together. Treatment may be needed if the teeth are so crooked or out of position that they don't chew properly, interfere with speech development, or are difficult to clean.

Causes
Malocclusion is often caused by the overcrowding of teeth. The condition is usually inherited and appears as the child's jaws and teeth develop. It may also occur when primary teeth are lost early, because of either decay or injury. When teeth are lost early, the remaining teeth move into the gaps, so that there is insufficient room for the permanent teeth. Overcrowded teeth may grow to be crooked, overlapping, or too prominent. A less common, inherited cause of malocclusion is misalignment of the jaws so that the upper or lower set of teeth is too far forward or too far back.

Dental treatment
Orthodontic treatment is usually carried out at 11–13 years of age, although early orthodontic work may start as young as 6 years. If the teeth are overcrowded, some may have to be taken out and your child may have to wear a special appliance. Appliances may be fixed (braces) or removable. They exert pressure on the teeth to move them into the right position. The length of orthodontic treatment depends on the extent of the malocclusion. Misalignment of the jaws may need to be corrected by surgery.

How to help your child
You should take your child to the dentist at regular intervals so that the growth of his teeth and jaws can be carefully monitored. If you are at all worried about your child's teeth, or if your child is concerned about his appearance, you should ask your dentist for advice. He may recommend that you wait to see if the malocclusion corrects itself as the jaws grow, or he may refer your child to an orthodontist.

GASTROINTESTINAL TRACT DISORDERS

INFECTIONS OF THE DIGESTIVE SYSTEM that result in diarrhea and/or vomiting are especially frequent in children. At an early age, they put all kinds of things in their mouths and can pick up germs easily with their unhygienic eating habits. Although diarrhea and vomiting may be troublesome for parent and child, they are rarely persistent enough to be a serious threat to health. Increasingly, children are developing reactions to cow's milk protein or fish, nuts, and eggs, but most children grow out of them in time. Some of the less common digestive disorders may cause chronic illness that can affect growth if not treated.

ANATOMY OF THE DIGESTIVE SYSTEM

▶ **DIGESTIVE SYSTEM**
The digestive tract consists of a long tube that extends from the mouth to the anus. As food passes along this tube, it is broken down into minute molecules that can be absorbed into the bloodstream. Associated organs secrete chemicals to assist the digestive process.

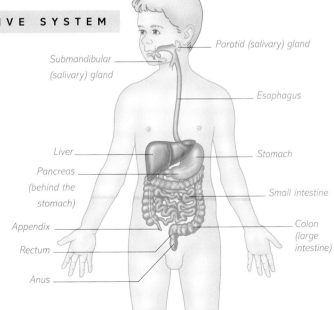

Parotid (salivary) gland
Submandibular (salivary) gland
Esophagus
Liver
Pancreas (behind the stomach)
Stomach
Small intestine
Appendix
Colon (large intestine)
Rectum
Anus

REACTIONS TO FOOD

Some children have adverse reactions to certain foods, such as cow's milk protein, lactose, sucrose, fish, eggs, and nuts. A food allergy is due to an inappropriate response by the body's immune system. Food intolerance or sensitivity produces similar symptoms but does not generally involve the immune system. A child who has adverse food reactions should see the doctor.

COW'S MILK PROTEIN ALLERGY

Cow's milk protein is a common cause of an adverse reaction to food. The cause of the allergy is unknown, but the problem usually begins during the first year of life, between a week and several months after starting to drink cow's milk formula. It usually disappears by the time the child reaches 3 years.

Medical treatment

If you suspect your child has an allergy to cow's milk protein, take her to the doctor. Provided the initial reaction was mild, the doctor may recommend that you exclude all products containing cow's milk from your child's diet for 2 weeks. If the symptoms disappear, your child will be given a small, trial amount of cow's milk. If symptoms come back, the diagnosis is confirmed.

If the initial symptoms were more severe, the reintroduction of the cow's milk should be carried out under the close supervision of a doctor.

How to help your child

Breastfeeding your baby is the best way to prevent the onset of milk allergy. If necessary, your doctor can suggest an appropriate formula. A dietitian can advise you on an appropriate diet for your child, one that is free of products containing cow's milk. The cow's milk trial will be repeated about every 3 months, until your child no longer has an adverse reaction to the protein. The amount of milk given can then be increased gradually. The dietitian can make sure that your child is receiving enough calcium for growth.

LACTOSE & SUCROSE INTOLERANCE

Children can be intolerant to two sugars: lactose, which is found in milk, or sucrose, which is found in many fruits. These same children may also be intolerant to other foods.

The intolerances are due to a deficiency of the enzyme responsible for breaking down lactose or sucrose in the small intestine. Both types of intolerance are usually temporary and may develop as a complication of an infection (see Gastroenteritis, p.254) or another intestinal disorder, such as celiac disease (see p.256). Some children with an allergy to cow's milk protein are also intolerant to lactose.

Permanent lactose intolerance of genetic origin is common in people of African, Hispanic, or Asian descent. Children up to 2 or 3 years tolerate an unlimited amount of milk, but when they grow older they may suffer from diarrhea after drinking only a small amount. Many individuals, however, can tolerate certain amounts of lactose before they have symptoms. Permanent sucrose intolerance may also occur occasionally as an inherited disorder.

Medical treatment

Your doctor may confirm the diagnosis of a food allergy by giving your child a special breath test.

If a child is lactose intolerant, a dietitian can design a lactose-free or reduced-lactose diet. Your child may tolerate milk products such as yogurt and cheese and possibly small amounts of milk. Sucrose intolerance is treated with a sucrose-free diet.

SPECIFIC FOOD ALLERGIES

Fish, eggs, and nuts are other foods to which children commonly have allergies. The reason an allergy to a specific food occurs is not known. In many children, no specific cause is found for the symptoms. However, the problem often clears up during the course of a "few foods" diet. In others, exclusion of between one and three foods eliminates the symptoms. Most children outgrow reactions to food.

Medical treatment

If you suspect your child has an allergy to a food, consult your doctor. She will examine your child and may carry out tests to exclude other causes. Your child may be put on a milk-free diet to rule out allergy to cow's milk protein or lactose intolerance. If symptoms persist, one of two methods may be tried to find out whether she has an adverse reaction to a specific food.

One method involves comparing your child's symptoms when the suspected food is included or excluded from her diet. In another method, your child is given a "few foods" diet, consisting of specific foods known to be unlikely to induce symptoms. Within a couple of weeks of following this diet, the symptoms usually stop. Then one new food is given every 3 days until symptoms occur or the diet has returned to normal.

APPENDICITIS

A small tubelike pouch that branches off the start of the large intestine, the appendix has no known function. It can become infected and inflamed, causing appendicitis. This cause of abdominal pain requires surgery.

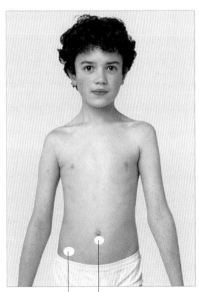

Usual first site of pain

Usual site of pain after a few hours

THE SITE OF PAIN *Pain usually begins around the navel, gradually becomes more severe, and migrates to the lower right-hand side of the abdomen. In some children, the pain is in the lower right abdomen from the beginning.*

Immediate action

If the abdominal pain is so severe it makes your child cry out, or if the pain continues, call your doctor immediately. Dial 911, call EMS, or take your child to a hospital emergency room if you are extremely concerned about the pain.

If appendicitis is not treated promptly, the appendix may burst, or perforate. Pain becomes continuous and pus enters the abdominal cavity, causing widespread infection and leading to a potentially fatal condition called peritonitis.

Medical treatment

If appendicitis is suspected, your child will be admitted to the hospital. If it is confirmed, the appendix will be removed as soon as possible. Your child will be given pain medications for about 24 hours after the operation. He may go home within a few days if the appendix was not perforated. If it was perforated, he will be given

🔲 SYMPTOMS

- Dull pain in the lower abdomen (*see illustration, left*). Any pressure on the painful area, movement, or deep breathing increases the pain, so a child with appendicitis often lies still.
- Nausea, which may or may not be accompanied by vomiting.
- Fever.
- Constipation or diarrhea.

antibiotics and will remain in the hospital until the infection has cleared up, which may take about 7 days. After leaving the hospital your child will be able to eat normally, but should avoid sports and strenuous physical activities for about a month.

How to help your child

If your child complains of abdominal pain, it is difficult to know at first how serious it is and how to help. A warm compress held against the site of the pain may be soothing. Try not to give acetaminophen or other medications because they may make the diagnosis more difficult. The child should not eat or drink anything in case an operation is necessary.

GASTROENTERITIS

Most children will have occasional attacks of gastroenteritis (inflamed lining of the stomach and intestines), causing diarrhea and/or vomiting. The most common cause is a virus transmitted by hand-to-mouth contact with infected stools. Bacteria in food or water may also cause gastroenteritis. Most attacks are mild but serious attacks can cause severe dehydration.

Medical treatment

Diarrhea is frequent loose or watery stools. If your child has vomiting and/or diarrhea that do not improve after 24 hours, call your doctor. If your child is 2 months old or less and you suspect gastroenteritis, contact your doctor immediately. Notify the doctor right away if your child is dehydrated (*see* Danger signs, *p.63 and p.172*); vomits material that is green, blood-tinged, or looks like coffee grounds; or has fever that lasts longer than 24 to 48 hours, bloody stools, a distended abdomen, severe abdominal pain, or jaundice (yellow coloration of the skin and eyes).

After an examination, your doctor may want to do further tests to determine the cause or to make sure your child is not becoming dehydrated. The doctor will also evaluate whether your child needs to be admitted to the hospital. If she can be treated at home, the doctor will explain how to care for her illness.

In most cases of dehydration, a child will be given rehydrating fluids by mouth before resuming a normal diet. In severe cases, intravenous fluids may need to be given.

There are no effective medications for treating intestinal infections caused by a virus. Prescription medications may be used to treat certain types of bacterial or parasitic intestinal infections, which are much less common. Over-the-counter diarrheal medications are not recommended for children under age two and should be used with caution in older children. Always consult your doctor before giving your child any medication for diarrhea.

How to help your child

If your child has mild diarrhea without dehydration and is active and hungry, you don't have to change the diet and can continue breastmilk or formula. If your child is also vomiting, give small, frequent amounts of an electrolyte solution. Once the vomiting has subsided (usually within 1–2 days), gradually restart the normal diet.

If your child has very frequent, watery bowel movements and/or has signs of dehydration, consult your doctor. She may advise you to withhold solid foods for about 24 hours and to avoid liquids that are high in sugar (soft drinks, full-strength fruit juices, or sweetened beverages), high in salt (canned soup), or very low in salt (water and tea). She may recommend giving only commercially prepared electrolyte solutions, which contain an ideal balance of salt and minerals. After 12–24 hours, as the diarrhea is decreasing, you may gradually expand the diet to include small amounts of foods such as applesauce, pears, bananas, and flavored gelatin or bland foods such as rice, toast, potatoes, and cereal for older children.

SYMPTOMS

- Diarrhea.
- Vomiting.
- Loss of appetite.
- Abdominal pain.
- Lack of energy.
- Fever.

PREVENTION

You cannot protect a child from becoming infected with the viruses that cause gastroenteritis, but after infection your child will be immune to that particular virus. You can protect a baby by breastfeeding.

The spread of gastroenteritis due to bacterial infections is prevented with sensible precautions:

- Promote personal hygiene (such as handwashing after using the toilet or changing diapers and before handling food) and other sanitary measures in your household and in your child's preschool or child care center.
- Avoid drinking raw (unpasteurized) milk or potentially unsanitary water (such as from streams or in developing countries) and eating foods that may be contaminated.
- Clean a baby's feeding utensils and pacifiers before use.
- Make sure all family members are scrupulous about personal hygiene.
- Wash hands with warm water and soap before preparing food and after handling raw meat.
- Defrost food in the refrigerator or microwave.
- Marinate meat in the refrigerator.
- Wash plates and utensils that have been used with raw poultry or meat before using them for cooked meat or other food.
- Refrigerate leftovers promptly.

TODDLER DIARRHEA

Toddler diarrhea affects children between the ages of 1 and 3 years. An otherwise healthy child passes watery stools that often contain recognizable pieces of food. The condition is often caused by excessive fluid (especially juice and sweetened beverages).

SYMPTOMS

- Passes watery stools with pieces of undigested food in them.
- Child is generally well, but may have a constant diaper rash.

Medical treatment

Toddler diarrhea is not serious, but it is a good idea to take your child to your doctor to make sure the condition is not the result of an infection or another disorder. The doctor will check whether your child's growth is normal by measuring her height and weight. Toddler diarrhea does not affect your child's growth, so failure to grow normally may suggest another disorder. As a precaution, the doctor may send a sample of a stool for laboratory analysis.

How to help your child

Reduce her intake of sweetened fluids. Mash or puree foods she finds hard to chew or digest. She will probably outgrow the problem by age 3.

CONSTIPATION

A child who passes hard, dry stools infrequently may be constipated. Just passing stools infrequently does not necessarily mean your child is constipated – the normal frequency for passing stools may vary from 4 times a day to once every 4 days.

SYMPTOMS

- Infrequent bowel movements.
- Pain when passing stools.
- Hard, dry stools.

Chronic constipation symptoms are:
- Liquid stools trickling from the anus, which may soil the underwear.
- Pain on trying to pass stools.
- Loss of appetite.
- Blood on the stools.

Causes

Temporary constipation may be due to dehydration brought on by an illness involving vomiting and fever. Changes in a child's diet may cause constipation. In older children, a lack of fiber-rich foods may be the reason. Chronic constipation may arise if an anal fissure (*see right*) develops after passing hard stools. It can also arise if a child deliberately withholds stools during toilet training or because of emotional problems.

Medical treatment

Consult a doctor if constipation lasts for more than a week, there is pain on defecation, or you suspect chronic constipation. She will ask about diet and recent illnesses. Dietary changes may solve the problem.

For chronic constipation, you may be given a prescription for stool softeners and stimulant laxatives, as well as dietary advice and a suggestion that your child sit on the toilet at the same time each day to restore a regular bowel habit. After about 2 months, when a regular habit has been reestablished, the drug dose may be reduced. The softened stools produced by laxatives allow an anal fissure to heal, usually within 6 weeks.

If no solution works, the doctor may refer your child to a gastro-intestinal specialist for further evaluation or a child psychiatrist to investigate possible emotional causes.

How to help your child

Give your child plenty of fluids to alleviate and prevent constipation. If your child is over 6 months, give more fiber in wholegrain cereals, vegetables, and fruit. If constipation is a problem, do not give more than 16 oz (500 ml) of milk a day. School-age children can drink skim or low-fat milk.

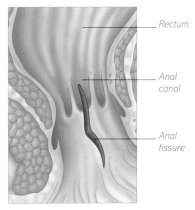

Rectum

Anal canal

Anal fissure

ANAL FISSURE *A tear in the anal canal may occur if a child strains to pass large, hard stools. It makes bowel movements painful and she may withhold stools deliberately.*

CELIAC DISEASE

Rare but serious, this disease is caused by sensitivity of the small intestine to the protein gluten, which is found in wheat, barley, rye, and perhaps oats. As a result, food is not absorbed properly, a condition known as malabsorption.

Medical treatment

If your child has any of the symptoms, take her to the doctor, who will check her weight and may do blood tests for anemia and antibodies. If the results indicate celiac disease, you may have

INTESTINAL DAMAGE *In celiac disease, the tiny fingerlike projections, or villi, in the lining of the small intestine become flattened, preventing proper absorption of nutrients.*

to take her to a specialist for a biopsy of the small intestine. If this shows changes in the intestinal lining (*see left*), the diagnosis is confirmed.

How to help your child

A child with confirmed celiac disease must follow a gluten-free diet. Many specially produced substitute foods are available, including gluten-free bread, crackers, flour, and pasta. Other foods, such as dairy products, eggs, meat, fish, vegetables, fruit, rice, and corn, can be eaten as normal. Check that everyone concerned with the care of your child knows that she can eat only certain foods.

As your child grows up and becomes increasingly independent, make sure she knows the importance of keeping to the diet. Children vary in how they react to renewed exposure

to gluten, and you will soon learn how much gluten is likely to cause an adverse reaction and how severe the reaction might be.

Outlook

The symptoms of celiac disease will clear up within a few weeks of your child starting a gluten-free diet, and she should begin to gain weight. Your child can remain in good health and grow as expected, but she will have to keep to a gluten-free diet throughout her life.

SYMPTOMS

Symptoms develop gradually a few months after a baby starts on solids. Generally caused by foods containing wheat, such as bread, breakfast cereals, and crackers, they include:

- Weight loss or failure to gain weight.
- Very pale, floating stools that have an unpleasant smell.
- Pale skin, breathlessness, and lack of energy due to anemia.

INTESTINAL OBSTRUCTION

This is a partial or complete blockage of either the small or large intestine. The passage of food is obstructed, causing cramping abdominal pain. Treatment is usually needed and complete obstruction of the intestine may be fatal if left untreated.

Causes

In children under 2, the condition is usually caused by a disorder known as intussusception, in which the intestine folds in on itself (*see illustration on opposite page*). Occasionally, it may be caused by a strangulated hernia (*see p.260*) or a congenital abnormality of the intestine.

In children of any age, intestinal obstruction may be caused by Crohn's disease (*see* Inflammatory bowel disease, *p.259*) and volvulus, or twisting, of the intestine.

Dehydration is a serious complication that may develop as a result of the frequent vomiting attacks that are symptomatic of the condition

SYMPTOMS

- Intermittent attacks of severe pain in the abdomen.
- Vomiting, which may produce greenish yellow fluid and occur at increasingly frequent intervals.
- Gas and failure to pass stools. In partial obstruction, passing gas and defecating usually bring temporary relief from pain.
- Bloodstained, jellylike mucus on the stools, in cases of intussusception.
- Fever and swelling of the abdomen, if treatment is delayed.

(*see p.63 and p.172, for signs of dehydration*).

There is a chance that the blocked part of the intestine may rupture, leading to peritonitis (inflammation of the lining of the abdominal cavity). Alternatively, the blocked part may lose blood flow and become gangrenous, which is potentially fatal.

Medical treatment
If you think that your child might have an intestinal obstruction, seek immediate medical care. Your child will be examined and fluids may be given intravenously to prevent dehydration from developing. To confirm the diagnosis and to find out the cause of the obstruction, she may have X-rays or other tests.

If intussusception is suspected, a special X-ray examination involving the use of an air or barium enema may be performed. The child may be given a laxative to clear her bowels. The enema is placed in the anal

passage and then, a short time later, an X-ray is taken. The procedure is completed in about half an hour, during which time the child may experience muscle spasms. The pressure exerted by the enema often forces the displaced intestinal tissue back into the right position.

If the enema does not correct the problem, an operation is performed. Other types of intestinal obstruction require surgery, which sometimes involves removing the obstructed part of the intestine.

Outlook
Your child should grow and develop normally once the obstruction has been treated and cleared, or if only a short section of bowel has been surgically removed. However, if the intestinal obstruction was due to an underlying condition (such as Crohn's disease), the blockage may recur unless the disorder that caused it is being effectively treated.

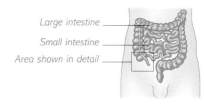

Large intestine

Small intestine

Area shown in detail

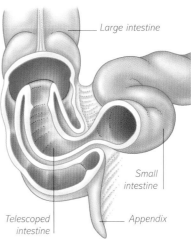

Large intestine

Small intestine

Telescoped intestine

Appendix

INTUSSUSCEPTION *A condition in which part of the intestine telescopes in on itself, intussusception tends to occur in the area where the large and small intestines meet.*

IRRITABLE BOWEL SYNDROME

Irritable bowel syndrome, also known as IBS, is a disorder of the walls of the large intestine. It causes recurrent bouts of abdominal pain which may be accompanied by diarrhea or constipation – sometimes both.

Causes
In this condition, the muscles in the walls of the large intestine act abnormally, leading to problems with digestion. The cause is not clear.

Stress and anxiety appear to trigger and aggravate the symptoms, perhaps by interfering with the digestive process. Intolerance of, or sensitivity to, certain foods, especially wheat, corn, cow's milk protein, nuts, and eggs, can cause abdominal cramps with some muscle spasms.

Irritable bowel syndrome is not common in children, but it is a condition that often persists. Symptoms may recur periodically throughout life.

Medical treatment
Take your child to the doctor if you think that she might be suffering from irritable bowel syndrome. A diagnosis is usually made on the basis of the symptoms combined with a physical examination. Sometimes,

further evaluation or referral to a specialist might be required to exclude another disorder, such as giardiasis (*see p.262*), reactions to food (*see p.252*), or inflammatory bowel disease (*see p.259*).

◻ SYMPTOMS

- Abdominal pain that is relieved by a bowel movement or passing gas.
- Persistent sense of fullness and distension of the bowel.
- Gas and diarrhea or constipation, or bouts of diarrhea alternating with periods of constipation.
- Nausea, headache, and general lack of energy.

In order to be diagnosed with irritable bowel syndrome, your child must display certain symptoms. Your child must have had abdominal pain or discomfort for at least 12 weeks within the past year. The 12 weeks don't have to have been consecutive. In addition, the pain or discomfort must have two of the following three features: pain relieved by having a bowel movement; pain accompanied by a change in the usual frequency of bowel movements; and pain accompanied by a change in the stool's appearance or consistency.

How to help your child

Certain foods may be making your child's symptoms worse, so it is a good idea to keep a diary of her diet so that you can attempt to identify and avoid the problem foods.

Stress and emotional factors can sometimes increase the severity of the symptoms. Try to identify situations that make your child feel anxious, and if they cannot be avoided, give her extra care and support.

Make sure your child eats plenty of fresh and dried fruit, green leafy vegetables, and oat bran. These are all good sources of water-soluble and easily digested fiber. Encourage her to drink plenty of water and to get regular exercise to help with digestion and the progression of food through the large intestine.

Giving your child a high-fiber diet is helpful in many cases of irritable bowel syndrome, especially if the main symptom is constipation.

Sometimes an attack of irritable bowel syndrome is triggered by a bout of gastroenteritis or by an overgrowth of the bacteria that normally inhabit the bowel. Prescription medicines are usually not helpful for irritable bowel syndrome. Consult your doctor before using any herbal remedies or homeopathic treatments.

Relaxation and correct breathing for older children may help manage stress and reduce anxiety. IBS sufferers may have more difficulty adjusting to life and may experience more stress. You should consult your doctor for specific advice about treatment for your child.

MALABSORPTION

Malabsorption is the result of the small intestine's failure to absorb adequate nutrients, such as vitamins, minerals, fats, and amino acids, from food. The problem is always associated with an underlying condition.

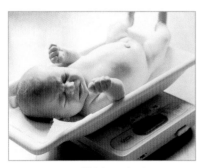

CHECKING WEIGHT *Malabsorption is one possible reason for a child failing to gain weight normally.*

Causes

Malabsorption is sometimes caused by damage to the lining of the small intestine, which interferes with the intestine's ability to absorb nutrients from food. Malabsorption may also be due to a deficiency of the enzymes involved in digestion, which prevents the breakdown of food into units small enough to be absorbed.

Malabsorption is always associated with an underlying disorder, such as Crohn's disease (*see* Inflammatory bowel disease, *p.259*), cystic fibrosis (*see p.315*), or celiac disease (*see p.256*), or adverse reactions to foods such as cow's milk protein or lactose sugar (*see p.252*).

Medical treatment

Take your child to see your doctor if she shows any of the symptoms of malabsorption. Her weight will be checked and compared to what is normal for her age. She may be referred to a specialist who can order

☐ SYMPTOMS

- Very pale, floating stools with an unpleasant smell. The stools contain undigested fat.
- Diarrhea.
- Loss of weight or a failure to gain weight.
- Listlessness.

In severe cases, malabsorption results in deficiencies of vitamins and minerals, such as calcium and iron. These deficiencies may, in turn, lead to malnutrition and anemia (see p.305).

tests to find the underlying cause of the problem. The doctor may also refer you to a dietitian to assess whether your child's diet is adequate for her needs. The underlying cause is treated and your child's diet modified or supplemented, usually ensuring that she grows and gains weight normally. Your child may, however, need to stay on a special diet for life.

INFLAMMATORY BOWEL DISEASE

Crohn's disease and ulcerative colitis both produce chronic inflammation of the intestine. They are rare in children under the age of 7 but more common in adolescents. Although the causes are unknown, genetic factors play a part.

CROHN'S DISEASE

Once a rare condition, Crohn's disease is becoming more common. It may cause inflammation of any part of the digestive tract, but generally affects only the last section of the small intestine (the ileum). As a result of chronic inflammation, the intestinal wall becomes extremely thick, and deep and penetrating ulcers may form.

Crohn's disease reduces the small intestine's ability to absorb nutrients from food (see Malabsorption, *opposite*). Thickening of the intestinal wall may also narrow the inside of the intestine to such an extent that the bowel becomes obstructed (see Intestinal obstruction, p.256). Complications in other parts of the body may include arthritis and inflammation of the eyes or mouth.

Medical treatment

Take your child to the doctor if any of the symptoms persist for more than a few days. Crohn's disease is less likely to be the cause of the symptoms than some other disorder, such as intestinal infection. If your doctor does suspect Crohn's disease, your child may undergo some tests, such as a barium enema X-ray and endoscopic examinations of the intestines, to look for evidence of the disease.

If Crohn's disease is diagnosed, your child may be given anti-inflammatory drugs. Alternatively, she may be given special liquid supplement drinks containing proteins that have been broken down into smaller components, making

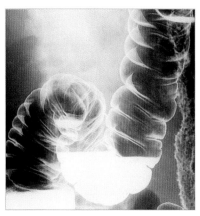

CROHN'S DISEASE *A barium enema X-ray may show narrowing of the intestine due to Crohn's disease.*

absorption easier. In severe cases, and if your child is badly malnourished, she may be given drugs and nutrients intravenously. Blood transfusion may also be needed. If the condition does not improve with medical treatment, or if complications occur, the damaged parts of the intestine may need to be removed surgically.

Outlook

Crohn's disease is a long-term condition and some children continue to suffer from flare-ups of the disease for many years. The symptoms may recur at intervals of a few months or a few years. For other children, Crohn's disease may subside after only one or two episodes.

ULCERATIVE COLITIS

This condition causes the colon and rectum to become both inflamed and ulcerated. The first attack of ulcerative

colitis is often the worst, and then the symptoms may come and go over a long period of time. Bloody diarrhea is the main symptom of this condition; repeated blood loss may cause anemia (see p.305).

Medical treatment

If your child has bloody diarrhea and abdominal pain, take her to see your doctor immediately. Bacterial infection is the most common cause of these symptoms, but if your doctor suspects ulcerative colitis, your child may need to have tests similar to those for Crohn's disease.

If ulcerative colitis is confirmed, your child may have to take anti-inflammatory drugs indefinitely. If drugs do not control the symptoms, or if the colon is badly damaged, the affected part of the colon may be removed surgically.

PYLORIC STENOSIS

An uncommon condition that affects babies under 2 months, pyloric stenosis is the narrowing of the outlet (pylorus) from the stomach into the small intestine. If it is severely narrowed, only a small amount of food enters the intestine; the rest is vomited.

Medical treatment

Call your doctor immediately if your baby shows any symptoms of pyloric stenosis or signs indicating dehydration (*see* Danger signs, *p.63* and *p.172*). Until she is examined by the doctor, you should feed your child small amounts frequently, so not too much undigested food is in her stomach.

The doctor will examine your baby's abdomen to feel for a swelling in the area of the pylorus. If pyloric stenosis seems likely, your child will be admitted to the hospital where she will have further evaluation. An ultrasound examination may confirm the diagnosis.

Intravenous fluids are given if your baby is dehydrated. The obstruction is relieved by a minor surgical operation to widen the pylorus. Your baby can probably leave the hospital after 1 or 2 days. After the operation, you will be advised to increase the amount of your baby's feedings gradually to the normal level (usually within 48–72 hours).

Outlook

Once pyloric stenosis has been treated, the condition will not recur and there are no permanent ill effects.

SYMPTOMS

The main symptoms of pyloric stenosis usually appear between 2 and 6 weeks after birth:

- Persistent projectile vomiting. This is vomiting that is produced forcefully, and projected from the mouth, often reaching some distance from the baby.
- Vomit usually contains milk curds but no bile.
- Dehydration caused by persistent vomiting.
- Constant hunger: the baby often wants another feeding immediately after vomiting.
- Infrequent bowel movements.
- Weight loss and listlessness if the symptoms have been present for more than a few days.
- Baby may appear to be distressed.

HERNIA

A hernia is the protrusion of a part of the intestine through the abdominal wall. Umbilical and inguinal hernias are the most common types in children. In an umbilical hernia, the intestine bulges through the muscle wall at or above the navel (umbilicus).

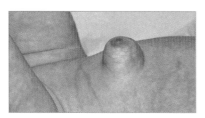

UMBILICAL HERNIA *Usually, an umbilical hernia is at the navel (umbilicus). Sometimes, it appears just above the navel.*

UMBILICAL HERNIA

This type of hernia results from a gap in the muscles of the abdominal wall and usually develops a few weeks after birth. It is more common in babies of African descent. In most cases, the hernia disappears without treatment before a child is 2 years old. However, it may persist up to the age of 5 years.

Medical treatment

Check with your doctor if the hernia is particularly large or if it has not disappeared by the time the child is 5 years old. Your child may need a minor operation to reposition the intestine in the abdominal cavity and stitch together the gap in the muscles of the abdominal wall. Hernias above a child's navel may be more likely to require surgery. An umbilical hernia is unlikely to recur after it has been treated.

SYMPTOMS

Umbilical hernia:
- A soft swelling, usually at the navel.
- Often not present in the morning but may reappear during the day.
- May increase in size if the child cries or tenses the abdominal muscles.
- Not painful.

Inguinal hernia:
- A soft swelling just above the groin crease or in the scrotum.
- Often not present in the morning but may reappear during the day.
- May increase in size if the child cries.

INGUINAL HERNIA

Inguinal hernias are present in about 3 in 100 children, most commonly in boys. They occur when the inguinal canal, which normally closes once the testis has descended, remains open. It forms a space through which a loop of intestine can pass into the groin or the scrotum.

Medical treatment

If you detect a swelling in your son's groin or scrotum which you think might be an inguinal hernia, contact your doctor. If the diagnosis is confirmed, your child will need an operation to correct the problem, since an inguinal hernia will not disappear without treatment.

If the hernia is painful or tender, your child may be admitted to the hospital immediately for emergency surgery. The operation will reposition the intestine in the abdominal cavity and will close the inguinal canal with stitches. An inguinal hernia is unlikely to recur once your child has had the operation.

Possible complications

A strangulated hernia develops when a loop of intestine becomes trapped in the canal, reducing or cutting off its blood supply. The swelling in the groin or scrotum will become hard, tender, or painful, and discolored, and your child may vomit.

If the swelling in the groin or scrotum is painless, you should take your child to the doctor within 24 hours. If the swelling is painful or tender, you should seek medical care immediately.

HEPATITIS

Hepatitis, or inflammation of the liver, is most commonly caused by viruses. Children are most often affected by the virus causing hepatitis A. The hepatitis B virus usually affects adults but can affect newborn babies if their mothers are carriers of the virus.

Causes

The hepatitis A virus is usually transmitted by swallowing water or food contaminated with infected feces. Hepatitis A rarely causes permanent damage to the liver and, after one infection, your child should be immune to further attacks of the disease. Immunization against the hepatitis B virus is routinely offered, and the hepatitis A vaccine may be recommended if you live in or plan to visit certain areas.

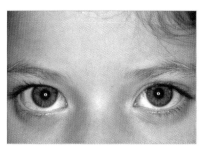

JAUNDICE *In hepatitis, a buildup in the blood of the waste product bilirubin may cause jaundice, a yellowing of the whites of the eyes and skin.*

☐ **SYMPTOMS**

In preschool children, most hepatitis A infections are mild and do not produce any symptoms. Older children usually do have symptoms, but these are rarely severe, and may include:

- Flulike symptoms of fever, headache, and weakness.
- Poor appetite.
- Nausea and vomiting.
- Tender upper right abdomen (where the liver is located).

About a week after the other symptoms have appeared, your child may develop jaundice (see photograph, left), often accompanied by dark urine and pale stools and, sometimes, diarrhea. Jaundice may last for up to 2 weeks.

Medical treatment

Make an appointment to see your doctor within 24 hours if your child has any symptoms of hepatitis. Hepatitis A is not treated with drugs, but the doctor will advise you on how to care for your child at home. Rarely, an attack may be serious enough for your child to be admitted to the hospital, where doctors can keep a close eye on her. The doctor may recommend that family members be immunized to prevent the spread of the disease. A child with hepatitis A is infectious for 2 weeks before, and for 1 week after, the onset of jaundice.

How to help your child

Let your child stay in bed if she wants. While she is vomiting or her appetite is poor, give her small amounts of rehydrating fluid (*see p.63 and p.172*) regularly during the day. As the jaundice decreases, your child's appetite should improve and she can start to eat normally.

Prevent the spread of the hepatitis A virus between family members by washing your hands carefully and by thoroughly washing food utensils. Your child should feel well enough to go back to school from 2–6 weeks after the onset of symptoms.

GIARDIASIS

Giardiasis is an infection of the small intestine caused by the parasite *Giardia lamblia*. Once a problem only in tropical areas, giardiasis now also occurs in temperate countries, where it affects mainly preschool children.

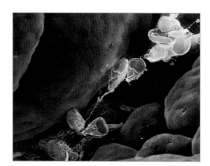

THE CAUSE OF GIARDIASIS *The parasite* Giardia lamblia *clings to folds in the lining of the intestine. It absorbs nutrients from the fluid in the intestine.*

Medical treatment

Children can develop giardiasis by swallowing food or water that is contaminated with the parasite, a protozoan that interferes with fat absorption from the small intestine. The condition is often seen in children who attend child care. Most cases are mild and clear up without treatment within 2 weeks. However, if your child has been suffering from diarrhea for more than 2 weeks, severe diarrhea for over 48 hours, or diarrhea with high fever, take her to the doctor, who will take stool samples and send them for microscopic examination. If your child has the single-celled parasite *Giardia lamblia*, a course of an antiparasitic drug will be prescribed.

How to help your child

Your child should drink plenty of fluids to replace those she loses through diarrhea and to prevent her from suffering from dehydration. Be very scrupulous about handwashing after going to the toilet or changing diapers and before preparing food. These precautions will help prevent the disease from spreading to other members of your family.

SYMPTOMS

About two-thirds of children who are infected have no symptoms. When they do occur, symptoms usually start between 1 and 3 days after the parasite has entered the body:
• Violent attacks of diarrhea accompanied by gas.
• Very pale stools that float on water and have an unpleasant smell. This symptom is the result of malabsorption (*see p.258*).
• Discomfort and cramps in the abdominal area.
• Swollen abdomen and nausea.

PINWORMS

The most common parasitic worms in temperate countries, these worms live in the intestines and resemble tiny white pieces of thread. Children who suck objects or eat food contaminated with worms' eggs are mostly affected.

Causes

The least harmful of parasitic worms, pinworms (*Enterobius vermicularis*) live in large numbers in the lower bowel. Females emerge from the rectum at night (*see illustration*) to lay as many as 10,000 eggs around the anus. This causes intense irritation.

Medical treatment

If you think your child may have pinworms, you should take her to your doctor, who may ask you to collect some eggs for microscopic examination. The whole family will need to be treated with an antiparasitic drug. One course should cure your child, but to prevent reinfection, the family may be treated again in 2 weeks. Wash hands thoroughly after using the toilet or changing diapers.

SYMPTOMS

• Itching in the anal region, especially at night when pinworms lay eggs.
• An itchy vulva in girls.
• Inflammation of the anus as a result of constant scratching.
• Sometimes, tiny white worms wriggling in the stools.

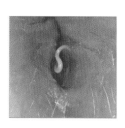

PINWORMS *Worms may be seen emerging from the anus. They usually come out while a person is sleeping. They are whitish gray and threadlike and are ¼ to ½in (6–13mm) long.*

INFECTIOUS DISEASES

CHILDREN ARE GENERALLY MORE SUSCEPTIBLE to the various infectious diseases than adults. This is because a child's immune system takes time to build up resistance to the bacteria, viruses, fungi, and parasites that are commonly found in the environment – in the air we breathe, the water we drink, and the food we eat. The body's defenses against infectious diseases range from the antiseptic solution that washes the eyes to the sophisticated white blood cells that destroy invading germs. Antibiotics can usually cure bacterial infections rapidly and completely, and routine immunization has rendered the contagious, serious viral and bacterial infections, such as measles, mumps, and rubella, much less common than they used to be.

MEASLES

Measles is a highly contagious childhood disease, but widespread immunization has now made it uncommon in Canada and other developed countries. A viral infection that is sometimes very serious, measles causes fever and a rash.

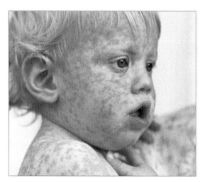

MEASLES RASH *At first, the rash is made up of separate spots, which then merge to give the skin a blotchy look.*

Medical treatment

If you think your child has measles, consult your doctor within 24 hours to confirm the illness. Call the doctor at once if he develops any of the following: earache, abnormally rapid breathing, drowsiness, seizures, severe headache, or vomiting.

How to help your child

Let your child stay in bed or be up and around, as he wants. He may feel very sick. Make sure he drinks plenty of fluids, and consult your doctor for the appropriate dose of ibuprofen or acetaminophen to reduce a fever. He will be contagious for 2 days before the rash appears and then for another 5 days. Try to keep him away from other people who have not already been immunized. Most children recover completely within about 10 days of the first signs. A single attack of measles usually gives lifelong immunity to the disease.

Possible complications

Complications are rare, but some children can develop infection of the middle ear (*see p.240*) or pneumonia (*see p.227*), in which case antibiotics may be prescribed. Serious complications may develop, especially in children who have chronic heart or lung disease or whose immune system is weak. About 1 child in 1,000 with measles may develop encephalitis, a serious illness caused by the infection reaching the brain or by an abnormal immune response to the measles virus.

SYMPTOMS

Incubation period: 10–14 days.
- Fever.
- Red, watery eyes.
- Runny nose.
- Dry cough.

These symptoms are followed by:
- Tiny white spots with a red base (Koplik's spots) may appear on the insides of the cheeks a couple of days after the first symptoms.
- A flat, blotchy, red rash appears (*see p.187*) 3–4 days after the start of the illness, first on the face and behind the ears, then over the whole body. The rash begins to fade after a few days, the fever drops, and your child should start to feel better. In most cases, the rash is gone within a week.

RUBELLA

Often called German measles, rubella is a mild viral infection that is now rare, since most children are immunized against it. It may cause a rash and swollen lymph nodes, but in about 25 percent of cases there is no rash and your child may barely notice the illness.

Medical treatment

Call your doctor if you suspect rubella but do not take your child to the office or emergency room because he could infect pregnant women. Rubella is serious if a woman contracts it early in pregnancy when it can cause damage to the developing baby.

Call your doctor immediately if your child shows any of the following symptoms: a rash of flat, dark red spots that do not fade when they are pressed; severe headache; vomiting; a general lack of energy; or unusual drowsiness. All of these may indicate a more serious illness than rubella.

SYMPTOMS

Incubation period: 2–3 weeks.
- Mild fever.
- Swollen lymph nodes at the back of the neck and behind the ears. Some children may have enlarged lymph nodes in other parts of the body, such as the armpits and groin.
- A nonitchy rash (*see p.187*) may develop after 2–3 days but usually disappears within about 3 days.
- Some children may complain of pains in their joints.

There is no specific medical treatment for rubella, but your doctor will examine your child closely and may confirm the diagnosis by taking a blood sample for laboratory testing.

How to help your child
Give him the recommended dose of acetaminophen or ibuprofen to reduce his fever, and encourage him to drink plenty of fluids. Keep him away from pregnant women and warn any who might be pregnant. Rubella is infectious from 1 week before the rash appears until about 4 days after the rash disappears. Children usually feel much better within about 10 days of the first symptoms appearing. Once he has recovered, your child should be immune to the disease for life.

Possible complications
Rare complications are possible and include inflammation of the brain (encephalitis) and thrombocytopenia (*see p.307*), a disorder in which the number of platelets (clotting agents) in the blood is abnormally low.

RUBELLA RASH *Tiny, flat pink spots appear first on the face and quickly spread to the trunk, arms, and legs. The spots merge as the rash spreads.*

CHICKENPOX

Chickenpox, which is also called varicella, is caused by a virus, and its main symptom is an itchy, irritating rash. It is most common in late winter and spring. Infection in children is decreasing with the increased use of immunization.

Medical treatment
Most children with chickenpox do not need to be seen by a doctor. Call your doctor immediately if your young baby contracts chickenpox, or if your child has reduced immunity or is prone to eczema and has been exposed to chickenpox. See the doctor if pus is coming from the child's rash or if the skin around the spots is red.

Call your doctor or seek medical care immediately if your child starts coughing or has seizures, rapid breathing, persistent or recurrent fever, abnormal drowsiness, or unsteadiness.

Your doctor may prescribe antibiotics for your child to treat a secondary infection caused by bacteria. Children with eczema may be given an antiviral drug such as oral acyclovir. If your child is at high risk of complications, your doctor may recommend a course of intravenous acyclovir or an injection of varicella zoster immune globulin.

How to help your child
Soothe itchiness with calamine lotion. Over-the-counter oral antihistamines may also help, as may a bath in warm water containing a handful of baking soda. Give the appropriate dose of acetaminophen or ibuprofen to reduce a fever (never aspirin, which can cause Reye syndrome, a disease that affects the liver and brain). Provide plenty of drinks. Keep his fingernails trimmed and keep him from scratching to prevent infection.

Chickenpox is infectious from the day before the rash has appeared until all blisters have formed scabs, so keep your child away from anyone at high risk of complications during this time.

Possible complications
A secondary skin infection with streptococcal bacteria, caused by scratching blisters, is the most common complication. Children with eczema (*see p.234*) are particularly prone.

Most at risk are children with a deficient immune system (because they may take oral corticosteroids or have chemotherapy) and newborn babies, who can develop chickenpox if the mother has it late in pregnancy.

Outlook
Your child should feel better 7–10 days after symptoms start. One infection usually gives lifelong immunity, but the virus remains dormant in nerve cells and may cause shingles in late childhood or adulthood.

FIFTH DISEASE (ERYTHEMA INFECTIOSUM)

Mildly contagious, erythema infectiosum is a viral illness that causes a red rash on both cheeks. Also known as fifth disease, it tends to be most common in the spring among children over the age of 2.

Medical treatment

There is no specific medicine for fifth disease; treatment is given to alleviate symptoms. You should call your doctor if you are worried about your child or if he has a blood disorder that can lead to complications. If possible, avoid taking your child to the doctor's office because of the risk of infecting others. Your child may need to have a blood test to check the diagnosis.

How to help your child

Give your child the recommended dose of acetaminophen or ibuprofen to reduce the fever and encourage him to drink plenty of fluids. He is unlikely to be infectious after the rash appears but, just in case, it is best to keep your child away from anyone who might be pregnant, especially someone in the first trimester of a pregnancy. The rash may recur over a period of several weeks or months.

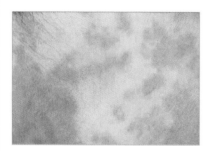

DISTINCTIVE RED CHEEKS *This infection is also called "slapped cheek" disease because of the bright red rash on the cheeks.*

SYMPTOMS

Incubation period: 4–14 days.
* Bright red cheeks, as if they have been "slapped."
* A pale area around the mouth.
* Fever.
* A rash that appears 1–4 days after the redness on the cheeks and lasts for 7–10 days. The rash usually appears on the arms and legs and sometimes on the body. Blotchy or with a lacy pattern, especially on the limbs, the rash can vary according to the temperature. It may, for example, seem worse after a warm bath or after spending time out in the sun.
* Joint pain – but this is rare.

HAND, FOOT, AND MOUTH DISEASE

Common in children up to the age of 4 years, hand, foot, and mouth disease usually occurs during the summer and early autumn. It is a mild viral infection that causes blisters to appear in the mouth and on the hands and feet.

How to help your child

There is no specific treatment for hand, foot, and mouth disease. However, you may try to ease the symptoms. For example, if your child is suffering from painful mouth ulcers, give him ibuprofen or acetaminophen in the appropriate dose. Mouth rinses may help soothe the pain (*see p.207*).

Make sure your child drinks plenty of fluids each day – water or milk are best. Avoid citrus juices, because these are acidic and may make the pain in his mouth worse. If your child is reluctant to eat solids, then offer smooth, soft foods.

The blisters on your child's hands and feet will usually clear up within about 3 or 4 days, and the fever should have disappeared by then, too. However, the ulcers in the mouth may last for as long as 4 weeks. Once your child has had a single attack of the disease he may be immune for life.

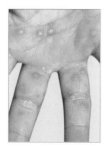

BLISTERS ON THE FINGERS *In hand, foot, and mouth disease, blisters commonly appear on the fingers, the palms of the hands, or the soles of the feet.*

SYMPTOMS

Incubation period: 3–5 days.
* Mild fever.
* Blisters on the inside of the mouth, which may develop into sore, shallow ulcers.
* Child has lost appetite and does not want to eat.
* Painless blisters on the hands and feet, which usually appear 1 or 2 days after those in the mouth. The blisters may also appear in the diaper area.

ROSEOLA INFANTUM

Most children will have caught roseola infantum by the time they are 4 years old. This viral infection causes a high fever, which comes on suddenly and lasts for about 4 days, followed by a rash of tiny pink spots.

Medical treatment

There is no specific treatment for roseola, but call your doctor immediately if your child has a

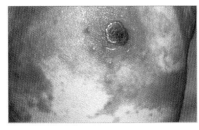

ROSEOLA RASH *In the second phase of roseola, a rash of tiny pink spots appears and lasts for about 4 days.*

temperature of 39°C (102°F) or above, has a febrile seizure (*see p.292*), or is drowsy or irritable. To bring down the fever, your doctor may recommend giving him acetaminophen or ibuprofen. Sponging with lukewarm water may give some comfort.

The doctor may want to do blood or urine tests to confirm the diagnosis and check for bacterial infections – meningitis, for example, can produce similar symptoms. Recovery is quick. Your child should feel completely better by the time the rash has gone. Complications are rare in otherwise healthy children, but a child with a

suppressed immune system could develop hepatitis (*see p.261*) or pneumonia (*see p.227*).

☐ SYMPTOMS

Incubation period: 5–15 days.
- A fever of 39–40°C (102–104°F), although your child may otherwise seem well.
- Sometimes, one or more febrile seizures (*see p.292*).
- Some children also have mild diarrhea, a cough, enlarged lymph nodes in the neck, and earache.

About 4 days after the start of the fever, the illness enters its second phase:
- Child's temperature suddenly goes back to normal.
- A rash of tiny pink spots appears (*see p.187*), usually on the head and trunk, and lasts for a few days.

SCARLET FEVER

Scarlet fever is caused by streptococcal bacteria. It usually occurs in association with streptococcal pharyngitis (strep throat). The most obvious feature of the illness is the red, sandpaper-like rash.

Medical treatment

Call your doctor within 24 hours of the symptoms appearing. Your doctor can confirm your child has scarlet fever by looking at his symptoms and doing a throat swab test. He will usually prescribe a course of antibiotics. Call your doctor immediately if your child's urine is red, pink, or brown, or if your child has a fever that lasts for 5 days.

How to help your child

Acetaminophen or ibuprofen in the recommended dose can help reduce

the fever and ease pain. Make sure that your child finishes the course of medication. Rheumatic fever can follow untreated or incompletely treated scarlet fever. Your child should feel better within a few days. Since there are many different serotypes (strains) of streptococcal bacteria, scarlet fever may recur.

Thanks to antibiotic treatment, the complications of scarlet fever are rare. However, they do include rheumatic fever, which can lead to permanent heart damage and glomerulonephritis (*see p.276*).

☐ SYMPTOMS

Incubation period: 2–4 days.
- Vomiting.
- Fever.
- Sore throat and headache.
- Rash which appears within 24 hours of the first symptoms developing (*see p.187*). The rash is slightly raised and may feel rough, like sandpaper. It is most dense on the neck and in the armpits and groin. It does not affect the face. The rash lasts about 3–5 days and the skin then peels.
- Cheeks are flushed and there is a pale area around the mouth.
- In the early stages the tongue has a thick white coating with projecting red spots. The coating peels by the fourth day, leaving a bright red "strawberry tongue," still with the spots.

MUMPS

A mild viral infection, mumps causes a fever and a swelling of one or both of the salivary (parotid) glands. These are in front of and below the ears, above the angle of the jaw. Mumps was much more common among children until routine immunization began.

Medical treatment

If you think your child has mumps, call your doctor to confirm the diagnosis. Phone immediately if your child has a severe headache (with or without vomiting) or has pain in the abdomen. A child suffering from a severe headache may require tests to rule out encephalitis (*see p.295*) or bacterial meningitis (*see p.294*).

How to help your child

Swollen glands may be painful but the recommended dose of acetaminophen or ibuprofen can reduce the fever and make your child more comfortable. Give plenty of fluids but avoid citrus juices: they stimulate the flow of saliva and may worsen pain in the glands.

Children generally feel much better in about 10 days. Problems affecting the testicles and pancreas do not usually have long-term ill effects and infertility as a result of inflamed testicles is rare. Your child is usually immune to mumps after one infection.

Possible complications

Occasionally, adolescent boys with mumps develop inflamed testes, a condition called orchitis (*see* Penis and testis disorders, *p.277*). This starts about a week after the mumps.

Very rarely, serious disorders such as pancreatitis (inflammation of the pancreas), encephalitis, and meningitis may develop, either before or after the salivary glands have become swollen.

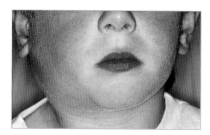

SYMPTOMS

Incubation period: 14–24 days.
- Fever.
- Tenderness and swelling of one or both sides of the face, giving your child a puffy, hamsterlike appearance. This usually comes on 1 or 2 days after the fever starts and may last 4–8 days.
- Pain in the jaw, ear, and abdomen.
- Swelling of other glands.

SWOLLEN GLANDS *The most obvious feature of mumps is the swelling of the salivary glands, just below the ears. The swollen glands may be painful.*

TETANUS

A serious illness affecting the nervous system, tetanus is now very rare in developed countries where children are immunized against it. Bacterial spores enter the body through a deep wound, particularly one contaminated by garden soil or animal manure.

Causes

Tetanus is caused by a poison produced by a bacterium called *Clostridium tetani*. Paradoxically, these bacteria inhabit the intestines of both humans and animals without ill effects. Because of this, clostridium bacteria can be found wherever stools contaminate the soil.

When a wound is contaminated by dirt, the bacteria can spread into the bloodstream and multiply. The

bacterial toxin causes the voluntary muscles of the body to contract and stiffen – first the jaws, then the face and neck. When the toxin causes the back muscles to contract, the body may suddenly arch backward.

Immediate action

Tetanus is a medical emergency. If you think your child is showing any of the symptoms of tetanus, you should call your doctor immediately or take your

SYMPTOMS

Incubation period: 3–21 days.
- Cannot open the mouth because of contractions in the muscles of the jaw. This gives the condition its alternative name of lockjaw.
- The child finds it hard to swallow.
- Muscles in the face contract, making the child look as though he has a fixed smile. This is known as *risus sardonicus*.
- Spasms of muscles in the neck, back, abdomen, and limbs. These spasms can be painful and may happen over a period of 10–14 days. The spasms may make it difficult for the child to breathe.

child to the nearest emergency room for urgent treatment.

Medical treatment

If your child has cut himself and you think the wound may have been infected with contaminated soil, consult your doctor immediately. If he suspects tetanus your child will need an evaluation. If the infection is mild – there is only stiffness around the site of infection and spasms, if any, are weak – he may need only sedative drugs and a light diet.

Severe cases of tetanus need more urgent treatment. A tube may be inserted into the trachea (windpipe) to help your child breathe and a mechanical ventilator will keep his breathing going. Muscle relaxants and sedative drugs will be administered to relieve the muscle contractions and spasms.

Outlook

Tetanus can be a fatal illness, but with prompt hospital treatment most children will recover from it completely. Many children feel better within 3 weeks but those who have suffered a severe attack of tetanus may take longer.

▢ PREVENTION

Your child will usually be immunized against tetanus starting as a baby. If he does sustain a deep wound, do not wait to see if any symptoms develop. Seek treatment immediately, even if he has been immunized against tetanus. To prevent the disease from developing, the doctor may clean the wound to clear away all the dirt and dead tissue. Your child may be given antibiotics, tetanus immune globulin, and/or a tetanus vaccine booster.

PERTUSSIS

Also known as whooping cough, this bacterial infection is most dangerous in babies under 6 months. Most young children in Canada are immunized against it, so it is uncommon. A cough is the characteristic symptom, sometimes followed by a whoop.

Medical treatment

Call a doctor within 24 hours if your baby is under 6 months and has a cough, or if your child vomits from coughing or has a cough that lasts more than a week. Call immediately if your child's tongue or lips turn blue during a coughing attack or if he has a seizure. Seek medical care immediately if your child has had a seizure or turns blue, especially if he is under 6 months old.

Your doctor may take a sample from your child's nose or throat to confirm the diagnosis. Antibiotics are usually given for 1–2 weeks. They are most effective when given early. They do not cure the cough but can lessen the severity of the illness and prevent complications such as pneumonia. Giving the infected child antibiotics can also prevent spreading the infection to others. Ask your doctor if other household members may need an antibiotic to prevent pertussis or a vaccine booster.

How to help your child

Let your child rest in bed and use a vaporizer to help soothe his lungs and loosen secretions. Ask your doctor about the best position to help drain those secretions and improve breathing. Give plenty of fluids to drink and soft food to eat.

Outlook

Your child may continue to cough for up to several months. If a child is generally ill, or the cough has not improved after 6 weeks, a chest X-ray may be obtained. Permanent lung damage is rare. Older children and adults usually have only mild symptoms and recover more quickly than infants and younger children.

▢ SYMPTOMS

Incubation period: about 7 days.
- Short, dry cough, often occurring only at night.
- Runny nose.
- Possibly a slight fever.
- Sore, pink, and runny eyes as in conjunctivitis.

The next stage of the illness may last between 8–12 weeks with the following symptoms:
- Bouts of 10–20 short, dry coughs that may happen during the day and at night.
- Long attacks of coughing followed by a sharp indrawing of breath, which may produce a "whooping" sound – babies may not "whoop."
- Vomiting brought on by the persistent coughing.
- Pauses in breathing (apnea) – i.e. for more than 10 seconds.
- Seizures.

Very occasionally, an air passage may become blocked by mucus, causing either part of a lung to collapse or pneumonia to develop.

INFECTIOUS MONONUCLEOSIS

Infectious mononucleosis is usually caused by the Epstein-Barr virus, which attacks the white blood cells that fight infection in the body. Also called "mono," the disease may be difficult to diagnose because of its similarities to other illnesses. It is most common in adolescents and young adults but can infect people of any age, including young children.

Causes

Infectious mononucleosis is most commonly caused by the Epstein-Barr virus, athough another virus called cytomegalovirus, or CMV, may sometimes be the cause. The Epstein-Barr virus is passed through contact with infected saliva, such as by kissing or sharing drinks. Sometimes the virus may be passed through respiratory droplets spread by coughs or sneezes. The incubation period (the time between exposure to the virus and showing symptoms) ranges from 1 to 6 weeks, typically about 10 days in children.

Medical treatment

If you think that your child may have infectious mononucleosis, you should consult your doctor as soon as possible. A specific blood test, called a mono spot test, may confirm the diagnosis. The test detects antibodies to the virus. Alternatively, your child may need other tests to diagnose infectious mononucleosis.

A positive test also rules out other possible infections that have similar symptoms. The muscular pains of infectious mononucleosis are the same as those associated with influenza (*see p.225*), and the sore throat and infected tonsils are similar to the symptoms of tonsillitis (*see p.223*). Occasionally, the illness starts with a rash that is similar to rubella (*see p.264*).

There is no treatment for mono, per se. Since the infection is caused by a virus, antibiotics do not help and may even bring on a rash that affects the whole body. The doctor may advise that your child rest until the fever is gone.

How to help your child

Since the disease cannot be treated, you and your child should accept that it needs to run its course. However, you may be able to help alleviate some of the symptoms. Make sure your child has plenty of cool drinks and does not get overtired. You may want to give him acetaminophen or ibuprofen in the recommended dose to help reduce a high fever and any pain. He may want to stay in bed or he may be happier playing in the house.

The infection is easily spread – one of its common names is the "kissing disease" because it can be spread by mouth-to-mouth contact – so you should make sure that your child avoids very close contact with other children while he is sick.

Encourage good handwashing practices for the whole family. Instruct your child not to share food, drinks, or utensils.

There are various measures you can take to boost your child's immune system so that he is better able to fight the virus. Encourage him to eat a healthy and balanced diet. Any

nutritional deficiency can make his fatigue worse, so you should consult your doctor about giving him a multivitamin and mineral supplement.

Possible complications

The most common complication is hepatitis (*see p.261*). Other, rarer complications may include pneumonia (*see p.227*) and rupture of the spleen. Problems of the nervous system, blood circulation, and breathing may also develop. Children with enlarged spleens will likely be advised to avoid contact sports.

Outlook

Most children will be able go back to school after a couple of weeks but some may need to rest longer. Once back at school your child should still avoid energetic sports for a few weeks so that he does not get too tired. Symptoms typically disappear completely within 4 to 8 weeks, and most people do not get sick with mononucleosis again.

▣ SYMPTOMS

Incubation period: about 10 days.

- Swollen lymph nodes, or "glands," in the neck and/or in the armpits or groin.
- High fever of about 39–40°C (102–104°F).
- The fever may last only a few days or several weeks.
- Extremely sore throat.
- Fatigue and lethargy.
- Weight loss and lack of appetite.
- Headache.
- Achiness.
- May have muscle pain.
- Possibly a rash.
- Tender, painful abdomen.

MALARIA

A serious health problem in tropical and subtropical areas, malaria is increasing elsewhere as more and more people travel to regions where the disease is prevalent. Malaria is caused by parasites that enter the blood after a bite by an infected mosquito.

Causes

Malaria is caused by a protozoan called *Plasmodium*, which is transmitted from one person to the next by mosquitoes that feed on blood. Once symptoms of the disease develop and take hold, the parasite periodically invades red blood cells and the liver.

Medical treatment

Call your doctor immediately if your child has traveled out of the country and has any symptoms of malaria. His blood will be tested for the parasites. He will be treated with antimalarial drugs if necessary.

Seek medical attention immediately if he has any of the following: seizures, drowsiness, or yellowing or extreme paleness of the skin. If there are complications, he may need treatment in an intensive care unit. If he is treated quickly he

PROTECTION

If you plan to visit a region where malaria is common, you and your family will need to take antimalarial drugs for several days before you depart, for the duration of your stay, and after you return. Ask which drugs to take since different ones are recommended for travel in different countries. Try to avoid mosquito bites by wearing protective clothing, applying insect repellent, and sleeping under mosquito nets.

SYMPTOMS

Symptoms of malaria usually develop 6–30 days after infection in an area of the world with malaria. They may appear as much as a year later if the child has taken only partly effective antimalarial drugs. The main symptoms are:
- High fever alternating with shivering.
- Headache.

Other symptoms include:
- Nausea and vomiting.
- Pain in the abdomen and back.
- Joint pain.

Falciparum malaria can result in very serious complications affecting the kidneys, liver, brain, and blood.

may be better in only a few days or up to 2 weeks, depending on the severity of the attack. The more severe form, falciparum malaria, may be life-threatening if complications affect the brain or the kidneys.

TYPHOID FEVER

Typhoid fever, also known as enteric fever, is caused by bacteria that infect the digestive tract. Children usually catch the disease by consuming food or water contaminated with bacteria from the stools of an infected person.

Causes

Typhoid fever is caused by a bacterium called *Salmonella typhi*. A similar but less virulent illness, paratyphoid fever is caused by the bacterium *Salmonella paratyphi*. Once inside the digestive tract, bacteria enter the bloodstream, causing a fever and other symptoms of blood poisoning. Typhoid is common wherever sanitation is poor and where flies carry the bacteria from human feces to supplies of food and water.

Medical treatment

You should call your doctor within 24 hours of the appearance of possible typhoid symptoms. If the doctor suspects that your child might have typhoid fever, the diagnosis can be confirmed by testing your child's urine or stools, or by carrying out a blood test. Your child will be treated with antibiotics, which may be given intravenously if his symptoms are severe.

SYMPTOMS

Incubation period: 7–14 days.
- Fever that rises to 102–104°F (39–40°C) and stays at that level without daily fluctuations for up to 4 weeks.
- Headache.
- Lack of energy.
- Decreased appetite.
- Pain in the abdomen.
- Constipation or diarrhea.
- Rash of pink spots on the abdomen and chest.
- Intestinal bleeding/perforation or other complications may develop by the third week if illness is not treated.

Children usually start to improve a few days after the start of treatment and recover completely in 2 or 3 weeks.

Possible complications

With prompt treatment, complications such as bleeding, pneumonia (*see p.227*), meningitis (*see p.294*), and cholecystitis (gall bladder infection) are rare.

Protection

The typhoid vaccine will give several years' protection against the disease although, in some cases, you may need a booster before traveling.

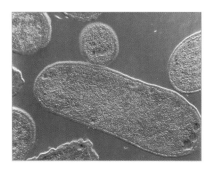

SALMONELLA TYPHI BACTERIA These bacteria are responsible for typhoid fever. They invade the wall of the small intestine before entering the bloodstream.

HIV INFECTION AND AIDS

Most of the children affected by HIV (human immunodeficiency virus) contract the virus from their mother before or during birth. Treating the mother during pregnancy reduces the risk of passing on the virus. Untreated HIV infection damages the immune system, leading to AIDS (acquired immune deficiency syndrome), so that illnesses such as pneumonia can develop.

Causes

HIV infection is transmitted via blood products, as in blood transfusion, or via other body fluids. The HIV virus particles attach themselves to the surface of white blood cells, destroying them and thus reducing the efficiency of the immune system.

The condition gradually debilitates the body, leading to full-blown AIDS when the immune system is so weak that potentially fatal illnesses such as pneumonia (*see p.227*) and tuberculosis develop unhindered.

Nearly all cases of HIV in children are due to transmission from their HIV-positive mothers, during either pregnancy or birth. This is called perinatal transmission.

Medical treatment

Children who are infected with HIV or who have developed AIDS require careful medical supervision. If the doctor suspects that a baby has HIV,

both parents are given counseling. With the parents' consent, the baby is given a blood test. If HIV antibodies are present, the baby has been exposed to the virus. This is not the same thing as infection. Although the mother's HIV antibodies may remain in the baby's blood for a year or more, a different test called HIV PCR can positively confirm or exclude the presence of the infection in the first 4 months of life.

The doctor or HIV physician specialist may prescribe drugs, such as zidovudine, in combination to attack the virus and to slow down the development and progress of the disease. Antibiotics can also help the child, by preventing or fighting infections, such as pneumonia.

How to help your child

If you are an HIV-positive mother, you are advised not to breastfeed your child because of the risk of

transmitting the virus in your milk. If you are treated while pregnant and during labor and avoid breastfeeding, the chances of passing on the infection are less than 5 percent. If your child has HIV infection or AIDS, you will be given advice on how to manage the illness.

Outlook

An increasing number of HIV-infected children are surviving into adulthood. Anti-HIV medications can help preserve or restore the health of most children infected with HIV.

SYMPTOMS

Most infants infected before or around the time of birth will have symptoms before they are 2 years old. But some may not develop symptoms until they are more than 5 years old, and a few cases have been diagnosed as late as 12 years. Some of the many possible symptoms in children are:

- Failure to gain weight.
- Recurrent diarrhea.
- Enlarged lymph nodes in the neck, armpits, and groin.
- Frequent infections, particularly of the ear and sinuses, often with fever.
- Episodes of pneumonia.
- Delay in normal development.

UROGENITAL PROBLEMS

Most urinary tract infections, such as cystitis and urethritis, clear up quickly with treatment. However, urinary infections and other disorders affecting the kidneys, the bladder, or the genitals may need medical attention to check for any structural defect that may be present. Most serious kidney disorders, such as glomerulonephritis, are now treatable, including the most common childhood kidney cancer, Wilms' tumor.

ANATOMY OF THE UROGENITAL SYSTEM

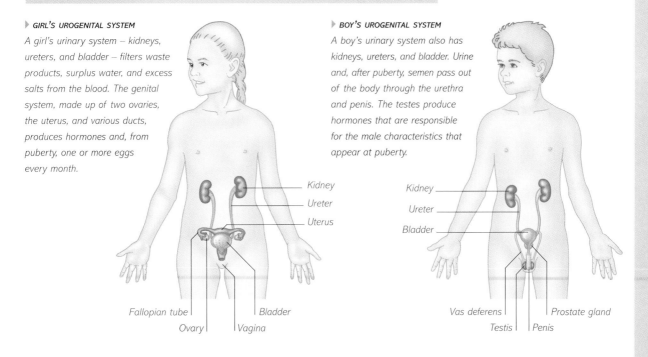

▶ **GIRL'S UROGENITAL SYSTEM**

A girl's urinary system – kidneys, ureters, and bladder – filters waste products, surplus water, and excess salts from the blood. The genital system, made up of two ovaries, the uterus, and various ducts, produces hormones and, from puberty, one or more eggs every month.

Kidney
Ureter
Uterus

Fallopian tube
Ovary
Bladder
Vagina

▶ **BOY'S UROGENITAL SYSTEM**

A boy's urinary system also has kidneys, ureters, and bladder. Urine and, after puberty, semen pass out of the body through the urethra and penis. The testes produce hormones that are responsible for the male characteristics that appear at puberty.

Kidney
Ureter
Bladder

Vas deferens
Testis
Penis
Prostate gland

NOCTURNAL ENURESIS (BED-WETTING)

Children vary greatly in the age they become dry at night, but few can control their bladders before the age of 3 and nocturnal enuresis, or bed-wetting, is common. Reliable control, day and night, may be gained any time between the ages of 3 and 5. There is usually no need for further evaluation unless your child continues to wet the bed after the age of 5.

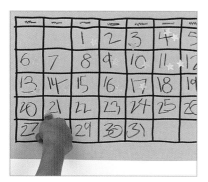

STAR CHART *Sticking a star on a chart after each dry night can be a satisfying way for your child to mark progress. The chart also allows parents to see how well the child is doing and to give praise for good results.*

Causes of nocturnal enuresis
Nocturnal enuresis usually happens because the parts of the nervous system that control the bladder are not yet mature. It may also develop if a child has a urinary tract infection (*see p.275*) or is anxious (*see* Anxiety and fears, *pp.131–132*). Rarely, a congenital defect of the urinary tract or diabetes mellitus (*see p.309*) is the cause.

Medical treatment
Consult your doctor if you are worried about your child wetting the bed, especially if she is 5 years old or over, or if the problem starts again after your child has been dry at night for at least 6 to 12 months and there is also daytime wetting.

The doctor will examine your child and will test a urine sample for infection or diabetes (*see p.309*). If a physical cause for the enuresis is found, treatment will be given; for example, antibiotics may be prescribed to treat a urinary tract infection. If no physical reason is found, follow the advice given here (*see also* Toilet training, *p.72*).

How to help your child
A child may be less likely to wet the bed if she is in the habit of urinating at regular times during the day and just before going to sleep. Never punish your child for a bed-wetting accident or you may increase her anxiety and make the problem worse. Always praise your child for dry nights.

A chart on which your child can stick a star after each dry night may help her motivation (*see left*). Some children become completely dry after using a star chart for a few weeks without having any other treatment. But if your child becomes discouraged because the chart reflects poor results, stop using it.

If methods involving praise and encouragement are unsuccessful, ask your doctor about an enuresis alarm. Available at many pharmacies, this device has a detector, which is placed under the bottom sheet or attached to pajamas or underwear and activates a buzzer if the child urinates. The alarm wakes the child, who stops the urine stream and gets up to go to the toilet. The amount of urine passed before the

HELPFUL TIPS

• Constipation may put pressure on the bladder, so try to help your child have regular bowel movements.
• Encourage your child to urinate at regular times throughout the day, and especially at bedtime.
• Praise your child for dry nights.
• Do not punish your child for bed wetting, as this may worsen the problem.
• Encourage your child to avoid drinks that contain caffeine, such as hot chocolate, tea, coffee, and cola.
• Limit your child's liquid intake in the evening.
• If your child has experienced an emotional upset or a significant change, such as moving to a new house or changing schools, or if she feels insecure after the birth of a baby brother or sister, spend more time doing one-on-one activities with her.

child wakes decreases. After a few months, most children wake up before the alarm starts or sleep through the night without wetting the bed. Alarms tend to be most helpful when children are starting to have some dry nights, and have some bladder control on their own.

Outlook
Most children stop wetting the bed without medical treatment. However, some benefit from using a medication such as desmopressin, which is made to be like a naturally occurring hormone that concentrates the urine. Those who are treated often improve within a few months. The older a child is, however, the longer it may take for the condition to improve.

URINARY TRACT INFECTIONS

In general, girls experience more infections of the urinary tract than boys, but newborn male babies are more susceptible to infections than female babies. An infection may affect the urethra (causing urethritis), the bladder (causing cystitis), and/or the kidneys (causing pyelonephritis). Prompt treatment may prevent scarring of the kidneys, which is most likely to affect children under 5. Scarring of the kidneys from recurrent infections may lead to high blood pressure or kidney failure in adult life.

Causes

The most common cause of urinary tract infections is bacteria which enter the urethra from the rectum. Girls are more prone to urinary infections than boys because their urethras are shorter.

Children who have urinary reflux are especially vulnerable to infection. In this congenital condition, when the bladder empties, some urine passes backward toward the kidneys. A tendency to reflux usually disappears during childhood without treatment.

Children with chronic constipation (*see p.255*), congenital malformations of the urinary tract, or kidneys scarred from previous infection are also more susceptible to infection.

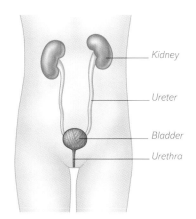

SITES OF INFECTION Infections of the urinary tract may affect only the urethra, but more commonly spread upward to affect the bladder or the kidneys.

- Kidney
- Ureter
- Bladder
- Urethra

Medical treatment

Your child should be seen by a doctor within 24 hours if she shows signs of having a urinary tract infection. Your doctor will probably collect a urine sample from your child or will ask you to do so.

A baby with urinary infection symptoms may have to have urine withdrawn from the bladder via a hollow needle passed through the skin or through a small tube (catheter) passed through the urethra. The urine is tested to rule out an underlying disorder and to confirm that infection is the cause of the symptoms.

If an infection of the urinary tract is confirmed, your doctor will prescribe oral antibiotics for your child, which may be given for up to a week. A seriously ill child may need to be treated in the hospital with intravenous antibiotics. A day or two after treatment for infection has ceased, your child's urine may be tested again and if there is still some infection, she may be given another course of antibiotics.

In some circumstances, further investigations may need to be carried out to see if your child's kidneys have been scarred or if there is a structural abnormality of the urinary tract. Some children may have special tests for urinary reflux. Because children with these conditions are often prone to

■ **SYMPTOMS**

In children under 2 years of age, the symptoms include:
- Fever.
- Diarrhea.
- Vomiting.
- Lack of energy or irritability.

In older children, symptoms are usually more specific, and may include:
- Burning sensation on urinating.
- Frequent urination.
- Pain affecting one side of the lower back or abdomen.
- Enuresis after being dry at night.
- Urine that is red, pink, or brown in color, due to the presence of blood.
- Fever.

recurrent infections, they may be prescribed a small daily dose of antibiotics for an extended period as a preventive measure or have surgery for correctable structural problems.

How to help your child

Give your child plenty of fluids to drink. A high fluid intake dilutes the urine, easing the pain and discomfort when urinating, and helps get rid of bacteria. It may also help improve her general health, and stimulate her resistance to infection.

To prevent further infections, you should encourage your child to urinate at least once every 4 hours (or before each meal) and before going to bed. Show your child how to wipe her bottom from front to back after going to the bathroom to prevent bacteria from spreading from her rectum to her urethra. You should encourage her to bathe or shower regularly, without irritants, such as scented soaps or bubble bath. Constipation should also be treated.

GLOMERULONEPHRITIS

This is an inflammation of the glomeruli, the filtering units in
the kidneys. The inflamed glomeruli produce less urine and leak
blood and protein into the urine. It usually affects both kidneys
and may follow an infection by streptococcal bacteria or viruses.

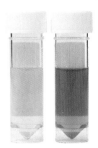

BLOOD IN URINE
*The presence of
blood gives urine
an abnormal
appearance. It looks
darker and cloudier
than normal clear,
pale yellow urine.*

Medical treatment
You should call your doctor
immediately if you think your child
has glomerulonephritis. She will need
to be evaluated. Her urine will be
tested and her kidney function may
be measured. If the diagnosis is
confirmed, she may need to stay in the
hospital for treatment. To lessen the
strain on the kidneys and prevent the
accumulation of fluids, your child may
be put on a diet that is low in sodium
and protein, and her intake of fluids
may be restricted.

If the condition was caused by
a bacterial infection, your child may
be given antibiotics. If she has high
blood pressure, this condition may
need to be treated as well until it
returns to normal.

With treatment, the condition
usually clears up within weeks.
Glomerulonephritis does not usually
have any lasting effect on a child's
kidneys and it does not usually recur.
Very rarely, it may be associated with
nephrotic syndrome (*see below*).

SYMPTOMS

*In postinfective glomerulonephritis, the
symptoms begin about a week after an
infection. Whatever the cause, the main
symptoms are:*
- Urine that is red, pink, or brown in
  color, caused by the presence of
  blood (*see photograph, left*).
- Urinating smaller amounts than
  usual.
- Sometimes, a headache.

*Fluid may also accumulate in the tissues,
leading to swelling, particularly of the
face and legs. High blood pressure is
a rare complication.*

NEPHROTIC SYNDROME

Nephrotic syndrome is an uncommon disorder, mainly affecting
children ages 1–6 years. A large amount of protein is lost via
the kidneys and the reduced levels of protein in the blood lead
to edema (accumulation of excess fluid in the body's tissues).

Medical treatment
Your child should be seen by your
doctor within 24 hours if parts of her
body are swollen. The doctor will
examine her and may test her urine
for protein. If nephrotic syndrome is
suspected, she will need to go to the
hospital for further tests and, if the
diagnosis is confirmed, to be treated
with corticosteroids.

Within 10 days, as the excess
fluid in the body is excreted by
the kidneys, there should be an
improvement in the edema, bringing
a rapid fall in weight. During your
child's hospitalization, you will learn
how to check her urine and how to
restrict salt in her diet.

How to help your child
Once your child is home from the
hospital, you will need to test a sample
of her urine regularly, using strips that
change color when protein is present.

If the test shows that protein has
reappeared in the urine, phone your
doctor for advice. Children who have
nephrotic syndrome are more
susceptible to infections and, rarely, to
the formation of blood clots in veins.

Outlook
Over time, most children recover fully
with no further problems. Those who
have frequent relapses are prescribed
corticosteroids and/or another
medication for a prolonged period.

SYMPTOMS

- Swelling of parts of the body, usually
  developing gradually over a period of
  several weeks.
- Reduction in the quantity of urine.
- Weight gain.
- Sometimes, diarrhea, loss of appetite,
  and unusual fatigue.

PENIS AND TESTIS DISORDERS

A variety of penis problems can affect young boys. These include a tight foreskin (phimosis), a tight foreskin stuck in the retracted position (paraphimosis), inflammation of the tip of the penis and foreskin (balanitis), and an abnormally placed urethral opening (hypospadias). The most common disorders of the testis are an abnormal collection of fluid around a testis (a hydrocele) and an undescended testis. Adolescent boys are prone to the disorders of testicular torsion and inflammation of the testes (orchitis).

TIGHT FORESKIN

In the first few years of life, an uncircumcised boy's foreskin usually cannot be pulled back over the tip of his penis. Never try to retract your son's foreskin by force or you may injure the tissues, resulting in bleeding, inflammation, and the formation of scar tissue.

In some boys, full retraction of the foreskin is possible by the age of 2, but in many boys it may not happen until about age 4. After this age, consult your doctor if you are unable to pull back the foreskin at all.

Causes

A tight foreskin may occur if strands of tissue that attach it to the penis at birth remain for longer than normal. It may also be due to phimosis, an abnormally narrow opening in the foreskin (*see below*). Phimosis may be congenital but is sometimes due to scarring caused by recurrent inflammation (*see* Balanitis, *p.278*) or by forceful attempts to retract the foreskin. A boy with phimosis is at increased risk of urinary tract infections (*see p.275*).

Medical treatment

Take your child to a doctor if he is older than 4 years and his foreskin cannot be retracted and/or he is having problems urinating. If your son has phimosis, the doctor may recommend circumcision, an operation to remove the foreskin (*see p.278*). If the foreskin is attached to the penis and the diameter of the outlet is normal, the tissues may be separated surgically. Both operations are performed using an anesthetic.

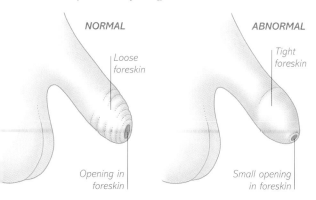

NORMAL

Loose foreskin

Opening in foreskin

ABNORMAL

Tight foreskin

Small opening in foreskin

PHIMOSIS *When there is an abnormally small opening in the foreskin, the foreskin becomes tight and is hard to retract over the glans of the penis. Urinating may also be difficult.*

PARAPHIMOSIS

This condition is the result of forcibly retracting a foreskin that is affected by phimosis (*see p.277*). In this situation, the foreskin becomes stuck in the retracted position, causing swelling and pain.

Medical treatment

If your child's retracted foreskin has become stuck, you should seek medical care immediately. He may be anesthetized or sedated so that the doctor can gently compress the penis and return the foreskin to its normal position.

In some cases, it is necessary to make an incision in the foreskin to free it. Paraphimosis may recur unless circumcision (*see below*) is performed to correct your son's phimosis.

BALANITIS

An inflammation of the foreskin and the head of the penis (glans), balanitis is usually caused by a bacterial or fungal infection. It is often the result of inadequate cleaning of the penis. Phimosis (*see p.277*) tends to make cleaning difficult and thereby increases the likelihood of inflammation occurring. Balanitis may also appear

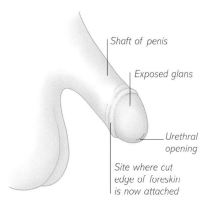

Shaft of penis

Exposed glans

Urethral opening

Site where cut edge of foreskin is now attached

CIRCUMCISION *This operation involves removing the part of the foreskin covering the glans. It may be recommended for a tight foreskin or in cases of recurrent balanitis.*

as a reaction to chemicals in detergents or soaps, or to irritating materials such as wool.

Medical treatment

If the balanitis does not clear up with self-help treatment (*see below*) within 3 days, take your child to see the doctor. He will probably be given either an antifungal or antibiotic cream or an oral antibiotic. These will usually clear up the infection within a week.

If your son suffers from recurrent attacks of balanitis, the doctor may recommend circumcision (*see below left*) to solve the problem.

How to help your child

In most cases, balanitis clears up when hygiene is improved. Make sure your son washes his penis and genital area twice daily. After the inflammation has disappeared, he should wash the penis thoroughly every day to prevent recurrence. If the balanitis is due to irritation by chemicals or material, make sure that your son wears cotton underwear and that his clothes are thoroughly rinsed after washing. He should also avoid using scented soaps.

HYDROCELE

This painless swelling of the scrotum occurs when fluid accumulates in the space around a testis. Hydroceles are common in newborn babies, and they usually disappear without treatment by the age of 6 months. The sudden appearance of a hydrocele in an older boy may be the result of an injury.

Medical treatment

If a scrotal swelling persists beyond the age of 6 months, or if it makes its first appearance after this age, you should take your son to your doctor. In these cases, the hydrocele may be associated with an inguinal

hernia (*see* Hernia, *p.260*), and will need surgical treatment.

A hydrocele that suddenly appears in an older boy should also be assessed by a doctor. It may be caused by an injury or other cause. Tests, including ultrasound scanning, may be done to exclude an abnormality of the testis.

UNDESCENDED TESTIS

In some boys, one or, less frequently, both testes fail to descend into the scrotum before birth. All newborn males babies are examined to determine whether the testes have descended normally. If a testis has not descended, he will be reexamined at each well-child visit; descent often occurs after a few months.

Medical treatment

If a boy's testis has still not descended at about 6 months he will probably need an operation to move the testis down into the scrotum. This is usually done by about 1 year. As long as the operation is carried out at the right time, his sexual development should not be significantly affected. However, there is a slightly increased risk of testicular cancer later in life. When there has been an undescended testis, monthly testicular self-examinations beginning in adolescence will be even more important.

TESTICULAR TORSION

This happens when a child's spermatic cord (the cord from which the testis is suspended) becomes twisted, cutting off or reducing the blood supply to the testis. Testicular torsion causes acute pain. If the torsion is not corrected within hours, the affected testis may be permanently damaged.

Medical treatment

If your son is experiencing a pain in one of his testes, you should seek medical attention immediately. An operation can be performed to untwist the spermatic cord and stitch both the testes to the scrotum to prevent torsion from recurring. If one of your son's testes has been irreversibly damaged by the testicular torsion, it will be removed.

Provided treatment is carried out in time, your son's testis should function normally. If a testis has been removed, the remaining testis should allow your son to have normal fertility as an adult.

ORCHITIS

This is an inflammation that affects one or both testes and can be a complication of mumps (see p.268). However, it can occasionally be caused by a bacterial infection that enters through the penis and spreads along the vas deferens. The affected testis is red and swollen, and can also be extremely painful.

Medical treatment

Consult your doctor or seek medical attention immediately in case your son

is suffering from testicular torsion (see p.278).

With immunization, mumps is now rare, but if your son has had this illness recently, take him to the doctor within 24 hours. Give him the recommended dose of ibuprofen or acetaminophen to relieve the pain.

If there is a bacterial infection, the doctor may prescribe antibiotics. Orchitis is not serious and usually disappears within a week. However, in some cases, the illness may lead to reduced fertility in adult life.

VULVOVAGINITIS

Vulvovaginitis is a usually minor inflammation of the vulva and vagina that is common in young girls. Typical causes include poor hygiene, tight clothing, bubble baths, or scented soap. In some girls, there may be no obvious cause for the symptoms; the vulva and vaginal lining are just particularly sensitive in prepubertal girls.

Causes

In addition to the causes given above, bacteria from the rectum may infect the vulva and vagina if your daughter wipes her bottom from back to front after a bowel movement. Less often, a bacterial infection may be due to the presence of a foreign body (such as a toy or a forgotten tampon) in the vagina. A possible cause of vulvovaginitis in young girls may be an infestation by pinworms (see p.262). After puberty, yeast is a common cause.

Medical treatment

If she is very uncomfortable, has a vaginal discharge, or experiences pain when she urinates, your daughter should see her doctor within 24 hours. You should also consult the doctor if your daughter has other

symptoms that persist for more than 2 weeks. The doctor will examine your daughter.

A vaginal swab may be taken to check for infection. If she does have a bacterial infection, an antibiotic cream or oral antibiotic may be prescribed. An antifungal cream or suppository (which is inserted into the vagina) may be used to treat yeast.

For persistent irritation when there is no infection, the doctor may prescribe an estrogen cream, which can thicken the skin of the vulva and the vaginal lining.

How to help your child

Vulvovaginitis that is not caused by an infection usually clears up with self-help treatment (see p.215).

Your doctor may recommend that your daughter sit in a bath (without

SYMPTOMS

- Inflammation, soreness, and itchiness affecting the genital area.
- Pain on urinating.
- Greenish or grayish yellow vaginal discharge, if bacterial infection is the cause. The discharge may have an odor if the infection is caused by a foreign body in the vagina.
- Thick, white vaginal discharge, if yeast is the cause.

using scented soaps or bubble baths) one to two times a day for a week to wash her genital area. Application of an emollient product such as zinc oxide ointment may also be recommended.

Your daughter should wear loose-fitting underwear made of cotton but not synthetics. These should be changed daily.

If possible, encourage her to expose her genital area to the air for a little while each day.

To keep the vulva and vagina free of irritating fecal material, make sure she wipes her bottom from front to back after a bowel movement.

MUSCLE & BONE
DISORDERS

CHILDREN ARE AT HIGH RISK for problems with their muscles, bones, and joints – fractures, sprains and strains, dislocations, and cramps are common. This is because they are generally very active yet their bones and joints are immature and still growing. Some disorders result from genetic abnormalities or birth defects and are more rare. Minor musculoskeletal disorders, such as in-toeing and out-toeing, are quite common in children.

ANATOMY OF THE SKELETON

▶ *HOW THE SKELETON WORKS*

The skeleton is the strong internal framework that provides support for the body. In addition to supporting the soft tissues, the skeleton also protects the organs and provides anchorage for muscles. During childhood, the skeleton is continually growing and changing shape. In childhood, most of the long bones contain cartilage. The cartilage in these areas grows and develops into bone. Limb, hand, and foot bones, the areas in which most growth occurs, are made up of a diaphysis (shaft), which is the main part of the bone, and an epiphysis (growing region) at one or both ends. During childhood, the epiphyses gradually turn to bone, leaving a cartilage plate where growth continues until adult height and size are reached in late adolescence.

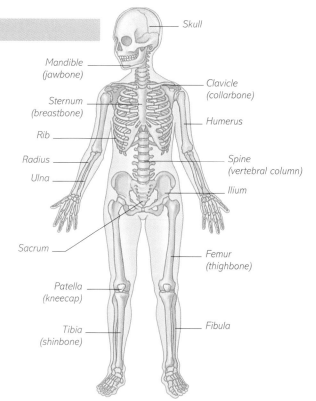

Skull

Mandible
(jawbone)

Clavicle
(collarbone)

Sternum
(breastbone)

Humerus

Rib

Radius

Spine
(vertebral column)

Ulna

Ilium

Sacrum

Femur
(thighbone)

Patella
(kneecap)

Tibia
(shinbone)

Fibula

LIMPING

A limp is usually caused by a minor injury that will get better on its own. It can sometimes, however, be caused by an underlying disorder that requires prompt treatment to prevent permanent disability. Never ignore a limp in a child.

Causes

Pain from disorders involving a joint, muscle, or bone around the hip or in the leg or foot may cause a limp. The site of pain can be misleading; an abnormality in the hip may cause pain in the thigh or knee.

The following are possible causes: a fracture (*see p.283*); irritable hip (*see p.285*); bone or joint infection (*see p.288*); Perthes disease (*see p.286*); muscle strain (*see below*); juvenile idiopathic arthritis (*see p.288*); plantar warts (*see warts, p.231*); or a sharp object in the sole of the foot.

A child may limp because his legs are unequal lengths. A bone may be short from birth or may fail to grow because of a spinal cord abnormality or cerebral palsy (*see p.295*), leading to muscle weakness on one side of the body. A limp may be due to apparent shortening of a leg, as a result of developmental hip dysplasia (*see p.286*) that was detected late or spinal curvature such as scoliosis (*see p.287*).

Children with a disorder of the muscles and/or the nervous system, such as muscular dystrophy (*see p.289*) or cerebral palsy (*see p.295*), may have muscle weakness or a lack of coordination, causing walking problems that resemble a limp. A limp may also develop as part of a behavioral problem in a child with emotional or psychological difficulties.

Medical treatment

Take your child to the doctor if he has a limp with no obvious cause or is old enough to walk but refuses to do so. Call your doctor immediately if your child also has a fever, rash, or hot, swollen joints – these could signal a bone or joint infection that requires immediate medical treatment.

The doctor will examine your child and may carry out X-rays, blood tests, and/or scans to help diagnose the cause of the problem. Your child may be referred to an orthopedic surgeon and may go to the hospital for further tests or observation. The treatment will depend on the underlying cause.

A limp due to a minor injury will probably get better within a few days. A limp due to most other causes should disappear once the underlying problem has been treated. In a few cases, the underlying cause, such as unequal leg length or muscular weakness, cannot be cured, and walking problems may remain.

STRAINS AND SPRAINS

Strains and sprains are often caused by falls or vigorous physical activity. If a muscle is overstretched and the muscle fibers are damaged, it may result in a strain. A joint is sprained when one or more of its ligaments is overstretched or torn. Unless they are severe, such injuries can usually be treated at home.

Medical treatment

Take your child to the doctor if the pain and swelling are severe just after the injury has occurred – for example, if the child cannot walk on an injured ankle. You should also take your child to the doctor if there are any milder symptoms that have shown no improvement within a few days.

The doctor will examine the injury and may arrange for an X-ray to be taken to rule out the possibility of fractured bones (*see p.283*).

The injured part may need to be wrapped in a compression bandage. Your child may also have to use crutches for a leg injury or wear a sling if the arm is affected.

> ### ☐ SYMPTOMS
>
> - Pain and tenderness, increasing with movement of the affected area.
> - Swelling in the injured spot.
> - Muscle spasm (tightness of a muscle produced by involuntary contractions).
> - Limping, if a leg is affected.
> - Bruising, which may appear within a few days after the injury.

For a very severe strain or sprain, nonsteroidal anti-inflammatory drugs (NSAIDs) may be prescribed to reduce the pain and swelling and to speed the healing process. Your child may have to wear a splint or plaster cast.

How to help your child

For the first 48 hours or so after the injury has occurred, you should treat a sprain by means of the four-step

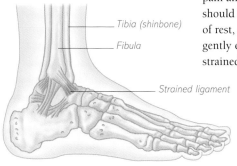

Tibia (shinbone)

Fibula

Strained ligament

process known as RICE – rest, ice, compression, and elevation (*see* First aid, *p.335*).

You should not apply heat to the injury for the first 48 hours. If your child needs pain relief, you should ask your doctor for the correct dose of ibuprofen or acetaminophen. The pain and swelling around the injury should begin to ease after 1 or 2 days of rest, and your child may begin to gently exercise the sprained or strained limb gently.

SPRAINED ANKLE *The ankle is the most commonly sprained joint. The injury may occur during a fall when the foot is twisted onto its outside edge.*

Outlook

A minor strain or a sprain should heal within 2 weeks. Once the pain has disappeared, your doctor may suggest exercises that will strengthen the affected part or refer your child to a physiotherapist. If the affected ligament or muscle is allowed to heal properly and is exercised, it will recover fully and not be permanently weakened.

Preventing strains and sprains

Teach your child to warm up appropriately before any sport or strenuous physical activity. A warm-up routine may include movements that mobilize the joints and warm up the muscles, followed by gentle stretches.

CRAMPS

A cramp is when a muscle strongly contracts and cannot relax. The pain is usually sudden and severe, but rarely lasts more than a few minutes. As well as being painful, the muscle feels hard and tight, and there may be a lump or distortion in the affected area.

Causes

An attack of cramps can be triggered by vigorous exercise, lying or sitting awkwardly, or continuously repeating a movement. Cramps can come on suddenly at night during sleep or while exercising soon after eating a meal.

Cramps are usually due to the inability of a hardworking muscle to remove the lactic acid produced when glucose is turned into energy. The muscle appears to lock and is only relieved when circulation is restored.

Exercise-related cramps may be partly caused by the loss of salt and water from the body through sweating. Low levels of nutrients such as calcium, potassium, or magnesium in the blood may also cause cramps.

How to help your child

As soon as your child feels an attack of cramps he will probably cry out, so help him as quickly as you can. Hold the affected limb – it is most likely to be the calf muscle below the knee – in your hand and gently massage and stretch the tightened muscle to relieve your child's cramp.

If it is the calf muscle, you can show him how to stretch it. First, you need to gently pull the toes of his affected leg toward you. Then push his foot back so that his toes are pointing upward. Hold each of these two positions for a few minutes. Repeat the exercise until the pain starts to subside.

If there is still some residual pain, fill a water bottle with warm water and

SYMPTOMS

- Cramps frequently affect the calf muscle in the legs.
- Muscle feels hard and tight.
- Lump may appear temporarily.

wrap it in a towel. Hold it to the affected area for a few minutes. Alternatively, you could give your child a warm bath or shower.

A cramp can be a very painful experience, so reassure your child that cramps are common, temporary, and not serious. To help relieve the pain, you can give him acetaminophen or ibuprofen.

To help prevent cramps, make sure that your child drinks plenty of fluids during exercise, particularly in hot weather. These will help him to preserve the electrolyte balance in his body. If the cramps continue, ask your doctor for specific recommendations.

FRACTURES AND DISLOCATIONS

Common causes of fractures and dislocations in children are falls, sports activities, and traffic collisions. The bones in the legs and arms and the collarbone break most frequently. Dislocation can happen when the ligaments that hold the bones of a joint, such as the elbow, are stretched or torn, so that the bones are displaced. When a joint is dislocated, bones may also be fractured.

Immediate action

If you think your child's neck or back may be injured, do not move him. Dial 911 or call EMS immediately. If you suspect a fracture or dislocation of another part of the body, seek medical help immediately. In the meantime, support or immobilize the broken limb (*see* First aid, *pp.334–335*).

Medical treatment

Once at the hospital, your child will be x-rayed to check whether the affected bone is fractured and/or dislocated, and to identify the site and severity of the injury.

Your child may be given a local or a general anesthetic to decrease the pain so that any displaced bones can be manipulated back into the correct position. In some cases, surgery may be needed to reposition the bones and repair any damage to surrounding tissues.

The affected limb may have to be put into a plaster cast or held in a splint to keep the bones in the correct position as they heal.

GREENSTICK FRACTURE Because children's bones are supple, the long bones of the arms and legs tend to bend and to crack on only one side.

In severe cases, your child may need traction, or have metal screws, rods, pins, or plates inserted to hold his bones in position.

Fractures in children generally heal more quickly than they do in adults. A small bone, such as a finger bone, that does not bear weight may heal in a few weeks. Large, weight-bearing bones such as the femur (thighbone) may take several months. Dislocations, such as the displacement of the curved end of the humerus from its normal position in the socket of the ulna, will usually heal within a week or two.

As soon as it is safe for your child to use the affected part, he may be given physiotherapy or recommended exercises to prevent the muscles and joints from stiffening up and becoming weak.

☐ SYMPTOMS

- Severe pain and unwillingness to move the affected part.
- Extreme tenderness if pressure is put on the area directly over the site of the injury.
- Swelling and skin discoloration at the site of the injury.
- Visible deformity (in a dislocated joint and some serious fractures).
- Damage to surrounding tissues. If the skin is broken, there may be infection.

A minor fracture may cause only mild symptoms and may be mistaken for a strain or sprain.

Outlook

As long as the fractured or dislocated bones are properly repositioned and kept in place while they grow together and heal, your child should make a complete recovery. Muscle stiffness may take several weeks or even months to disappear entirely. Fractures of a joint may slightly increase the risk of arthritis in later life. Fractures of the growth plate may arrest growth. Close monitoring will be necessary.

☐ BONE HEALTH

Childhood is the most important time to lay the foundations for healthy bones and joints. A child's diet needs to include essential nutrients – for example, calcium, vitamin D, vitamin K, magnesium, and other minerals, such as boron, zinc, manganese, and copper.

The recommended daily intake of calcium is 500 milligrams for toddlers, 800 milligrams for children ages 4–8, increasing to 1,300 milligrams a day for children up to the age of 11.

Encourage your child to drink plenty of milk and eat enough cheese, yogurt,

nuts, and legumes to ensure adequate calcium supplies. Fatty fish, such as herring, salmon, and tuna, are rich in vitamin D, which is also made by the body when the skin is exposed to ultraviolet rays in sunlight. Many breakfast cereals and milk products have been fortified with vitamin D.

Regular exercise, such as running, tennis, and walking, helps build a strong bone mass. The exercise is even more beneficial if it is weight-bearing. Children who exercise regularly are more likely to do so as adults.

MINOR SKELETAL PROBLEMS

When your child begins to stand and then walk, it is a very exciting time. Sometimes, you may find yourself worrying that the positions of his legs and feet are not quite right. Many children walk pigeon-toed or splay-footed (in-toeing and out-toeing), or appear to have bowlegs, knock-knees, or flat feet. Generally, these problems are caused by the position of the baby in the uterus or are a normal variation. Rarely, they may indicate an underlying disorder.

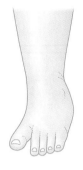

IN-TOEING *Inward curving of the front part of the foot (known as metatarsus adductus) is a common cause of in-toeing. The web space between the big and second toes is often increased.*

PIGEON TOES AND SPLAY FEET

Inward rotation of the whole leg from the hip (called femoral anteversion) can cause a child to have pigeon toes, known as in-toeing. Other causes are curving of the front part of the foot (*see top right*), inward rotation of the shinbone (tibial torsion), and bowlegs (*see below*). Outward rotation of the whole leg at the hip causes splay feet, or out-toeing.

Medical treatment
Consult your doctor if you are worried about the inward or outward position of your child's legs or feet. Inward-curving feet usually improve without treatment by the age of 3 or 4 years.

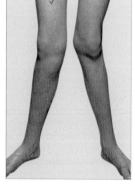

BOWLEGS *Outward-curved legs prevent the knees from touching; the shinbone is rotated inward.*

KNOCK-KNEES *The legs are curved inward so that the knees touch and the feet lie apart.*

Otherwise, they can be treated by gentle manipulation of the feet and immobilization in casts. Surgery is rarely needed in this situation. Hip rotation usually corrects itself by the age of 8 years and, again, the need for surgery is rare.

Walking splay-footed almost always corrects itself within a year of the child starting to walk. There are no long-term problems from in-toeing or walking splay-footed.

BOWLEGS AND KNOCK-KNEES

A slight outward curving of the leg bones is normal in toddlers. However, in bowlegs, the outward curve is exaggerated and the tibia (shinbone) is rotated inward. In knock-knees, the legs curve inward so that the knees seem to be trying to touch each other. Bowlegs usually correct themselves by the age of 3 or 4 years; knock-knees are usually outgrown by the age of 11.

Medical treatment
Check with your doctor if you are concerned about your child's legs. There is probably no

problem but, very rarely, a child may need an operation to correct a severe or persistent deformity, which can be the result of a disorder of bone growth, such as rickets.

FLAT FEET

If a child has flat feet it means that the soles of his feet rest on the ground, as if the normal arch of the foot does not exist. You may see this in the footprint – instead of the usual line where the instep touches the ground, the foot leaves a broad impression from the heel to the toes. An affected child may feel some pain beneath the ankle and along the instep.

Flat feet are normal in children up to the age of 2 or 3. Some children may have flat feet longer than this but they usually do not cause problems. In rare cases, flat feet are caused by an underlying abnormality of the bones or joints that makes the feet painful, stiff, and weak.

Medical treatment
If you are worried that your child may have flat feet, consult your doctor. She will probably check their mobility, appearance, and strength. If all these are normal, the feet are normal and require no treatment. If there is an underlying disorder, treatment may include immobilizing the feet in casts and, rarely, surgery.

CLUBFOOT

This is a congenital deformity, also known as talipes equinovarus, in which the foot is twisted out of shape or position. Clubfoot affects three times more male babies than female babies, and both feet may be affected.

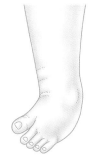

FEATURES OF CLUBFOOT
The heel of the foot is turned inward and the rest of the foot is bent downward and inward. In some cases, the tibia (shinbone) is turned inward and the leg muscles are underdeveloped.

Causes

Clubfoot is usually detected during a baby's routine examination at birth. There are two main causes of clubfoot. Postural clubfoot is caused in the uterus when the position of the baby's foot forces it to be compressed. Structural clubfoot is caused by a congenital abnormality of the bones in the foot.

Medical treatment

Clubfoot may be diagnosed during a newborn examination or noticed during a prenatal ultrasound. If the mobility in the foot is normal, your child has postural clubfoot and needs no treatment. The problem will usually correct itself within a few weeks of birth.

If the mobility is restricted, your child may have structural clubfoot and will need treatment. In mild cases, this may involve some physical therapy combined with exercises to stretch the ligaments. Following some instruction, you will be able to perform these on your child at home.

In more severe cases, your doctor will probably refer your child to a pediatric orthopedic surgeon. The foot may need manipulation and casting to hold the bones in position. If the bones have not straightened by the age of 3–6 months, your child may need to have an operation to straighten it.

After the operation the foot is put in a plaster cast for at least a few months. In most cases, this is successful. A small number of children may need a series of operations over a 5-year period to improve the function and appearance of the foot, which may never be completely normal, or may differ in size from the other leg or foot.

IRRITABLE HIP

For an unknown reason, irritable hip (also called transient or viral synovitis) often develops within about 2 weeks of a mild upper respiratory tract infection, such as a cold. The lining of the hip joint becomes inflamed and fluid accumulates inside the joint, causing symptoms to develop suddenly. Children between 2 and 12 years of age are most susceptible to irritable hip.

☐ SYMPTOMS

- Limping.
- Pain in the hip, groin, thigh, or knee.
- Sometimes, a mild fever.

Medical treatment

Take your child to the doctor within 24 hours if he has a pain in the hip, groin, thigh, or knee, and/or a limp without an obvious cause.

If the doctor confirms irritable hip to be the diagnosis, a nonsteroidal anti-inflammatory drug (NSAID) such as ibuprofen can soothe your child's discomfort. Encourage him to rest in bed until the condition improves, usually between 1 and 7 days. However, if the pain is very severe, your child may need to have blood tests to rule out a bacterial infection.

His hip may also be x-rayed and scanned to rule out conditions such as Perthes disease (*see p.286*) or joint infection (*see p.288*). In some cases, traction may be applied to the hip to relieve both the muscle spasm and the pain.

Outlook

Your child should make a complete recovery, but if he becomes too active too soon after the treatment, the problem may flare up again and he may need to take nonsteroidal anti-inflammatory drugs (NSAIDs). If pain recurs in the hip despite the treatment, the problem may be due to Perthes disease (*see p.286*) or juvenile idiopathic arthritis (*see p.288*).

PERTHES DISEASE

This condition affects children, particularly boys, ages 4–8 years. Poor blood supply causes progressive softening, followed by reforming and hardening, of the head of the thighbone, or femur. Perthes disease will get better spontaneously within 2–4 years, but a child should have treatment as early as possible in order to prevent the hip joint from becoming deformed.

SYMPTOMS

- Limping.
- Pain in the hip or knee.
- Restricted movement at the hip.

Medical treatment

If your child is suffering from pain in the hip or knee and/or a limp, you should take him to your doctor within 24 hours. After examining your child, your doctor may obtain an X-ray of the hip joint to check what is causing the problem.

Treatment depends on the severity of the disease. Less severe cases of Perthes disease may be treated by resting in bed for a week or two until the pain subsides, with regular monitoring by X-ray. But if the joint is at risk of becoming deformed, your child may have to wear a brace, splint,

or plaster cast to keep the joint in position while the condition improves. In very severe cases, an operation may be needed to align the head of the femur within the pelvic socket.

Outlook

Children age 6 and under as well as children with less severe disease have the best results and are most likely to function normally. In some very severe cases, it is impossible to prevent the joint from becoming deformed and, as a result, there is a chance that the child will suffer from arthritis of the hip later in life.

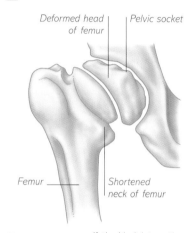

FEMORAL DEFORMITY *If the hip joint continues to bear a child's weight while he has Perthes disease, the head and neck of the femur may become deformed.*

DEVELOPMENTAL HIP DYSPLASIA

One in every 250 babies is born with a hip dysplasia, in which the head of the thighbone, or femur, lies outside the socket of the pelvis or is unstable and likely to slip out of position. All babies are screened soon after birth and again in checkups during the first year of life. Developmental hip dysplasia runs in families and is more common in girls and babies born by breech delivery.

Causes

The underlying cause is not known, but one or both of a baby's hips may be dislocated or unstable because the fibrous capsule surrounding the hip joint is weak or because the pelvic socket is abnormally shallow.

Developmental hip dysplasia is usually spotted when the doctor

checks a baby soon after birth and manipulates the newborn baby's thighs and hips. If a hip is dislocated, the doctor may feel a "clunk" as the head of the femur moves into the socket of the hip. An ultrasound examination will confirm the diagnosis.

If developmental hip dysplasia is not detected at birth, or during one

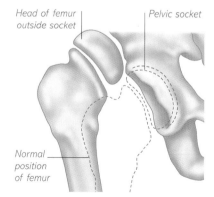

A DISLOCATED HIP *In a newborn child with a hip dysplasia, the rounded head of the femur (thighbone) does not sit in the cup of the pelvic socket as it should. Instead, it lies above the socket but usually moves into the correct position soon after birth.*

of the routine checkups during a child's first year, it may not be discovered until your child begins to walk. At this point, you may notice that your child has a limp or that the back of the affected leg has a different appearance or more skin folds below the buttock than the unaffected leg.

Medical treatment

You should consult your doctor if you suspect your child may have developmental hip dysplasia. If your baby's hip abnormality has not corrected itself by about 3 weeks of age, he may need to wear a Pavlik harness brace to move the head of the femur into the socket and to keep it in position.

The Pavlik harness is usually worn for 2–4 months and your doctor will give you advice on how to care for your baby during this period. When it is removed, the hip joint should be normal.

If your baby's developmental hip dysplasia is not discovered until later in life, the head of the femur may have to be reduced into the socket and held in place by a cast for several months. If the problem is not discovered until your child starts to walk, he may need a series of operations to correct the disorder.

Outlook

The sooner your child receives treatment, the better. If he is treated in early infancy, he should be able to walk normally and is unlikely to suffer any ill effects later in life. However, if treatment is delayed, or if your child has no treatment at all, there may be a risk of a permanent limp and the early onset of arthritis in the affected hip.

SCOLIOSIS

This condition causes an abnormal sideways curvature of the spine. Scoliosis can be due to a structural abnormality of one or more vertebrae or to a local muscle weakness. It is most common in girls, starting around the time of the adolescent growth spurt.

Causes

One reason for scoliosis is that a child's legs are of unequal length so that, as she grows, her pelvis tilts over to one side and the shoulder is raised on the opposite side. This alters the line of the head and shoulders. As the spine tries to bring the line back to the horizontal, it starts to curve.

Scoliosis is rarely noticeable at birth and is usually so mild that it only becomes apparent when a child grows or when his back is x-rayed for an entirely unrelated reason.

In true scoliosis, the vertebrae become narrower on one side of the spine, forcing it to lean to one side and to twist back again higher up toward the neck.

Medical treatment

If your child seems a little crooked, watch her bare back when she stands up and bends forward. If you think you can see a curvature, consult your doctor. He may obtain X-rays or refer your child to an orthopedic surgeon for monitoring and to check if the curvature worsens over time. A mild curvature that is not progressive does not usually need any treatment.

However, in progressive cases, a child may need to be fitted with a body cast or spinal brace to prevent the curvature of the spine from becoming worse. Sometimes, the deformity of scoliosis is severe enough to warrant surgery.

Outlook

If scoliosis is treated promptly, it should not get worse and your child is unlikely to have any long-term ill effects. But left untreated, progressive scoliosis may, in some children, cause severe deformity of the ribcage and spine, leading to breathing difficulties and recurrent chest infections.

☐ SYMPTOMS

- Sideways curve of the spine.
- Pelvis tilts to one side.
- One shoulder is held higher than the other.
- Chest may be more prominent on one side than the other.

The curvature of the spine may be accentuated when your child bends forward to touch her toes with her knees kept straight.

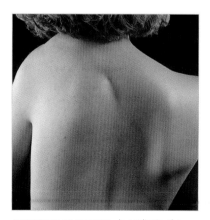

APPEARANCE OF SCOLIOSIS *In scoliosis, the spine curves to one side, usually the right, and one shoulder is higher than the other.*

JUVENILE RHEUMATOID ARTHRITIS

Juvenile rheumatoid arthritis (JRA or JA) is a chronic inflammation of the joints. The underlying cause of this disease is unknown, but genetic factors play a part. It may be triggered by a viral infection.

Medical treatment

You should take your child to see your doctor within 24 hours of the onset of severe joint pain or stiffness, a limp, or a rash with a fever. After your doctor has examined your child, he may arrange to have blood tests carried out to try to determine the cause of the symptoms.

If four or fewer large joints, such as the knee or shoulder, are affected, the child may have oligoarticular arthritis. If many small joints, such as those of the hands and feet, are affected, he may be suffering from polyarticular arthritis. If the small joints are affected but there are additional symptoms of general illness, the child may have systemic juvenile arthritis.

Whichever diagnosis is confirmed, your child will need to receive some physiotherapy to maintain his muscle strength and joint mobility. He may need to wear splints at night to prevent joint deformity or during the day to rest the joints.

Your doctor may prescribe nonsteroidal anti-inflammatory drugs (NSAIDs), such as ibuprofen, to relieve the pain and swelling. If these are ineffective, your child may need stronger medication such as methotrexate.

Your child's eyes will probably need to be tested regularly for iritis (*see p.244*), an inflammation of the iris and the muscular ring around it that may affect children with juvenile rheumatoid arthritis.

Outlook

Fifty percent of children who have juvenile rheumatoid arthritis become healthy adults without active arthritis or disabilities.

☐ SYMPTOMS

- Pain, redness, swelling, stiffness, and decreased function of affected joints.
- Limping, if feet or legs are affected.
- In polyarticular arthritis, a mild fever.

Systemic juvenile arthritis affects the whole body, causing the following symptoms, which may appear several weeks or months before the joints become affected:

- Temperature above 39°C (102°F).
- Swollen glands throughout the body.
- Blotchy, transient rash.

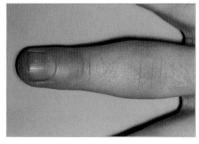

ARTHRITIS AFFECTING THE HANDS *In cases of polyarticular arthritis, the joints of the fingers are red, inflamed, and swollen. The neck and jaw may also be affected.*

BONE AND JOINT INFECTION

Bacteria carried through the blood from an infected site, such as a wound or a boil elsewhere in the body, is the most common cause of bone or joint infection. In some cases, the infection spreads directly from nearby tissue.

BONE INFECTION

Without prompt treatment, infection of a bone (osteomyelitis) may become chronic and difficult to eradicate. It is most common in the long bones of the arms and legs – the humerus and femur. Young children and premature babies appear to be more susceptible.

Medical treatment

Call your doctor immediately if you suspect a bone infection. He will evaluate your child and may admit her to a hospital for a blood culture, bone scan, and treatment. Antibiotics are used to treat a bone infection; rarely, some bone may be surgically removed.

☐ SYMPTOMS

In bone infection the symptoms may be:
- Severe pain in the affected arm or leg.
- Child is unwilling to move the affected limb or let it be touched.
- Fever.
- Swelling and inflammation of the skin over the bone if treatment is delayed.

If the infection is caught early enough, your child should recover completely without permanent damage.

JOIN INFECTION

In this condition (also called septic arthritis) bacteria infect the tissues in a joint, causing the joint to become inflamed and fluid to collect within it. If the infection is not identified and treated promptly, the cartilage that covers the surface of the bones inside the joint may be damaged, causing the joint to become stiff and deformed.

Joint infections are most common in children up to the age of 2 years and in adolescents. With prompt treatment, sufferers of joint infection can make a complete recovery.

Medical treatment

If you suspect your child may have a joint infection, you should contact your doctor for an evaluation. To confirm the diagnosis of a bacterial infection, fluid may be removed from the joint with a syringe and sent for microscopic analysis. Your child may also need blood tests to identify the source of the infection.

Your child will likely be admitted to the hospital for a course of antibiotics to treat the infection. She may also need an operation to drain the infected fluid from the joint.

SYMPTOMS

In joint infection, the symptoms may be:
- A hot and swollen joint.
- Severe pain in the affected joint.
- Fever.

Once the infection has cleared up completely, your child may need to receive physiotherapy, which will help keep the joint flexible. As long as the infected joint is identified early enough and treated promptly, your child should make a full recovery.

DUCHENNE MUSCULAR DYSTROPHY

Progressive weakness and the wasting away of muscle are the main features of this congenital disorder. Of the several types, the most common and serious is Duchenne muscular dystrophy, which affects only boys.

Causes

Duchenne muscular dystrophy is linked to a gene on the X chromosome and affects about 1 in 3,500 boys worldwide. The condition usually appears before 5 years of age.

The gene in question is responsible for producing the protein dystrophin, which is thought to be essential for structural support inside muscle cells. When the gene is defective, the protein is not produced and the muscle cells degenerate and waste away.

A boy born to a woman who is a carrier of Duchenne muscular dystrophy has a 50 percent chance of developing the disorder. If he has sisters, they would have a 50 percent chance of becoming carriers.

Medical treatment

Consult your doctor if you think your child might have muscular dystrophy. After examining him, your doctor may send him to a neurologist, who may request tests in order to confirm the diagnosis.

As yet, there is no substantial treatment or cure for the progressive weakness and wasting of muscles experienced by sufferers of the various muscular dystrophies. Your child may receive treatments such as physiotherapy to prevent contractures, in which the shortened muscles around the joints cause the joints to be positioned abnormally and painfully. The physiotherapy will allow your child to maintain some form of mobility. You can learn how to help him with these exercises.

Genetic testing

A woman with a family history of Duchenne muscular dystrophy can be tested to find out if she is a carrier. If she is, and she wants to have a baby, she will be offered genetic

SYMPTOMS

- Weakness in the leg muscles, which may cause your child to walk late (over the age of 18 months) and waddle, climb stairs with difficulty, fall easily and roll onto his front, and climb or "hand walk" up his own legs.
- Enlarged calf muscles.
- Inward curvature of the lower spine.

counseling to explain the risks of the baby being affected. Tests can also be performed during pregnancy to see if the fetus has been affected with the abnormal gene.

Outlook

The muscle weakness of a child with Duchenne muscular dystrophy increases and gradually spreads to affect more and more of the muscles that control his movements. As a result, it may not be long before he is unable to perform simple tasks or to walk. He may need a wheelchair, and he may become increasingly vulnerable to chest infections during the teen years.

NERVOUS SYSTEM DISORDERS

THE BRAIN IS THE CONTROL CENTER of the nervous system and most of its development is complete by the time a child is about 5 years old. A brain injury or infection may have serious long-term consequences, so early recognition and treatment are vital. Generally, a child's brain recovers from injury or infection better than an adult's. A few nervous system disorders are permanent but can be helped by treatment.

ANATOMY OF THE NERVOUS SYSTEM

▶ **THE BRAIN AND NERVOUS SYSTEM**

Composed of the brain, spinal cord, and many millions of nerve cells, the nervous system is the control center for all voluntary activities and involuntary bodily functions. Nerves are responsible for the perception of sensations, such as touch, taste, smell, vision, and hearing.

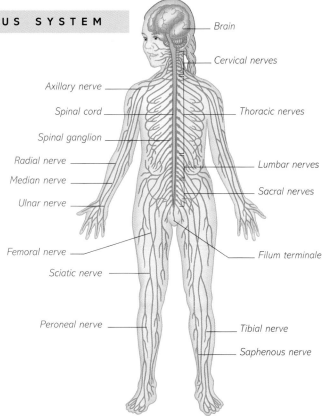

Brain

Cervical nerves

Axillary nerve

Spinal cord

Thoracic nerves

Spinal ganglion

Radial nerve

Median nerve

Lumbar nerves

Ulnar nerve

Sacral nerves

Femoral nerve

Filum terminale

Sciatic nerve

Peroneal nerve

Tibial nerve

Saphenous nerve

HEAD INJURY

Most children suffer some bangs or knocks to the head, and these are rarely serious or have any long-lasting effects. The main risks are swelling of the brain and bleeding inside the skull, which can lead to brain damage, resulting in physical or mental disability.

Immediate action

If your child falls down and hits her head – for example, when trying to get out of the crib or while playing on a jungle gym – she may be knocked unconscious. Dial 911 or call EMS and check her airway, breathing, and

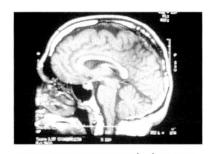

MAGNETIC RESONANCE IMAGING (MRI) OF BRAIN
A scan can show bleeding inside the skull causing a blood clot, which may cause damage to the brain tissues.

circulation (*see* First aid, pp.326–328) while you wait. If she is confused or abnormally drowsy, vomits persistently, or has fluid or watery blood leaking from her nose or ears, call for medical attention right away.

Medical treatment

A doctor will examine her and take any necessary action. A cut on her scalp or forehead may require stitches. If a fracture is suspected, her head may be x-rayed or scanned (*see left*).

If the scan shows signs of a brain hemorrhage, your child may need an emergency operation to stop the bleeding and remove a blood clot. If your child has a fracture of the skull or a severe head injury, she will be admitted to the hospital for observation and treatment if needed.

> ▢ **SYMPTOMS**
>
> *Mild head injury symptoms include:*
> • Slight headache.
> • Bump or swelling.
> • Vomiting.
>
> *More serious head injuries involve:*
> • Brief or prolonged unconsciousness.
> • Confusion.
> • Inability to remember what happened just before the injury.
> • Dizziness.
> • Blurred vision.
> • Vomiting.

How to help your child

After hospital treatment a child with a head injury needs rest. If it is a minor head injury, let your child rest for 2–3 days. Watch her for the first 24 hours and seek medical attention immediately if any of the following develop: difficulty speaking; persistent drowsiness; irritability; vomiting; confusion; or fluid or watery blood leaking from the nose or ears.

RECURRENT HEADACHES

Most children have headaches from time to time but some children suffer recurrent ones, which may interfere with daily activities and schoolwork. The two main types are migraine and tension headaches.

MIGRAINE

Children who have frequent migraines usually have a family history of the disorder. Emotional stress is the most common trigger, but other triggers may include: foods, such as oranges, peanut butter, chocolate, or cheese; hunger; too much sun; and fatigue. Children rarely have more than one or two migraine headaches a month.

Medical treatment

If your child develops the symptoms of a migraine, take her to the doctor, who may help identify and eliminate the potential trigger factors.

Antiemetic medicine may be prescribed to prevent vomiting during the attacks. Drugs to prevent a migraine may be prescribed if your child has frequent attacks. During a

> ▢ **SYMPTOMS**
>
> *Migraine causes some children to have a sudden onset of pain, affecting one or both sides of the head. Other symptoms of migraine follow and may include:*
> • Sparkling lights as a warning sign of the migraine attack.
> • Vomiting.
> • Sensitivity to light and noise.
> • Lightheadedness or dizziness.
> • Tingling, weakness, or numbness of an arm or hand.
> *An attack may last from about 2 hours to as long as 2 days.*

migraine attack, you can give her the recommended dose of acetaminophen or ibuprofen and let her rest in a darkened room to help relieve the pain.

Frequent attacks may be followed by long periods in which no migraines occur. Certain prescription medications may help reduce the frequency of migraine attacks.

TENSION HEADACHE

Muscular tension in the face and neck – for example, from clenching or grinding the teeth – may cause tension headaches. Emotional stress is the most common trigger.

How to help your child

To relieve the pain, give your child the recommended dose of acetaminophen or ibuprofen. Try to identify and reduce any causes of stress. If the headaches continue, your doctor may refer your child to a pediatric neurologist.

OTHER CAUSES

Other causes of headaches, such as tumors, are extremely rare. If your child shows any symptoms or you suspect a problem, have your doctor examine her and arrange tests if necessary. Treatment and outlook will depend on the nature of the problem.

◻ SYMPTOMS

Tension headaches include the following symptoms:
- Pain that can affect any part of the head.
- Sometimes, other signs of tension, such as abdominal pain.

Rarely, headaches include the following symptoms:
- Pain that wakes a child at night, is present on waking in the morning, or is made worse by coughing.
- Seizures.
- Changes in behavior.

FEBRILE SEIZURES

These seizures are triggered when a child's body temperature rises abruptly, often during a viral illness or ear infection. The convulsions tend to run in families and usually occur during the first few hours of a fever.

Immediate action

You should call your doctor immediately if your child has a seizure that is accompanied by a fever. If your child has a seizure that lasts more than a few minutes, you should dial 911 or call EMS.

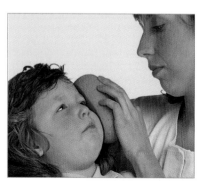

REDUCING YOUR CHILD'S TEMPERATURE Sponge your child with lukewarm water to reduce a fever. Give the recommended dose of acetaminophen or ibuprofen.

Medical treatment

The doctor will examine your child and may check for infections such as meningitis (*see p.294*). She may take a throat swab and carry out blood and urine tests. The doctor may give your child antibiotics for a bacterial infection. The doctor will also explain how you should deal with any future attacks, should they occur.

How to help your child

Febrile seizures are most common in children between 6 months and 5 years of age. Although frightening, they are rarely serious and cause no long-term problems. About a third of children who have had one attack will have a second seizure with a fever. A few children do go on to develop epilepsy (*see p.293*), but most will not have any future seizures. Try to bring down your child's high temperature to

◻ SYMPTOMS

The first stage of the seizure, which lasts about 30 seconds, involves:
- A loss of consciousness.
- Rigid body.
- Breathing stops for up to half a minute; when it starts again, breathing may be shallow and barely detectable.
- Possible temporary loss of bowel or bladder control

The second stage of the seizure, which may last less than 5 minutes, involves:
- Child remains unconscious.
- Limbs and/or face twitch.
- Rolling back of the eyes.

At the end of the second stage, the child regains consciousness and may then fall into a deep sleep for an hour or two. She may be confused, sleepy, or irritable when she wakes up.

prevent convulsions (*see p.59 and p.171*). Give your child the recommended dose of ibuprofen or acetaminophen. After any seizure stops, place your child in the recovery position (*see p.326*).

EPILEPSY

Around 1 in 200 children has recurrent seizures – a condition called epilepsy. A single seizure does not mean a child has epilepsy. Two types of epileptic seizure are most common in children – generalized tonic-clonic and absence seizures.

Causes

Children with epilepsy sometimes have a structural abnormality in the brain, but usually there is no obvious cause. Individual attacks may be brought on by a trigger, such as flashing lights.

During a seizure, there is chaotic and unregulated electrical activity in the brain, which causes an alteration in consciousness and sometimes uncontrollable movements of the limbs and/or head. There are many causes of seizures other than epilepsy, including nervous system infections and metabolic disorders.

Medical treatment

If your child has never had a generalized tonic-clonic seizure before, call your doctor immediately. If she remains unconscious longer than a few minutes, whether the attack is her first one or not, dial 911 or call EMS, or take your child to the nearest emergency room. While you wait for help, you should check her airway, breathing, and circulation (see First aid, pp.326–328).

If your child has any other type of seizure for the first time, consult your doctor right away. The doctor will probably ask you to describe your child's behavior and symptoms before, during, and after any seizure.

Tell your doctor what your child was doing just before the seizure to help pinpoint possible triggers. Your child may need to have an electroencephalogram (EEG) to measure the electrical activity of the brain and identify the type of epilepsy.

Your child may also have a brain scan to determine whether a structural brain abnormality might be the cause of the problem. Blood tests may be carried out in order to rule out other possible causes, such as low blood sugar.

Children with epilepsy usually require anticonvulsant drug therapy until 1–2 years have passed since their last seizure. In selected cases, a ketogenic diet, vagal nerve stimulator, or surgery may be possible treatments.

How to help your child

If your child has experienced a generalized tonic-clonic seizure, place her in the recovery position (see First aid, p.326) when the convulsions stop and stay with her until she has fully regained consciousness.

If your child has another type of seizure, sit her down quietly and stay with her until she is fully recovered and alert. Reassure your child calmly and quietly, and do not try to stop the seizure by shaking her.

Outlook

More than three-quarters of children with generalized tonic-clonic epilepsy who have been free of seizures for 2 years do not have them again. Many children with partial (focal) seizures outgrow the condition and may be able to discontinue medications. Absence seizures are not as easy to predict and the outlook varies with the individual.

Most children with epilepsy, even those who do not outgrow the

condition, are able to attend school and participate in sports. Your doctors can advise you on what precautions you or your child should take, and what activities should be avoided.

MENINGITIS

Meningitis is an inflammation of the membranes, or meninges, that cover the brain and spinal cord. Bacterial meningitis can be life-threatening, although antibiotics given in the early stages usually lead to a full recovery. Viral meningitis is less serious.

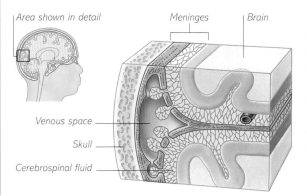

Area shown in detail | Meninges | Brain

Venous space

Skull

Cerebrospinal fluid

THE MENINGES *Three layers of protective membranes, known as the meninges, cover the brain and spinal cord. Meningitis is caused by infection of the meninges by viruses or bacteria.*

Bacterial meningitis

This is most common in children under the age of 5, although it can occur at any age. It usually appears in isolated cases and is most often caused by *Streptococcus pneumoniae*, *Neisseria meningitidis* (called meningococcal meningitis), and, rarely, *Haemophilus influenzae*. The neisseria bacteria are normally present in the nose and throat, where they are usually harmless. Why they cause meningitis in some children is not understood.

Viral meningitis

Outbreaks of viral meningitis, which is most common in children over the age of 5, occur most often in summer and fall. The viruses responsible for meningitis are usually spread through contact with respiratory secretion or infected stools. It is unclear why the viruses infect the meninges.

Immediate action

If your child is abnormally drowsy or develops at least two of the symptoms of meningitis, you should seek medical care immediately.

Your child may be given a lumbar puncture to test for either viral or bacterial meningitis and try to identify the organism responsible. Blood and stool samples and throat swabs may also be obtained from your child to determine the cause.

Medical treatment

If bacterial meningitis is suspected, your child will be started on a course of antibiotics immediately. As soon as the laboratory results are available, the antibiotic treatment will either be continued or changed to target the particular bacterium that has been identified.

Your child may also need to be given intravenous fluids. If she is having seizures, she may also receive anticonvulsant drugs.

If the diagnosis of viral meningitis is confirmed, the antibiotics can be discontinued. Pain medications may be prescribed. Your child's infection should clear up within 5–14 days, depending on the particular virus involved. Viral meningitis rarely has any lasting effects.

□ SYMPTOMS

Bacterial and viral forms of meningitis are similar in the early stages. But symptoms of bacterial meningitis are usually more severe and tend to develop rapidly, sometimes within a few hours.

Infants *may have vague early symptoms, which may include:*
- Abnormal drowsiness.
- Fever.
- Vomiting.
- Reluctance to feed.
- Increased crying; restlessness.

Older children *may have the above and the following symptoms:*
- Severe headache.
- Dislike of bright light and loud noise.
- Neck stiffness.

Later symptoms in children of all ages with bacterial meningitis include:
- Increasing drowsiness and, occasionally, loss of consciousness or seizures.

Some children who have meningitis develop:
- A characteristic rash consisting of flat, red or purple spots that do not fade when they are pressed (see p.187).

Protection

Immunization protects against *Haemophilus influenzae* and some strains of streptococcal and meningococcal meningitis. People in close contact with an affected child, especially in the same household, may receive antibiotics to help prevent the spread of bacterial meningitis.

Outlook

A few children may have some brain damage, resulting in deafness, seizures, or learning difficulties, especially if treatment is delayed. Rarely, the illness may be fatal, even if treated promptly.

ENCEPHALITIS

A rare condition, this inflammation of the brain is caused by any number of viruses. For unknown reasons, the viruses spread via the blood to the brain from elsewhere in the body. In newborn babies, the herpes simplex virus is the most common cause.

Causes

Rarely, encephalitis can develop after herpes simplex (the cause of cold sores), measles, rubella, or chickenpox. Encephalitis can vary in severity from mild and harmless to serious and life-threatening.

Most children make a full recovery, but very rarely, encephalitis can prove to be fatal. In a few cases, there is permanent brain damage, which may cause weakness of an arm and/or leg, learning difficulties, behavioral problems, or epilepsy (*see p.293*).

Medical treatment

Seek medical care immediately if your child is abnormally drowsy or if she has a fever plus any two encephalitis symptoms. Tests and brain scans may be needed. In the early stages of the illness, the tests may show nothing, even if the disease develops later. A lumbar puncture will look for bacterial or viral infections.

If the encephalitis is due to the herpes simplex or chickenpox viruses it will be treated with an antiviral drug. There are no drugs to treat other viral infections. Mechanical ventilation may be needed if your child develops breathing difficulties.

> **■ SYMPTOMS**
>
> - Fever.
> - Abnormal drowsiness.
> - Irritability.
> - Vomiting.
> - Double vision or strabismus (*p.245*).
> - Weakness of muscles.
> - Seizures.
>
> *In mild cases, symptoms may be barely noticeable. For example, a child with chickenpox encephalitis may have only slight unsteadiness on walking. In severe cases, there may be pupils of different size, loss of consciousness, or confusion.*

CEREBRAL PALSY

Cerebral palsy is the term for a condition that involves any abnormalities of limb movement and posture resulting from damage to the brain. Cerebral palsy is particularly common in babies born prematurely or weighing less than 1.5 kg (3 lb 5oz).

Causes

Brain damage can occur during pregnancy, at birth, in the newborn period, or in early childhood. Damage usually happens before birth, but cerebral palsy may not be recognized until a child is several months old.

Some children have stiff muscles in one or more limbs, making normal movement difficult. This problem may first appear from the age of 6 months. Other children may make irregular and involuntary writhing movements.

Children with cerebral palsy may have varying degrees of learning difficulties, epilepsy (*see p.293*), and hearing and vision problems. Speech

and language problems are common due to slow learning, poor hearing, and poor coordination of the muscles used in speech. A child may also have behavioral or feeding problems.

How to help your child

If your baby is not developing properly, see your doctor, who may consult specialists and do various tests and scans. Even then, a precise diagnosis may be difficult.

Encourage your child to complete tasks he can handle. Medical and educational professionals can evaluate your child and assist him in reaching his goals.

> **■ SYMPTOMS**
>
> - Stiffness of the arms and legs on being picked up.
> - Reluctance to use one or more limbs.
> - Feeding difficulties.
> - Abnormal muscle tone.
> - Delayed motor milestones.

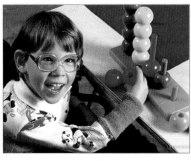

OCCUPATIONAL THERAPY *Puzzles and games involving fine hand movement can improve concentration and coordination.*

NEURAL TUBE DEFECTS

The neural tube is the part of an embryo that develops into the brain and spinal cord, and the back of the skull and vertebrae. If it fails to develop properly, a baby may be born with defects in any of these parts. The most common type of defect is spina bifida.

PREVENTION

The risk of having a baby with a neural tube defect is substantially reduced if a woman takes the recommended dose of folic acid before becoming pregnant and during the first few months of pregnancy.

Folic acid is a B vitamin that can be found in enriched grain products and vitamin supplements. All women considering pregnancy should consume 400 micrograms of folic acid daily. Women who have had previous children with a neural tube defect may be advised to take a higher dose before future pregnancies.

Consult your doctor to determine the appropriate amount of vitamins needed. Be sure that you do not take more than the recommended dose.

Causes

Spina bifida and other neural tube defects occur during the first four weeks of pregnancy. Varying parts of the neural tube fail to close in these conditions. It is unclear why there is improper cell growth and development causing these neural tube defects. Known risk factors include an insufficient maternal intake of folic acid and already having a child with a neural tube defect. Maternal heat exposure from prolonged high fever or the use of hot tubs or saunas early in pregnancy may also increase the risk. In addition, maternal diabetes and the use of certain medications used to treat seizures may be associated with neural tube defects in infants.

Medical treatment

A child with a mild defect may have no symptoms and need no treatment. More severe defects and associated complications may need surgery; with hydrocephalus, for example, a tube may be inserted into the brain to

SYMPTOMS

- The spinal cord, the brain, or the membranes (meninges) that cover them are exposed, to a greater or lesser degree. This makes these vital nerve tissues vulnerable to damage and infection.
- A dimple or a tuft of hair on the lower back may be the only indication that a defect is present.
- A large, fluid-filled swelling, covered by a thin membrane or by skin, may indicate a more severe defect.

Symptoms, if there are any, depend on the severity of the neural tube defect and may include:
- Weakness or paralysis of the legs.
- Deformity of the legs.
- Urinary and/or bowel incontinence.
- The skin below the level of the abnormality is insensitive to pain.
- Sometimes, hydrocephalus (excess spinal fluid in the brain).
- In some cases, the child may experience learning difficulties.

drain off excess fluid, which puts pressure on the brain. Despite treatment, a child with a neural tube defect may have some permanent disabilities. He will receive physical therapy and help with learning to live with his condition.

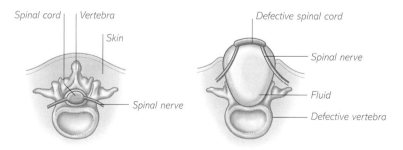

Spinal cord | Vertebra
Skin
Spinal nerve

NORMAL

Defective spinal cord
Spinal nerve
Fluid
Defective vertebra

ABNORMAL

SPINAL SECTION *In this severe neural tube defect (right), a fluid-filled sac covered by a thin membrane has developed between a vertebra and the skin.*

DYSLEXIA

Between 4 and 10 percent of children have dyslexia, so in an average class, at least one or two will be affected. Reading is usually the most obvious difficulty, and problems with spelling are also common.

Causes
There is often a family history of dyslexia or reading difficulties. Boys and girls are equally likely to have dyslexia. A child's language environment also plays a part.

Medical treatment
About half of those affected need help. Children at risk can be identified as young as 3. Usually, teachers detect the problem when a child is learning to read at school at around 6 or 7. Once identified, a child is assessed by a psychologist or specially trained teacher to gauge his strengths and weaknesses, and whether he needs extra support. If he does, the next step is to develop an educational program to help him develop the skills and best strategies for effective learning as well as boosting his morale.

How to help your child
It is easy for a child with dyslexia to feel discouraged, so be positive about your child's achievements, and help him build on his strengths. Read to him even when he can read himself to help improve his vocabulary, and work with his teachers to ensure he has the best possible support. As your child grows, he might find that using a computer is easier than relying on handwriting.

With the right support and help, he should be able to reach his full academic potential.

SYMPTOMS

- Able to recognize individual letters and numbers but has trouble getting them in the right order.
- May have difficulty recognizing different sounds, holding information in his short-term memory, and processing language at speed.

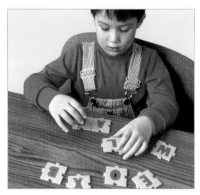

A CHILD WITH DYSLEXIA *Recognizing letters is not difficult but using them to spell words can be a particular problem.*

DYSPRAXIA

This developmental coordination disorder affects between 5 and 6 percent of children, most commonly boys. Broadly speaking, it is a motor learning problem in which a child has difficulty planning and organizing smoothly coordinated movement.

Causes
The exact cause is unknown but it is often linked with premature birth or low birth weight. Children are affected to varying degrees and other family members may have similar problems.

Medical treatment
Dyspraxia often goes unrecognized and children may be labeled as being lazy or not trying. Dyspraxia can be associated with educational, social, and emotional problems that continue into adult life. Sometimes, physiotherapy or occupational therapy can help.

How to help your child
He may easily lose self-esteem, so avoid criticism and comparisons with more able children. He should take part in activities he is good at and do as much as he can for himself. Praise his efforts and successes. Before he starts school,

SYMPTOMS

- Typically, a child may be late reaching developmental milestones such as sitting, crawling, and walking.
- Later, he may find it difficult to learn activities such as hopping, skipping, and pedaling a bike; tying shoelaces; or fastening buttons.
- He may have speech difficulties or problems with handwriting.

explain his difficulties to the teachers. He should improve with age as he learns to deal with specific things he finds difficult.

BEHAVIORAL PROBLEMS

THE MAJORITY OF CHILDHOOD HABITS are so common that they should be considered normal. Infants often suck their thumbs, bang their heads, and hold their breath for an alarming length of time. School children may be affected by tics and compulsions, while children of all ages may bite their nails or pull or twirl their hair. Most of these habits do little harm and may provide a child with comfort in times of stress and anxiety, or else become an expression of anger, boredom, or frustration. However, parents often find it hard to know whether a condition needs attention or not. Children usually grow out of their behavioral problems or their upsetting and odd habits, but some disorders, such as attention deficit hyperactivity disorder (ADHD) and autism, require expert help. Talking to your doctor can help address parental concerns and determine whether treatment is likely to be needed.

ADHD (ATTENTION DEFICIT HYPERACTIVITY DISORDER)

A child who is particularly restless and unable to concentrate and performs poorly at school may have attention deficit hyperactivity disorder. It is best diagnosed by a child psychologist or psychiatrist, or a pediatrician, with input from teacher, family, and friends.

SYMPTOMS

- Lack of concentration.
- Excessive restlessness.
- Impulsive and excitable behavior.
- Hyperactivity
- Being easily distracted.
- Forgetfulness.

Causes

It is not known why children have ADHD, but some possible causes may be genetic factors and environmental influences. More boys than girls are diagnosed with ADHD. The condition tends to appear between the ages of 3 and 7 years. Children with ADHD may be predominantly inattentive (this is more commonly the case with girls), predominantly hyperactive/impulsive (more commonly boys), or a combination of both.

The diagnosis of ADHD is based on strict criteria, and children must meet the criteria before being appropriately diagnosed with ADHD. A child with ADHD must have had symptoms for at least 6 months, the symptoms must affect the child's functioning, and some symptoms must have started before age 7 years.

Medical treatment

Consult your doctor if you suspect your child's behavior is abnormal and shows symptoms that might be related to ADHD. The doctor may want him to visit a psychiatrist, psychologist, or other specialist for assessment. Tests, including brain scans, are almost always normal and the diagnosis is most often made on the child's symptoms and on the evaluation by the specialist. The observations of the child's parents and teacher will also be taken into consideration.

Treatment depends on the severity of the disorder. A consistent routine, clear expectations of behavior, and specialized educational advice may be helpful.

Severe ADHD may be treated with stimulants, which can help children and improve concentration while decreasing their impulsivity. Research shows that 70–80 percent of children with ADHD respond well to medication. Behavior therapy combined with medication has shown positive results.

Outlook

Symptoms of ADHD may go unnoticed until a child goes to school and his restless behavior can be compared with that of other children. Some school-age children with ADHD may have oppositional behavior or depression.

Most children with ADHD improve with treatment as they get older.

AUTISM

Autism affects a child's ability to relate to other people. Usually noticeable before the age of 3, it tends to affect boys more than girls. The cause is unknown, but there are genetic factors. Asperger syndrome is the mildest form of autism.

SYMPTOMS

- Child may fail to make eye contact or point to objects in order to draw people's attention to them.
- Repetitive behavior, such as flapping the hands or spinning toy wheels.
- Delay in developing speech or language skills.
- Apparent indifference to the presence of other people.
- Preference for solitary activities.
- Little interest in creative play.
- Dislike of changes in routine.
- Learning difficulties.

Medical treatment

Check with your doctor if your child seems to have difficulty relating to others, if you are concerned about his speech or language development, or if he has learning difficulties. If autism is suspected, your child may need to see a psychologist or psychiatrist who will assess his condition. There is no known cure for autism, but your child may be helped by speech and language therapy and by special education.

Children with autism may attend schools for children with learning difficulties or go to mainstream schools where they receive specialized support. Parents can add to their education by teaching their children as many self-help skills as possible.

Outlook

Children with autism who receive speech and language therapy and appropriate educational interventions tend to improve gradually throughout their childhood and adolescence. Some achieve a degree of independence as adults, but almost all continue to have certain limitations and find relating to other people difficult. Children with the milder form of autism known as Asperger syndrome have normal intelligence and are able to form relationships with people.

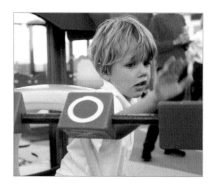

ASSESSING CHILDREN WITH SPECIAL NEEDS
Specialists watch a boy playing in order to assess his motor skills and sensory-processing abilities.

DEPRESSION

Depression is usually considered an adult problem, but it affects up to 1 in 10 children and adolescents. While feeling unhappy is normal from time to time, depression is a persistent feeling of unhappiness that may lift briefly but does not go away.

Causes

There is evidence that depression is linked to chemical changes in the part of the brain that controls mood. These changes prevent the brain from working normally and may cause many of the symptoms.

Depression can be triggered by experiences, such as the loss of a loved one, bullying at school, family breakdown, or adapting to a chronic illness. It can be related to prolonged stress – for example, if a child feels under pressure to do well at school – or can begin for no apparent reason.

Family history is also important. Studies show that children are more likely to become depressed if a parent or close relative suffers from depression. A child's environment also plays a role. The rate of mental health disturbance among children is twice as high in inner cities as in rural areas.

Depression can be hard to detect. Children often internalize feelings and may appear fine to the outside world. If your child does not want to do things, seems sad and irritable, and is approaching or going through puberty, it may be easy to assume it is just a normal part of growing up.

Medical treatment

For most children, identifying the cause of the problem and working together on coping strategies will help. However, if things do not get better or if depression is causing serious difficulties, your doctor may refer your child to a child mental health professional. Individual treatment should start with a psychological approach. Medication can be effective, but this is not a first-line treatment, particularly before adolescence.

How to help your child

Spend time talking together. At first he may seem irritable and push you away. But finding time to do something regularly together every day can help. It could be as simple as washing and drying the dishes together, cooking, or walking the dog. Try to find out what is making him feel sad and explore ways of coping. Make an effort to understand how he is feeling. Keep talking about it. If he is having a hard time at school and things do not improve after telling you, he may stop talking about it. Do not assume the problem has gone away.

Outlook

Depression can affect a child's whole life, leading to a loss of confidence; problems making decisions; difficulties in getting along with family and friends; an inability to study, work, and pass exams; and difficulty getting up to face the day.

SYMPTOMS

- Moody, irritable, tearful, easily upset.
- Seems miserable and unhappy a lot of the time.
- Becomes withdrawn and avoids friends and family.
- Self-critical about everything.
- Feels guilty about things.
- Feels persistently hopeless.
- Difficulty concentrating.
- Does not look after appearance.
- Difficulty getting to sleep or waking.
- Fatigue and lack of energy.
- Frequent minor health problems such as headaches or stomachaches.
- Change in weight or loss of appetite.
- Threatens self-harm or suicide.

TICS

Tics are rapid, repetitive movements of the body. They are not voluntary, and they cannot be controlled by the child. Tics usually affect the muscles of the face and neck and may appear as an eye twitching, shoulder shrugging, face grimacing, cough, or sniffling.

Causes
Tics have no known cause but seem to have a genetic component. They may run in families and tend to affect boys more than girls. Children are usually affected, although some adults also have tics. Up to 1 in 5 school-age children may have tics. Tics may appear during periods of stress and have an irregular pattern – they may occur frequently at some times and occasionally at others.

How to help your child
Since stress appears to worsen tics, it is best to ignore the movements and

not call attention to the behavior. Try to minimize pressure and commitments in your child's life. Talk to your child in a sensitive manner to see how she feels about the tics. Help her develop ways to deal with friends who may comment on her behavior. Seek help from your doctor if you have questions or concerns.

Medical treatment
Contact your doctor if your child has tics that are persistent, frequent, or very intense or if you suspect Tourette syndrome (see sidebar). Tics are diagnosed with a physical

examination. In most cases, medication is not necessary to reduce tic movements.

Outlook
Most tics disappear within several months without any special treatment.

TOURETTE SYNDROME

Tourette syndrome is a tic disorder that can cause motor tics in all parts of the body as well as vocal tics such as snorts or coughs or other noises. It occurs more commonly in boys and appears to be inherited. Children with Tourette syndrome may also have ADHD (see p.299) or learning disabilities. Medication may help relieve the tics.

CONDUCT DISORDERS

All children misbehave every now and then, whether it's being impudent, disobedient, or simply mischievous. But a conduct disorder constitutes a more serious problem. It means persistent disobedience and aggressive and disruptive behavior to a degree that affects a child's development and interferes with the ability of the child and his family to live a normal life.

Causes
One sign of a child who may have a conduct disorder is that he is experiencing problems at school. Antisocial behavior can result in a child being rejected by his peers.

Boys are twice as likely as girls to have a conduct disorder. Half do get better, but half get worse and as they grow these children are at risk of developing a hostile and defiant attitude, ignoring rules, getting into

physical fights, being prone to stealing and lying, and skipping school. They could begin to take risks with their own health and safety – for instance, by taking illegal drugs.

A number of factors could be present in a child with a conduct disorder. Factors may include a naturally "difficult" personality, a learning problem such as difficulty with reading or writing, depression (see p.300), and/or a history of

being bullied or abused. Children with attention deficit hyperactivity disorder (see p.299) and conduct disorder are also more at risk of experiencing learning disabilities such as reading disorders and verbal impairment.

SYMPTOMS

- Problems at school.
- Breaking rules – either at school or at home.
- Lack of self-esteem.
- Destruction of property.
- Aggression toward people and animals.
- Stealing and lying.
- Hostile attitude.

Medical treatment

If your child has serious problems for more than a few months, in which he makes life difficult both at home and at preschool or school, it would be worth consulting your doctor. He may decide that the best course of action is a referral to a child and adolescent mental health professional.

Treatment often consists of individual, group, and/or family therapy. A professional would work with your child to see what could be causing the problems and suggest practical ways of improving your child's difficult behavior. This could include helping your child learn how to limit and control his behavior as well as training in social skills.

Helping your child identify with a suitable role model might be helpful. Support would also involve family work – perhaps including education and information about the condition, help with giving your child's life a firm structure and setting and sticking to a consistent and clear set of rules.

How to help your child

There is a great deal that parents can do for their child at home. Discipline that is fair and consistent, along with praise and rewards for good or improved behavior, may help. Giving your child your attention when he is behaving well will give him a clear message about the sort of behavior you would like to see.

Talk to your child's teacher and agree on a code of conduct at school, clearly setting out the behavior you both expect within the context of the school rules. Discuss this with your child and agree on what will happen if he breaks any of the rules, along with what reward he may receive if he sticks to the agreed code for a set time. It is important that you implement your agreed course of action if he breaks the rules.

It might also be worth talking to the school's personnel to see if any further ideas might help or whether your child could be offered any particular support.

Outlook

If your child's conduct problems are recognized at an early stage, and if appropriate and comprehensive treatment and support are given, there is a good chance that he will outgrow them. Most children with mild conduct disorders improve markedly in a short time if they receive help – perhaps with counseling and practical support offered to their parents.

OBSESSIVE-COMPULSIVE BEHAVIORS

School-age children may have obsessive or compulsive behaviors. Obsessions are recurring ideas; compulsions are recurring actions. These are usually anxieties and habits that are normal for young children. However, about 1 in 200 children and adolescents have behaviors that are severe enough to interfere with daily living. This condition is called an obsessive-compulsive disorder.

Causes

Certain behaviors are considered normal for a child's given age and stage of development, and will disappear as the child matures. The cause of obsessive-compulsive disorder is unknown. The disorder may be associated with other problems such as depression or anxiety and may also run in families.

How to help your child

It is normal for children to be preoccupied with thoughts about certain things, such as always wanting to talk about particular dolls or toys. Children may also become accustomed to routines, habits, or other preferences. For example, they may consistently prefer certain clothing or arrange their belongings in a particular way. It may be best to ignore behaviors that are not harmful or extremely frequent. Often the child will outgrow these minor obsessions and habits, but some children continue to exhibit irrational and uncontrollable behaviors as they get older.

Medical treatment

If you have concerns about your child's excessive obsessions or compulsions, such as constant anxiety about fires or overly frequent handwashing, consult your doctor, who may refer you to a child psychiatrist or psychologist. Counseling may address any anxieties causing your child to have obsessive thoughts. Behavior therapy may be able to stop your child's rituals, and in some cases, medication may be used to treat him.

CARDIOVASCULAR
& BLOOD DISORDERS

A FULLY FUNCTIONING CARDIOVASCULAR system is essential for a child's health and vitality. The most common serious birth defects affect the heart, but many are now treatable. The blood vessels or blood cells may also develop abnormalities. Blood disorders may be present from birth (*see* Genetic Disorders, *p.312*) or acquired at any age. Early diagnosis and intervention may maximize the chances of successful treatment.

ANATOMY OF CIRCULATION

▶ **HOW THE CIRCULATION WORKS**

The heart pumps blood through the arteries, veins, and capillaries. Oxygen and nutrients are delivered by the blood to all parts of the body and waste products are removed. Blood is returned to the lungs for reoxygenation and elimination of carbon dioxide.

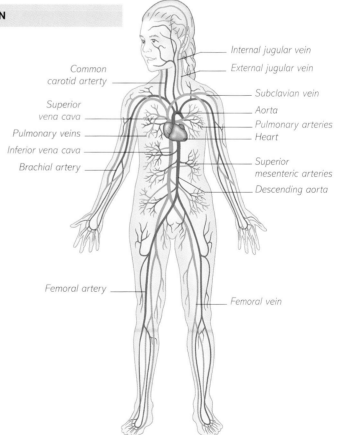

Common carotid artery

Superior vena cava

Pulmonary veins

Inferior vena cava

Brachial artery

Internal jugular vein

External jugular vein

Subclavian vein

Aorta

Pulmonary arteries

Heart

Superior mesenteric arteries

Descending aorta

Femoral artery

Femoral vein

CONGENITAL HEART DISEASE

Congenital heart disease means that a child is born with one or more malformations of the heart. About 1 child in 125 is born with a heart defect. Some children get better without treatment, but others need surgery. The risk of having a child with a heart defect is increased if a woman has poorly controlled diabetes, takes certain drugs during pregnancy, has previously had another child with a heart defect, or, in rare cases, has been infected with rubella in early pregnancy.

Types of heart defect

The more common heart defects are:
• Ventricular septal defect: an opening in the wall (septum) between the ventricles (heart pumping chambers).
• Patent ductus arteriosus: a bypass in a baby's circulation before birth, the blood vessel fails to close after birth.
• Atrial septal defect: an opening between the atria (upper heart chambers).
• Aortic stenosis: narrowing of the aortic valve.
• Pulmonary stenosis: narrowing of the pulmonary valve.
Rarer defects include:
• Transposition of the great arteries: the position of the aorta and pulmonary artery are reversed.
• Coarctation of the aorta: a narrowing of the aorta.

• Tetralogy of Fallot: a combination of four defects – pulmonary stenosis, thickened right ventricle, ventricular septal defect, and displaced aorta.

Medical treatment

The problem may be detected during a prenatal ultrasound or a newborn's routine examination. Symptoms of heart disease may not be apparent until later childhood or even adult life.

Take your child to the doctor if you suspect a congenital heart abnormality. You may be referred to a pediatric cardiologist, who may arrange for an electrocardiogram (ECG), an ultrasound (echocardiogram), and a chest X-ray, to determine if she has an abnormality and how severe it is. Medication to strengthen the heart may be needed.

□ **SYMPTOMS**

Symptoms vary with the nature and severity of the defect or defects. There are three possible signs of congenital heart disease:

Heart murmur:
• Abnormal heart sounds can be heard when a doctor listens to an affected child's heart through a stethoscope. Most murmurs are not a sign of congenital heart disease but are due to high blood flow. However, they may be due to a narrowed pulmonary or aortic valve, or to another form of heart defect.

Feeding problems and loss of weight:
• In some babies with congenital heart disease, the heart is unable to pump efficiently, causing them to feed slowly and to have difficulty finishing feedings.
• Affected babies may also breathe rapidly and sweat, especially after feeding.
• Children with congenital heart disease may grow at a slower rate than children who have healthy hearts.

Poor oxygenation of the blood:
• Bluish discoloration of the tongue and lips (cyanosis). Some defects prevent blood from circulating effectively through the lungs so the blood going to the body carries less oxygen than it should.
• Breathlessness on exertion.

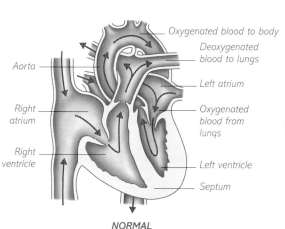

VENTRICULAR SEPTAL DEFECT *An opening in the septum allows blood to flow from left to right ventricle. Some oxygenated blood that should flow into the aorta and out to body tissues instead returns to the lungs.*

Aorta

Right atrium

Right ventricle

Oxygenated blood to body

Deoxygenated blood to lungs

Left atrium

Oxygenated blood from lungs

Left ventricle

Septum

NORMAL

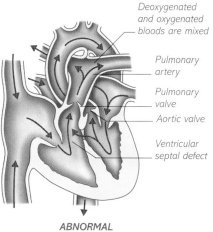

Deoxygenated and oxygenated bloods are mixed

Pulmonary artery

Pulmonary valve

Aortic valve

Ventricular septal defect

ABNORMAL

In many cases, the defects improve on their own. Some need urgent treatment or interventional catheterization, but others can go untreated until later childhood. Preventive antibiotics may be prescribed before dental treatment or surgery to minimize the risk of bacterial endocarditis – an infection of the heart valves.

How to help your child

Unless advised otherwise, encourage your child to lead a completely normal life, with a normal amount of exercise. In rare cases, particularly if your child has a heart abnormality that causes bluish discoloration of the tongue and lips, the doctor may tell you to restrict the amount of exercise she gets.

If you know that your child has congenital heart disease, always notify a doctor if your child develops a fever, lacks energy, and has a poor appetite – these symptoms could be signs of bacterial endocarditis.

If your child is prescribed antibiotics to prevent bacterial endocarditis, always make sure she takes all the medicine. Also make sure that your child always carries a card or wears a bracelet stating that she has congenital heart disease.

Outlook

The outlook depends on the type of defect and its severity. In many children, ventricular septal defects close on their own before age 5. Those that do not close may be treated by surgery. Other heart abnormalities, such as atrial septal defect, patent ductus arteriosus, and narrowing of an aortic or pulmonary valve, may be treated by catheterization or surgery. Due to great advances in treatment, children with heart disease, even those with severe defects, usually lead normal lives.

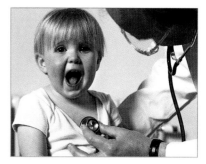

LISTENING TO A CHILD'S HEART *The doctor will use a stethoscope to listen to your child's heart. Abnormal sounds may indicate the presence of a defect.*

CHOLESTEROL AND HEART DISEASE

There is growing evidence that children who are genetically susceptible to heart disease as adults can be helped to reduce the risks if they are encouraged to follow a healthy lifestyle.

Atherosclerosis, which occurs when a high-cholesterol diet causes fatty substances to accumulate on and thicken the linings of artery walls, may develop over 30 or more years. By encouraging your child to be physically active and eat a healthy diet, you are helping reduce her risk of heart disease when she is older. Lifestyle changes are best applied to the whole family.

Here are 5 tips for a healthy lifestyle:
- Eat plenty (5 servings) of fresh fruit and vegetables every day.
- Restrict the amount of fatty meats and full-fat dairy products in the diet – they are high in saturated fats and raise cholesterol in the blood.
- Encourage regular exercise.
- Prevent smoking in your home and make sure your child understands the risks of smoking.
- Help your child manage stress and tension. If she tends to be anxious or worry a great deal, you should consult your doctor.

IRON-DEFICIENCY ANEMIA

A child with anemia has insufficient hemoglobin in her red blood cells. Her heart must work harder to deliver sufficient oxygen to the body. Mild anemia may have no symptoms. Iron-deficiency anemia is the most common form of anemia affecting children.

SYMPTOMS

- Pale skin.
- Lack of energy.
- Breathlessness on exertion.

Causes

Red blood cells are manufactured in the marrow of bones such as the femur (thighbone). They normally circulate in the blood for about 120 days before they are removed from the circulation. Anemia can develop if not enough red blood cells are made or too many are destroyed or from blood loss. If not enough red blood cells are made, it may be because the child lacks a substance, such as iron, which is an essential ingredient of hemoglobin and vital for healthy red blood cell formation. A child may not have enough iron in her diet or she may not be absorbing or using it effectively.

Long-term iron-deficiency anemia may impair mental development and function. If too many cells are being destroyed, there may be a genetic cause as in sickle-cell anemia (*see p.313*) and thalassemia (*see p.314*).

Medical treatment

Take your child to the doctor if you suspect she has symptoms of anemia. The doctor will ask about your family history and your child's general health and diet.

If the doctor suspects anemia, your child's blood will be analyzed to determine the number, shape, size, and color of the red blood cells – in iron-deficiency anemia, for example, they appear smaller and paler than normal. Subsequent tests, such as measuring

the level of iron in the blood, may be needed to make a precise diagnosis.

The doctor may give you advice on what sort of foods your child should be eating. She may also need to take iron supplements, usually for about 3 months, to build up her iron reserves.

If your child is under 6 months and was premature, she will probably already have been prescribed iron supplements. If not, the doctor may prescribe them at this time. Premature babies often do not have sufficient iron reserves to compensate for the usual iron content of a milk-only diet during the first 6 months of life, before they start on solids.

How to help your child

Iron-deficiency anemia is seen most often during phases of rapid growth such as infancy or adolescence. Loss of menstrual blood may cause iron deficiency in adolescent females. Iron deficiency can be prevented by a varied diet. Make sure your child's diet contains iron-rich foods – dark green leafy vegetables, iron-fortified cereals, and red meat. The iron in nonmeat foods is best absorbed by the body when eaten with sources of vitamin C, such as orange juice. If your child will not eat iron-rich foods, you should talk to your doctor about iron supplements.

LEUKEMIA

Leukemia is a form of cancer in which the bone marrow produces many abnormal (leukemic) white blood cells, and fewer normal white blood cells, red blood cells, and platelets. The leukemic cells infiltrate the liver, spleen, and lymph glands and undermine the immune system. The most common form of leukemia in children is acute lymphoblastic leukemia.

NORMAL   LEUKEMIA

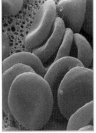 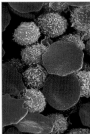

ACUTE LYMPHOBLASTIC LEUKEMIA *Seen under a microscope, blood taken from a person with leukemia (above right) shows a large number of abnormal white blood cells.*

Medical treatment

If you think your child might have leukemia, see your doctor, who will examine her and may obtain blood

tests. Your child may also need a bone marrow test, in which cells are removed from the bone marrow and analyzed. The care of a child with leukemia should be coordinated by a pediatric hematologist/oncologist.

Treatment for acute lymphoblastic leukemia is divided into two phases. In the first phase, which usually lasts weeks, your child will be given drugs to destroy the leukemic cells. This treatment continues until a bone marrow test shows that there are no abnormal cells. At this point, your child is said to be in remission.

The next phase of treatment lasts for about 2 years. During this phase your child will undergo periods of intensive drug treatment to destroy

leukemic cells left in the body. Much of this treatment is given on an out-patient basis. Help your child lead as normal a life as possible, but keep her away from anyone with a viral infection, particularly chickenpox or measles, because the drugs increase susceptibility to infection.

Outlook

With the medical treatments currently available, there is full recovery in about 70 percent of children who have been diagnosed as having acute lymphoblastic leukemia.

HENOCH-SCHÖNLEIN PURPURA

This immune system disorder causes inflammation of small blood vessels, which leak blood into the skin to cause a rash. The joints, kidneys, and digestive tract are also affected. It is most common in children ages 2–10 and affects boys more often than girls.

Medical treatment

Consult your doctor within 24 hours of any symptoms appearing that might indicate your child has Henoch-Schönlein purpura. The doctor may obtain blood tests to rule out other possibilities. Your child's urine will also be tested: the presence of red blood cells and protein in the urine indicates that the kidneys have become inflamed.

If symptoms are mild, no treatment is needed. If your child has severe abdominal pain she may be given corticosteroids, which should cause rapid improvement. If the kidneys are affected, the doctor may repeat the urine and blood tests to ensure the condition is improving.

How to help your child

If your child's symptoms are causing pain or discomfort, try giving her acetaminophen. Let her stay in bed if she wants. Henoch-Schönlein purpura may last a few days or up to a month and symptoms may come and go.

Most children who have the illness make a complete recovery, and there are no long-term ill effects. Any inflammation of the kidneys usually disappears in a few days, but in some children the kidneys remain inflamed for up to 2 years.

> **SYMPTOMS**
>
> - Rash, which is present in all cases, is made up of pink, red, or purplish spots that are filled with blood and do not fade when pressed.
> - The rash first appears on the buttocks and the backs of the arms and legs, especially around the ankles and elbows, and then spreads to the front parts of the limbs.
> - Joint pain and swelling.
> - Abdominal pain, often with vomiting and diarrhea.
> - Blood in the stools.

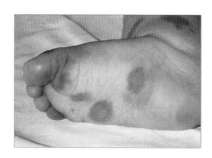

A TYPICAL RASH The spots of Henoch-Schönlein purpura may be pink, red, or purplish, and either flat or raised. Individual spots vary widely in size.

THROMBOCYTOPENIA

Individuals with this condition have an abnormally low number of platelets in the blood. In children, it generally develops as part of a disorder called idiopathic thrombocytopenic purpura (ITP), which usually follows within 2 weeks of a viral infection.

Medical treatment

Consult your doctor immediately if your child has the rash and symptoms of bleeding that might be caused by ITP. The doctor will need to obtain blood tests to confirm that she has ITP and not another illness with similar symptoms.

Some children with ITP do not need treatment, but they should avoid strenuous activities until symptoms clear up, usually within a few weeks.

Platelets are essential for blood clotting, so if your child has bleeding from the nose or mouth, or has a very low blood platelet count, she may be treated at the hospital. The doctor may prescribe a short course of corticosteroid drugs or intravenous gamma-globulin in order to speed recovery and reduce the risk of severe bleeding.

A brain hemorrhage, in which there is bleeding around or within

> **SYMPTOMS**
>
> - A widespread, flat purple rash caused by bleeding into the skin; the rash does not fade when pressed.
> - Bruising from only minor pressure.
> - Nosebleeds.
> - Bleeding in the mouth.
> - Blood in the urine as a result of bleeding in the kidneys.

the brain, is a rare complication of thrombocytopenia. Most children are free of symptoms within about 2 weeks. In some cases, however, blood platelet levels may take 6 months or more to return to normal.

HORMONAL PROBLEMS

SECTION CONTENTS

HORMONES ARE CHEMICAL MESSENGERS that are released directly into the bloodstream by the glands of the endocrine system. They all have different but vital roles to play in the way the body functions. They control growth, the production of energy, biochemical activities such as digestion, and sexual development and function. They also help the body deal with stress, danger, and fatigue.

ANATOMY OF THE ENDOCRINE SYSTEM

ENDOCRINE SYSTEM
The pituitary gland is found at the base of the brain. This master gland controls the release of many of the body's hormones into the bloodstream, which distributes them to all parts of the body. Some glands, such as the testes and ovaries, are inactive until puberty.

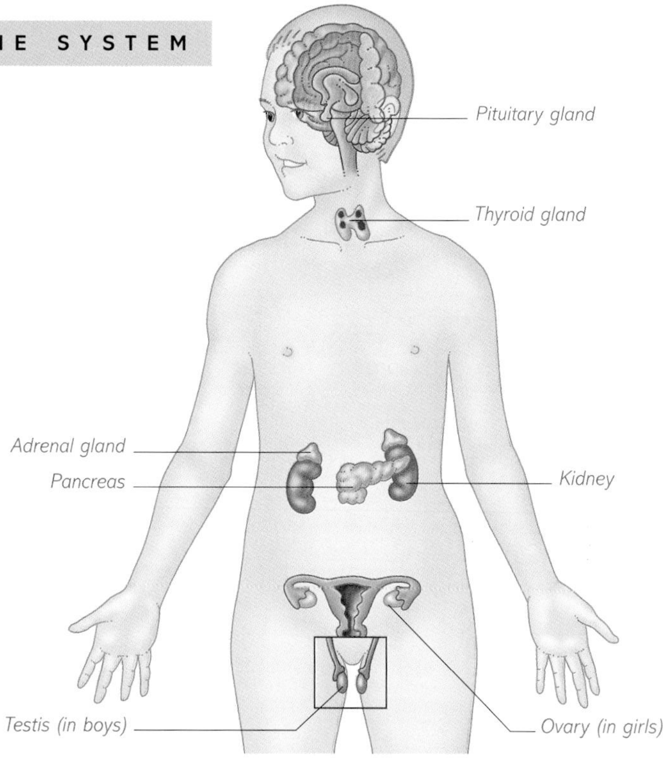
Pituitary gland
Thyroid gland
Adrenal gland
Pancreas
Kidney
Testis (in boys)
Ovary (in girls)

DIABETES MELLITUS

Insulin is a hormone that enables body cells to use and store the sugar glucose. In type 1 (juvenile) diabetes, cells in the pancreas suddenly stop making insulin and the lack of this hormone causes a buildup of glucose in the blood and a disturbance of the body's chemical processes. Unused glucose is excreted in large volumes of urine passed frequently, causing thirst. Children with this type of diabetes mellitus will need insulin replacement throughout their lives.

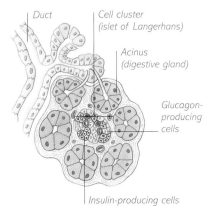

Duct

Cell cluster
(islet of Langerhans)

Acinus
(digestive gland)

Glucagon-
producing
cells

Insulin-producing cells

CELLS IN THE PANCREAS *The pancreas has several types of cells. Some secrete insulin to lower the blood glucose level; others secrete glucagon to raise it.*

Immediate action
Call your doctor immediately if you think that your child might have diabetes mellitus. If your child has already been diagnosed with diabetes mellitus, check with the doctor or endocrinologist if you ever have any concerns about your child's condition. Phone as soon as possible if your child has an infection or case of gastroenteritis, because these conditions may make it difficult to control the blood glucose level.

Medical treatment
If your child displays symptoms that suggest he might have diabetes mellitus, your doctor will arrange for

his urine and blood to be tested for glucose and other levels. If the results show abnormally high glucose levels, your doctor may recommend that your child go to a hospital immediately for further investigations and to begin insulin treatment. If your child is dehydrated from urinating in large amounts, intravenous rehydrating fluids may be given as well as insulin. The length of time your child will have to stay in the hospital will depend on his age as well as the severity of his condition.

The long-term control of your child's diabetes mellitus will be carried out under medical supervision. The aim is to provide enough insulin to keep his blood glucose level within the normal range, so that he is able to lead a normal life. To do this he will need to eat regular, balanced meals and receive insulin at least twice a day via injections or an insulin pump.

If your child's blood glucose level falls too low because of too high a dose of insulin, missing a meal, or a sudden burst of exercise, he may have a hypoglycemic attack. The doctor caring for your child's diabetes (your doctor or endocrinologist) will explain how to recognize the hypoglycemia and what to do if your child has an attack. The doctor will also prescribe glucagon, which can be injected to stop an attack.

How to help your child
Your doctor will show you how to test for the amount of glucose in your child's blood and record the results. These measurements allow you to adjust the amount of insulin your child is to be given by injection to the correct level. You will also need to learn how to give injections and how to store and dispose of used bottles and syringes. Some children may be able to use an insulin pump, which delivers insulin through a tube inserted in the abdominal skin.

You can also help your child by making sure he has properly planned meals, with consistent proportions of fat, protein, and carbohydrates, served at regular times.

A child 5 years or over should have a diet of about 30 percent fat, about 15 percent protein, and the rest carbohydrates. Children younger than 5 may eat more fat. The diet should be high in soluble and insoluble fiber. Soluble fiber is found in beans and oat-based foods; insoluble fiber is found in wholegrain breads, pasta, and cereals. Your doctor or a dietitian can advise you on appropriate food choices. You do not have to make special meals for a diabetic child. A similar healthy, well-balanced diet will benefit all members of the family.

Exercise can trigger an attack of hypoglycemia, so you may have to adjust your child's diet and dosage of insulin if he is taking part in a sports event or strenuous exercise. Ask the doctor who is supervising your child's treatment for advice.

Your child should carry a medical identification card or bracelet that indicates that he has diabetes mellitus and shows the medication that he is taking. Everyone involved in caring for your child, such as teachers, needs to know what to do if he has a hypoglycemic attack.

As your child gets older, encourage him to take as much responsibility as possible for the control of his own diabetes mellitus. Even quite young children can understand the need to eat regularly and to watch for and treat the symptoms of hypoglycemia. They can learn to inject themselves and to test and record their own blood glucose levels.

The main signs of hypoglycemia
• Lethargy.
• Sweating or shaking.
• Dizziness, and/or confusion.
If your child shows any of these signs, immediately give him a sweet drink or sweet food, such as glucose tablets or hard candy. If your child will not eat or drink, or his blood glucose drops so low that he becomes drowsy or loses consciousness, give an injection of glucagon in order to bring the glucose level back to normal.

Outlook
A well-controlled blood glucose level should let your child live a normal life, with a normal amount of exercise. It should also reduce the chance of any complications developing.

The complications that can affect people with diabetes, such as problems with the heart, circulation, kidneys, eyes, and nervous system, may begin to develop several years after the onset of the disease, especially in cases where the blood glucose level is poorly controlled.

DIABETES INSIPIDUS

Diabetes insipidus is due to a deficiency of an entirely different hormone than diabetes mellitus and is not related to glucose balance or energy use. The main symptoms, however, are similar to those of diabetes mellitus.

Causes
In most cases, diabetes insipidus is caused by the failure of the pituitary gland to secrete antidiuretic hormone (ADH). ADH normally acts on the kidneys to cause them to concentrate the urine and thereby restrict the amount of fluid that is excreted from the body via the bladder.

Failure of the pituitary gland to produce ADH results in the passage of large amounts of urine and excessive thirst. The failure may be due to an injury to the gland or, less commonly, a tumor. In rare cases, the disorder develops because the kidneys fail to respond to normal levels of ADH.

Medical treatment
Call your doctor immediately if you notice your child has the symptoms of diabetes insipidus or if he has any of the following signs of dehydration: sunken eyes, abnormal drowsiness, or weight loss.

The doctor will take a sample of urine and arrange for it to be analyzed. Diabetes insipidus is a possibility if the urine is not adequately concentrated. Your child may need further tests at a hospital to confirm the diagnosis and to find out the cause.

If your child's pituitary gland is not producing ADH in sufficient quantities, he will need to take synthetic ADH. If

> ### SYMPTOMS
>
> • Excessive thirst.
> • Frequent passing of large quantities of very pale urine.
>
> *Dehydration can occur as a result of the excessive fluid passed as urine.*

his kidneys are failing to respond to normal levels of ADH, your child will be treated with a low-sodium diet and, paradoxically, a diuretic drug.

Outlook
A damaged pituitary gland may heal and return to functioning normally, but sometimes the diabetes insipidus continues throughout life. However, treatment will enable the person to live a normal, active life and there are no long-term complications.

HYPOTHYROIDISM

The hormones of the thyroid gland are essential for a child's normal physical and mental development. In hypothyroidism, insufficient hormones are produced, and if the condition is not treated, it may affect a child's growth and learning abilities.

Causes

A child may have hypothyroidism from birth, usually caused by a thyroid gland that did not develop normally. A disease of the thyroid gland or an underactive hypothalamus or pituitary gland (both of which stimulate the thyroid gland to produce thyroid hormones) may also cause the condition. Hypothyroidism tends to run in families and may be associated with autoimmune diseases such as vitiligo, rheumatoid arthritis, diabetes mellitus, and pernicious anemia.

Medical treatment

All babies have their blood tested for hypothyroidism within a week of birth as part of the newborn screen. If your child has an underactive thyroid gland, he will be given treatment before any symptoms appear.

Take your child to the doctor if you suspect hormone problems. The doctor will probably take a blood sample to measure hormone levels. If these tests confirm hypothyroidism, your child will be given tablets of synthetic thyroxine (the main hormone produced by the thyroid gland), which he will then have to take for the rest of his life.

SYMPTOMS

In older children, the symptoms of hypothyroidism include:
- Reduction in the child's growth rate.
- Poor concentration.
- Lack of energy, poor appetite, and weight gain.
- Goiter (enlarged thyroid gland).
- Constipation.

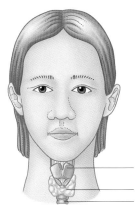

THE THYROID GLAND
This gland is located at the base of the neck in front of the trachea. The gland helps regulate the body's energy levels and growth.

Thyroid cartilage

Thyroid gland
Trachea

GROWTH HORMONE DEFICIENCY

All children need growth hormone for their bodies to grow normally. The hormone is produced by the pituitary gland, which is located at the base of the brain. If there is a deficiency of growth hormone, the child will grow slowly.

SYMPTOMS

- Slow rate of growth.
- Short stature and chubbiness.
- Delayed development of sexual characteristics in older children.

Causes

Normally, the growth hormone from the pituitary gland stimulates the development of the bones of the skeleton and the production of proteins of which the body's other tissues are composed.

If the pituitary gland is affected by a congenital abnormality or a tumor, or if a child has a head injury, then the production of growth hormone may be insufficient to stimulate normal development.

Medical treatment

Take your child to your doctor if you are worried about the rate at which he is growing. The doctor will measure his height at regular intervals so that his growth can be plotted on a chart.

If your child's rate of growth is slower than normal, he may need to have X-rays of some bones and tests such as an analysis of the growth hormone levels in the blood. If your child is diagnosed as having a growth hormone deficiency, he may need to take synthetic growth hormone, which you will need to inject daily or a few times per week until he reaches the end of puberty.

Outlook

Treatment improves a child's growth rate. Your child may reach the normal adult height expected for your family if treatment begins before puberty.

GENETIC DISORDERS

THE BIOCHEMICAL INFORMATION NEEDED for the normal growth and development of a fetus is carried on around 35,000 pairs of genes packed in 23 pairs of chromosomes. This is the human genome. If any of these genes, or indeed a whole chromosome, is abnormal then a baby may be born either with an immediately apparent defect or with a condition that manifests itself later in life. Genetic counseling and analysis allows couples with a family history of one of the roughly 4,000 inherited diseases to assess their chances of having an affected child. Tests during pregnancy and routine blood screens performed on every newborn may detect the presence of a disorder. The Human Genome Project and other discoveries have generated advances, not only in our understanding of DNA, genes, and how genes work but also in the technology that may be used to manipulate them.

SICKLE CELL ANEMIA

Sickle cell anemia is a serious, inherited blood disease most common among, although not exclusive to, people of African descent. The red blood cells become distorted into a sickle shape and can block narrow blood vessels. The cells are also destroyed more easily than normal red blood cells, producing anemia. Children who have sickle cell anemia are at increased risk of certain infections. Occasionally, blood flow is reduced to the kidneys, spleen, or brain, causing damage to these organs.

Causes

The red blood cells become distorted because they contain an abnormal type of hemoglobin (the oxygen-carrying protein) known as hemoglobin S. The sickle cells are more fragile than normal red blood cells. Because of their shape they sometimes block the narrow blood capillaries, causing extreme pain and preventing oxygen from reaching the cells of the body. The decreased blood flow that develops may cause some areas of tissue to be damaged.

If a child inherits the abnormal gene responsible for producing this hemoglobin S from each parent, the child will develop sickle cell anemia. If a child inherits the abnormal gene from one parent and a normal gene from the other, the child will have sickle-cell trait and will be a carrier but otherwise completely healthy. However, carriers can pass on the abnormal gene to their children.

Medical treatment

Check with your doctor if you are unsure whether your child might be at risk or if she is showing any of the symptoms of sickle cell anemia. The diagnosis can be confirmed by blood tests. Treatment includes taking folic acid supplements, which may reduce the severity of the anemia. Penicillin can help prevent infections, immunization will be given against pneumococcal and other infections, and analgesics may help if your child is in pain.

How to help your child

To reduce the likelihood of painful attacks, your child should drink plenty of fluids (to prevent dehydration) and make sure she does not become chilled. Call your doctor or sickle cell disease specialist immediately if your child has the following symptoms:

- Fever.
- Sudden paleness.
- Persistent vomiting or severe diarrhea.
- Pain not responsive to acetaminophen or ibuprofen.

- Abnormal drowsiness or lack of energy, or difficulty breathing.

If your child has severe abdominal pain or tenderness, you should seek urgent medical attention. She may need to be admitted to a hospital for pain relief and treatment of dehydration or any infection.

Outlook

With good medical care, most affected children survive into adulthood. If symptoms are severe, a child with sickle cell anemia may be considered for bone marrow transplantation if a suitable donor is found. A successful transplant provides a complete cure.

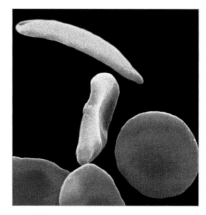

RED BLOOD CELLS IN SICKLE CELL ANEMIA
Seen through a microscope, blood taken from a person affected by sickle-cell anemia shows distorted, sickle-shaped red blood cells.

THALASSEMIA

This form of anemia is most common among people of African, Mediterranean, or Asian origin. Thalassemia minor usually has no symptoms; thalassemia major causes an enlarged spleen, jaundice, slow growth, and deformity of some bones if left untreated.

SYMPTOMS

- Pale skin.
- Chronic fatigue.
- Shortness of breath.

Causes

Thalassemia is due to an abnormality in the gene responsible for producing hemoglobin. A child who inherits the abnormal gene from both parents develops thalassemia major and cannot make normal hemoglobin. Her red blood cells are small, fragile, and rapidly destroyed, leading to severe anemia. A child who inherits a single abnormal gene develops thalassemia minor; her red cells are slightly smaller than normal but she has no symptoms.

Medical treatment

Thalassemia is diagnosed by blood tests. Thalassemia minor requires no treatment. Thalassemia major is treated with blood transfusions, which may damage internal organs due to iron overload. Regular injections of an iron-bonding agent reduce this risk. Bone marrow transplantation may cure the disorder. With treatment, the prospects for normal growth and development are good, and many people survive into middle age.

CONSIDERATIONS

Consult your physician for more information about thalassemia. Parents or other close relatives of a child with thalassemia, and any prospective parent with thalassemia, can have genetic counseling to establish the risk of having an affected child. Prenatal tests are also available.

FRAGILE X SYNDROME

This inherited chromosomal abnormality affects approximately 1 in 3,600 boys and 1 in 5,000 girls. Its name comes from the fact that these children have a fragile area on the long arm of the X chromosome in every one of their cells. It is a relatively common cause of learning difficulties and also causes a slightly abnormal physical appearance.

SYMPTOMS

- Relatively large head.
- Delay in mental development, which is usually slight in girls and moderate to severe in boys.
- Delayed speech development, which is usually more severe in boys.
- Hyperactivity and attention deficit hyperactivity disorder (see p.299).
- Features of autism (see p.299).
- Square jaw, long face, large ears, and large testes in boys at puberty.

Causes

The mutation of a particular gene on the X chromosome can affect the development of the brain, leading to difficulties in learning and behavior. Fragile X syndrome is the most common cause of congenital learning difficulties. Boys are more severely affected than girls, because the latter have 2 X chromosomes, one of which is normal, and boys have only one.

Medical treatment

A woman without any symptoms is able to carry the defective gene on an X chromosome and pass it on to some of her children. For mothers known to have fragile X syndrome, prenatal diagnosis is possible by DNA analysis of cells taken during amniocentesis.

If you think your child may be exhibiting some symptoms of fragile X syndrome, see your doctor. The disorder may be suspected only after puberty, when the physical features are more apparent. After examining your child, the doctor will assess his learning ability and may arrange for chromosome and DNA analysis of a blood sample. If the tests show your child has the defective chromosome, you will be referred for genetic counseling to discuss the risks of further children being affected.

There is no specific treatment. If your child is not already receiving help for speech or learning difficulties, the doctor may have her be assessed by a speech therapist or psychologist.

HEMOPHILIA

This genetic disorder affects about 1 in 5,000 boys and causes spontaneous bleeding. It is due to deficient activity of a clotting factor in the blood, most commonly factor VIII. Women who carry the abnormal gene may pass the disorder to their sons.

Causes

In hemophilia, the blood either takes a long time to clot or it does not clot at all. This is because the boys who develop the disorder are born with an abnormal gene that prevents them from producing factor VIII, one of a number of key ingredients in the process of clotting the blood.

Hemophiliacs should take care to avoid cuts and injuries because they can start the bleeding that is hard to stop. However, individuals are affected in different ways – bleeding may, in fact, start without any apparent cause.

Since the gene is sex-linked and is found on the X chromosome, nearly all hemophiliacs are males, while females in hemophiliac families are carriers. A daughter can have the disease if her father has hemophilia and her mother is a carrier.

Medical treatment

If your son shows signs of abnormal bleeding, see your doctor, who will ask about symptoms. If hemophilia seems possible, she will arrange for blood tests to assess the blood's ability to clot. If your son has hemophilia, his bleeding episodes may be treated with infusions of factor VIII, which you can learn to administer.

Severe bleeding may require a hospital stay. If a boy bleeds frequently, parents may be taught to infuse factor VIII as a prevention. The frequency and severity of bleeding varies greatly from boy to boy. Some hemophiliacs suffer from only occasional episodes of minor bleeding. When the condition is more severe, recurrent internal bleeding can damage muscles and joints, but appropriate therapy can prevent this from occurring.

SYMPTOMS

- Prolonged bleeding after an injury or even minor surgery, such as tooth extraction or circumcision.
- Painful swelling of muscles and joints as a result of internal bleeding.

Outlook

It is best for children with hemophilia to avoid possible hazards, such as contact sports. Provided an affected child has prompt treatment with factor VIII when bleeding occurs, or has regular infusions, the muscles and joints may not be damaged, and life expectancy should be normal.

CONSIDERATIONS

Women with a history of hemophilia in their family can be tested to find out if they have the hemophilia gene. If they do, they can receive genetic counseling to assess the risk of having an affected child.

CYSTIC FIBROSIS

Cystic fibrosis is a serious inherited disease affecting about 1 in 2,000 children. For a child to have the disorder, the abnormal gene must be inherited from both parents, who may be carriers and have no symptoms of the disease.

Causes

A defective gene causes the secretion of sticky mucus that cannot flow freely through the airways and so leads to recurrent chest infections, which can cause progressive lung damage. It also causes deficient secretion of pancreatic enzymes (which help in the digestion of food), leading to an inability to absorb nutrients properly from the intestines (see Malabsorption, p.258) and diarrhea.

Medical treatment

Although cystic fibrosis is present from birth, it may not be diagnosed for some months or even years, during which time damage to the lungs may

SYMPTOMS

- Failure to grow normally and to gain a normal amount of weight.
- Persistent coughing.
- Chronic diarrhea, typically with pale, greasy, strong-smelling stools.

have already begun. The screening of newborn children for cystic fibrosis is now being introduced in some areas.

If your child has any of the symptoms of cystic fibrosis, take her to your doctor, who will obtain tests if cystic fibrosis is considered possible. Your child's sweat will be analyzed and she may also have genetic tests.

If the tests confirm cystic fibrosis, your child will need to take special enzymes to help her digest her food properly. A diet that is high in calories and protein is usually recommended, along with vitamin supplements. The doctor may prescribe antibiotics and recommend regular physiotherapy for

◻ **CONSIDERATIONS**

Consult your physician for more information about cystic fibrosis. A prospective parent who already has a child with cystic fibrosis or who is a carrier may desire genetic counseling or prenatal testing.

treatment of chest infections and to help prevent chronic lung disease.

How to help your child
You will be shown how to give chest physiotherapy exercises (*see right*) to help loosen the thick mucus that obstructs the bronchi in your child's lungs. Do these exercises twice a day (more when your child is ill). Call your doctor or pediatric respirologist at the first sign of any illness so that your child can be treated quickly. To absorb enough nutrients for normal growth, she will need to eat high-calorie snacks.

Outlook
There is no cure for cystic fibrosis, but earlier diagnosis and new methods of treatment allow most affected children

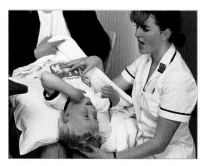

CHEST PHYSIOTHERAPY *This is a demonstration of the exercises that a parent needs to practice in order to help loosen the thick mucus that accumulates in the lungs of a child with cystic fibrosis.*

to survive well into adulthood. In rare cases, severely affected children may have a heart-lung transplant, which may improve their quality of life and increase their life expectancy.

PHENYLKETONURIA

This inherited disorder affects about 1 baby in 10,000. Babies are routinely screened for phenylketonuria by a blood test soon after birth. A defect in body chemistry causes a buildup of the amino acid phenylalanine (a component of protein) in the blood.

Causes
If it is left untreated, phenylketonuria will cause severe brain damage. This is because the body does not possess the enzyme necessary for breaking down phenylalanine. As a result, this amino acid accumulates and affects the function of the nervous system.

Medical treatment
At birth, affected babies show no signs of any abnormality, but if the condition is not quickly diagnosed, symptoms may soon develop.

A special diet, which must be continued throughout life, is the main treatment for phenylketonuria and should be started in the first weeks

after birth. The main reason for this is that the amino acid phenylalanine, which is present in most protein foods, must be restricted while at the same time making sure the child still eats enough protein for growth. The recommended diet is mainly vegetarian and special food supplements will be prescribed. Affected babies will need to be given special milk substitutes.

Outlook
The majority of children who have been treated for phenylketonuria attend normal schools and have normal intelligence. However, a few do exhibit behavioral problems and experience learning difficulties.

◻ **SYMPTOMS**

Without treatment:
• Severe learning difficulties.
• A tendency to seizures.
• A characteristic musty odor.
• Rash like that of eczema (*see p.234*).

With treatment:
• No symptoms or mild learning or behavioral difficulties.

◻ **CONSIDERATIONS**

Consult your physician for further information about phenylketonuria. If a couple give birth to an affected child, there is a risk that any further children they have will also be affected. Parents may be offered genetic counseling. Prenatal testing and diagnosis are also available.

DOWN SYNDROME

This is the most common chromosomal abnormality, affecting about 1 in every 700 babies. The risk of giving birth to a baby with Down syndrome increases sharply in women over 37 years old, and a third of all babies with Down syndrome are born to women in this age group. The risk is also greater in women who have already had an affected child.

Medical treatment

After examining your child for features of Down syndrome, the doctor will arrange for chromosome analysis of blood samples to confirm the diagnosis. Ultrasound examination of the heart may be performed to look for defects; X-rays of the abdomen may be taken if an intestinal defect is suspected. Surgery may be required to correct any defects. Your child may have follow-up care from speech and occupational therapists as well as special educational help.

Possible complications

Many children with Down syndrome have a heart defect, and some have an intestinal abnormality. Children with Down syndrome are at higher risk of developing an underactive thyroid gland and acute leukemia (*see p.306*). They are likely to have unstable neck joints (which may mean restricting some activities). They may also have hearing problems and be susceptible to infections.

Outlook

Many children with Down syndrome survive into early middle age, but a small proportion die before they reach the age of 5, usually because of severe heart problems. Adults who have Down syndrome are susceptible to the early development of Alzheimer's disease and arteriosclerosis.

Advances in educational methods have meant that more children with Down syndrome reach their full potential than in the past, and most are educated at mainstream schools.

SYMPTOMS

- Upward-sloping eyes, which have prominent skin folds at the inner corner of the eyelids.
- Small, round face and full cheeks.
- Large tongue that tends to protrude.
- Flat back of the head.
- Floppy limbs.
- Slow physical development.
- Learning difficulties.
- Short stature.

CONSIDERATIONS

Consult your physician for further information about Down syndrome. Pregnant women generally have a screening blood test to determine the risk of having a baby with Down syndrome. A prenatal ultrasound may also detect if the fetus has physical characteristics typical of Down syndrome.

Women who have an increased risk are offered amniocentesis, in which a sample of amniotic fluid is taken from the uterus and analyzed for abnormal chromosomes.

MCAD DEFICIENCY

MCAD deficiency is a rare inherited disorder, affecting about 1 in 8,000 children. MCAD is an enzyme that is essential for the breakdown of fats. For a child to have this disorder, both parents must carry the abnormal gene.

Causes

When levels of the enzyme medium-chain acylCoA dehydrogenase (MCAD) are very low, fat is not properly broken down, blood sugar falls, and the liver starts to malfunction. If the child is ill or fasting, she may lose consciousness.

Medical treatment

The child is unaffected if eating normally. Fasting should be avoided. During illnesses the child should have regular glucose drinks. If vomiting, she will need intravenous glucose. Long-term neurological damage or other complications may result if the disorder is not treated properly.

This is a lifelong condition but it can be prevented by avoiding fasting. Newborn screening, allowing detection of the condition shortly after birth, is being introduced in some areas.

COMPLEMENTARY
THERAPIES

Many families are interested in complementary therapies to use as an adjunct to traditional medicine. Some doctors practice holistic health care and consider complementary and alternative therapies when making treatment recommendations.

FREQUENTLY ASKED QUESTIONS

The answers to the following questions may give you a clearer understanding of what is involved in complementary therapies, holistic health and integrative medicine.

What is complementary therapy and why is it popular?

Complementary therapies, such as herbs, massage, and acupuncture, are treatments not traditionally used in many conventional Western medical settings. When complementary therapies are used along with conventional care, it is called integrative medicine. When a therapist focuses on all aspects of the child's wellness (mind, body, and spirit) instead of just the condition, it is called holistic care.

A holistic therapist aims to bring your child to optimal health by restoring his body's natural balance and maximizing his ability to heal himself. After taking a thorough history, listening and talking to you and your child, the therapist will normally offer carefully monitored treatment.

Complementary therapies are becoming more popular. Many parents want to take more responsibility for their children's health, as well as their own. Parents and doctors are concerned about the overuse of some medications and may choose to explore additional treatment options. There are aspects of conventional Western medicine that may unfortunately be limited in the scope of care provided. For example, chronic medical problems such as pain, chronic disease, and quality-of-life issues are sometimes not adequately addressed by conventional medicine.

Can complementary therapies be used alongside conventional medicine?

In general, complementary therapies work well alongside conventional treatments – indeed, this is why they are called complementary. It is important that your doctor and complementary therapist work well with each other. You should ask them to establish communication between them regarding your child's care.

Complementary therapies may have adverse reactions or drug interactions with traditional medicines. Always notify your doctor of any home remedies, nonprescription medications, vitamins, or herbs your child is taking. Your pharmacist may also be able to give you information about side effects and interactions.

Some doctors have additional training in complementary therapies such as osteopathy, acupuncture, and hypnosis. Many take a holistic view on health and are able to offer advice on complementary therapies.

How can I find a complementary practitioner?

To learn more about complementary therapies, ask your doctor, nurse, local hospital, or medical society. Some insurance companies cover complementary treatments, so you may also want to contact your carrier for a referral.

The professional regulatory bodies for complementary practitioners

"Always notify your doctor of home remedies, nonprescription medications, vitamins, or herbs your child is taking."

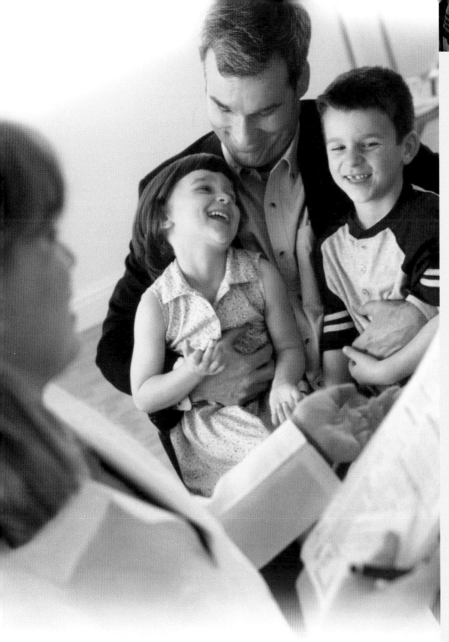

vary by province, so find out in advance what certification a potential practitioner in your area should have. Chiropractors are licensed in all provinces of Canada. Acupuncturists are licensed in some provinces, and naturopaths may be licensed in your area.

Choose a practitioner who is certified and in good standing with the provincial licensing agency. Your therapist should have experience with patients similar to your child and know the limits of his training and experience. It can be very confusing trying to learn about and understand the various qualifications, so don't hesitate to ask – it is important for you to feel comfortable.

Your therapist should clearly tell you at the outset what to expect, how long the treatment should take and how much it might cost, what you might reasonably expect to achieve within a certain time frame, and what the plan is for dealing with problems.

Some complementary therapists provide brochures or web sites with their services and prices clearly marked. Always find out how much the treatment will cost you before scheduling an appointment, and make sure you find out how many appointments your child will be expected to attend.

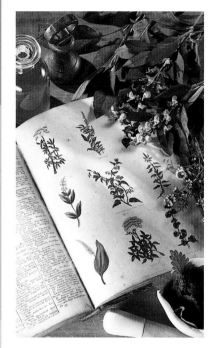

EXAMPLES OF COMPLEMENTARY THERAPIES

The following therapies might be considered for your child. Always review complementary therapies with your doctor before using. The majority of complementary therapies have not been studied in children and many studies suffer from poor design or insignificant numbers. Studies in adults cannot and should not be assumed to be similar to children.

Acupuncture and acupressure

These ancient Chinese therapies are based on the belief that the energy of life circulates throughout the body in a number of channels called meridians. Along each meridian lie several points (acupoints) that, if stimulated, can affect the flow of energy and rebalance the harmony of the body.

In acupuncture, fine, hairlike needles are placed in acupoints to create a balance in the body's energy.

It may be used to treat pain, nausea and vomiting, and other conditions. The needles are solid, sterile, and disposable. Complications are rare and may include bleeding, infection where the needle was inserted, or retained needle in the skin and soft tissue.

Acupressure involves stimulation of acupoints by squeezing, pushing, or kneading, often using the thumb. There is no data on the effectiveness of acupressure in children. In adults, acupressure may be useful for relieving dental pain, postoperative pain, and nausea.

Aromatherapy

Aromatherapy uses essential oils, which are highly aromatic oils extracted from specific plants. The oils can be used in massage, baths, and foot baths, and, in certain circumstances, in steam inhalation. An example of an oil used in massage is lavender, which can be calming and relaxing.

"Hands-on" techniques

Osteopaths and chiropractors are practitioners of "hands-on" techniques that diagnose and treat disorders of the spine, joints, and muscles. Osteopaths (doctors of osteopathic medicine) are most concerned with the body's framework and how well it is functioning. They attend osteopathic medical schools and undergo similar training to that given to medical doctors (allopathic or MD) but with an emphasis on manipulating the joints to treat illness.

Chiropractors view the spine as the key support that protects the nervous system and links the brain with the body. Both types of practitioners use manipulation of the spine and may treat back, neck, and joint pain.

Before seeking chiropractic treatment, consult your doctor to exclude or treat a serious disease. Remember that not all chiropractors are experienced in treating children, and there are no studies demonstrating the effectiveness of chiropractic for most pediatric problems.

Herbal medicine

Herbal remedies are prepared from leaves, flowers, and other parts of plants. They are available as extracts (tinctures), capsules, tablets, and teas (infusions). Examples of herbal remedies include echinacea and chamomile. Herbal remedies may be used to treat conditions such as headaches, stomach pains, eczema, and asthma.

There are very few pediatric herbalists in North America. Most herbalists are not trained to treat children and do not have to undergo any type of licensing process. Most herbs are self-prescribed by individuals, although they may be recommended by naturopaths, chiropractors, traditional Chinese medicine practitioners, or doctors.

If you chose to purchase herbs, make sure you use a good-quality supplier. Since herbal remedies are not regulated, there is also a chance that substances may be contaminated or tampered with, and their potency may also vary. Avoid Chinese patent medicines and herbs prepared in pill form because many are contaminated. Some herbal treatments can be harmful if they are used incorrectly.

Exercise caution when taking herbals and any medications since herb-drug interactions may have serious side effects. Always contact your doctor before your child takes any herbal remedies in order to avoid the herb-drug interactions.

Homeopathy

Homeopathy is a form of natural medicine that works on the principle of treating "like with like." The concept involves using a substance that can produce symptoms in a healthy child to cure the same symptoms in a sick child. If, for example, your child suffers from hay fever caused by grass or flower pollen, a "mixed pollen" remedy may be considered under this approach.

Homeopathic remedies are diluted substances that are carefully regulated; however, homeopathy remains controversial.

Hypnotherapy

Hypnotherapy is viewed as a natural way of making contact with the inner (subconscious) self. The process of hypnosis involves a pleasant state of relaxation, rather like a daydream, which in itself provides a feeling of well-being. While your child feels this sense of calm, negative images can be replaced with positive ones through suggestion or visualization. Hypnotherapy may be used to treat many conditions, but it is not usually recommended for use in the pediatric age group.

Massage

Therapeutic massage has been used for hundreds of years to treat the aches and pains in muscles and stiff joints. Massage may be good for improving mobility and for bringing about a feeling of well-being. Massage may help treat stress-related conditions in older children – conditions such as anxiety, sleeplessness, and depression.

Nutritional therapy

For children it is important to consult a registered pediatric dietitian since adult nutritional requirements and problems are very different than those of children. A dietitian will take a dietary history and perhaps ask you to keep a food record for 3 or more days for your child. This will tell the dietitian if your child is eating and drinking nutritious, age-appropriate foods and whether your child is meeting her nutritional requirements for her age. Based on this information the dietitian will make recommendations to improve your child's diet. Most pediatric dietitians use household foods, rather than dietary supplements for children.

If your child has a serious medical problem such as celiac disease (intolerance to gluten), inflammatory bowel disease, liver disease, or other illness the dietitian will work with your doctor to be sure your child is receiving a diet that will provide for normal growth and development. If your child has a medical condition, specific supplements may be needed. In that case the dietitian will work with your doctor to monitor blood levels of those nutrients to be sure your child receives the correct amount of that nutrient for him.

Because obesity is a problem for children and is associated with long-term health risks, a pediatric dietitian can also assist with weight problems.

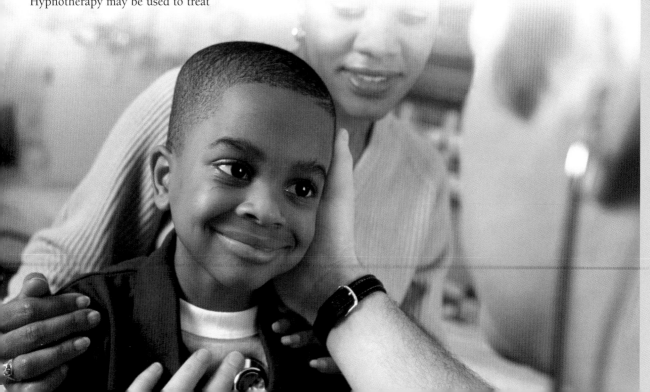

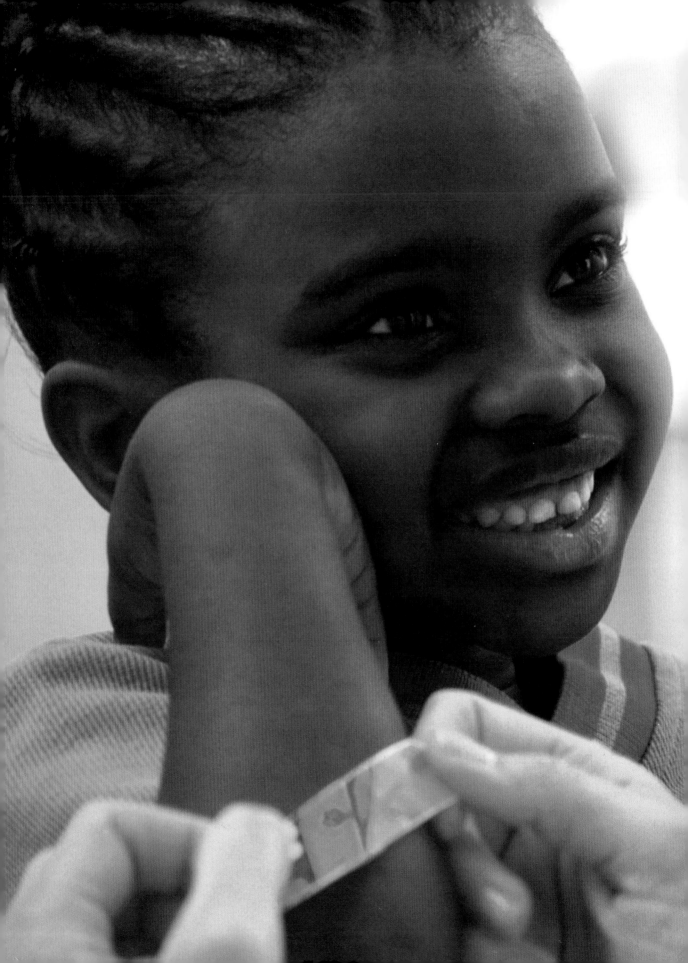

FIRST AID

CARING FOR YOUR SICK CHILD

Most illnesses do not require specialized care. For many conditions, it is helpful to know how to take a temperature and give medications to your child. It is also useful to have a first aid kit available. Always contact your doctor if you have any questions or concerns about your sick child.

CHECKING A PULSE

In certain circumstances, it may be useful to check your child's pulse. All you need to learn is where to place your fingertips. Where an artery lies just below the skin, you can feel the pressure of the blood as the heart pumps it around the body. The two easiest places are on the wrist and at the neck. In babies, check the pulse in the upper arm, near the elbow.

Press lighty with your fingertips – not your thumb – until you feel the pulse. Count the number of beats in one minute and try to tell if the pulse is weak or strong, regular or irregular. A pulse that is abnormally fast or slow may be a sign of an illness. In beats per minute, a baby's pulse is about 140, a toddler's pulse is about 120, and the pulse of an older child is about 100. (*See also* Checking breathing rates, *p.195*.)

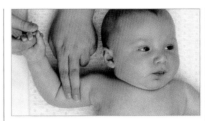

TAKING YOUR BABY'S PULSE
Place the tips of your two forefingers on the inside of the upper arm.

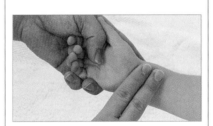

TAKING YOUR CHILD'S PULSE
Place two fingers in a line just below the wrist creases at the base of the thumb.

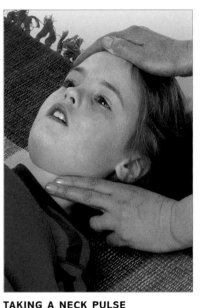

TAKING A NECK PULSE
Place two fingers in the hollow between the windpipe and the large neck muscle.

TAKING A TEMPERATURE

If your child seems sick and you suspect a fever, take her temperature with a thermometer (*see right*) periodically until it returns to normal. An oral temperature of 38°C (100.4°F) or above is a fever. Different methods may have different "normals."

A child over the age of 5 can probably hold a digital thermometer under her tongue. For a younger child, there are other ways to check her temperature. Your child's age will often determine which method is the best to use. Learn how to take your child's temperature *before* she gets sick, so that you are prepared.

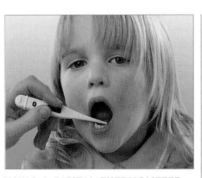

USING A DIGITAL THERMOMETER
With your child sitting still, hold the digital thermometer either in her mouth, under her tongue, or in her armpit. Wait for the thermometer to "beep," then remove it and read your child's temperature from the digital display.

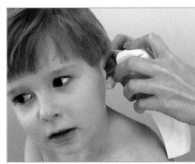

USING A TYMPANIC THERMOMETER
Place the tympanic thermometer in your child's ear. Hold the tip gently in position for the recommended time and then remove to read the temperature. The disposable tip should be replaced with a new one after every use.

GIVING MEDICINE

Liquid medicines are usually prepared in a sweet syrup to make the taste more agreeable to a child. Measure medicines carefully to ensure that you give the correct dose and administer them to your child with a spoon, medicine dropper, or syringe (*right*).

Gently shake the bottle before you give your child the medicine and follow the storage directions carefully; some liquid medicines must be stored in a refrigerator to prevent deterioration. You can use a measuring spoon or medicine cup to give medicine to older children.

Children often find it difficult to swallow pills, so a type that dissolves, can be chewed, or can be crushed and mixed with fruit juice or purée is preferable. Giving liquid medicine to young children with a syringe (without a needle) avoids spillage and ensures that the proper dose is given. An antibiotic course should always be completed.

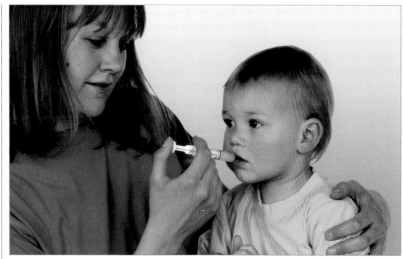

USING A SYRINGE

Pour a small amount of the medicine into a clean cup or other container. Place the tip of the syringe in the medicine and then slowly fill the syringe by pulling out the plunger until the syringe contains the correct dose as shown by the marked lines on the side.

Carefully remove the syringe containing the medicine from the cup. Place the tip of the syringe in your child's mouth so that it points toward one of his cheeks and slowly press the plunger. Be careful not to aim the syringe at your child's throat because this may cause him to choke or gag.

First aid kit

Every home needs a first aid kit to cope with the minor emergencies that can happen at any time. You never know when your child might need a cut cleaned or an arm bandaged. Keep a kit in the car, too.

You can buy a basic kit from a drugstore and add extra dressings, bandages, and disposable gloves. Or you may prefer to assemble your own kit to suit the needs of your family. Remember to keep the kit in a clean, waterproof, and readily identifiable container, and to make sure everything is regularly checked and ready for use. Try to avoid collecting too many items – just stick to the basic materials (*see right*).

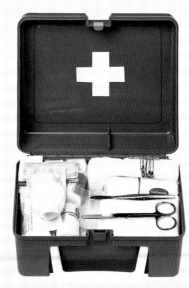

USEFUL ITEMS FOR A FIRST AID BOX:

- *scissors*
- *tweezers*
- *safety pins*
- *waterproof bandages*
- *hypoallergenic tape*
- *sterile dressing with bandage*
- *small roller bandage*
- *large roller bandage*
- *sterile, nonadhesive pad*
- *pack of gauze swabs*
- *calamine lotion*
- *antibiotic ointment*
- *disposable gloves*
- *two triangular bandages.*

UNCONSCIOUS BABY OR CHILD

If your baby or child becomes unconscious, you or a helper should call 911 or EMS. Then carry out the ABC of resuscitation – the Airway–Breathing–Circulation check. The aim is to ensure that the vital organs receive oxygen until medical assistance arrives.

THE ABC SEQUENCE

This sequence is similar in babies and older children. Your first aim is to open the airway and check for breathing. If breathing is evident, put your child in the recovery position (*see below*). If there is no breathing, give rescue breaths – the air you exhale contains enough oxygen to sustain a child's vital organs. After 2 rescue breaths, look for a pulse and other signs of circulation, such as movement, breathing, or coughing. If there is no pulse, start cardiopulmonary resuscitation (CPR) – chest compressions with rescue breaths – to keep the vital organs supplied with oxygen until medical treatment can be given. If your child is breathing and shows signs of circulation, treat other problems in this order: bleeding, burns, fractures. Also watch for signs of shock (*see p.332*). Finally, treat any other injuries.

> ### ▣ WARNING
>
> If you suspect that an unconscious child has an injury to the spine:
>
> - **Do not move the child unless** either of you are in immediate danger; the child's breathing is obstructed; or you must perform CPR. Always suspect a spine injury if there is a head injury.
> - **If you must move the child,** keep his head aligned with his body and avoid bending the neck.
> - **Do not tilt the head to give rescue breaths**. Lift the chin gently.

▣ IF YOUR CHILD IS BREATHING

Recovery position

This position allows fluids to drain out of the child's mouth so they are not inhaled. If your child has a fracture, support the injury. A child with a spinal injury (*see* Warning, *above*) should be turned only if the child's breathing is obstructed. Keep your child's head, neck, and back aligned at all times.

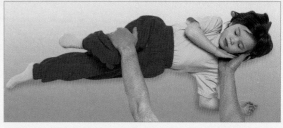

IF YOUR CHILD IS BREATHING, place her in the recovery position (above). First, grasp the thigh farthest from you, and roll your child over by pulling the bent leg toward you. As you roll, keep her hand held against her cheek.

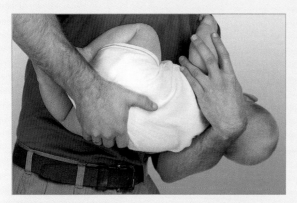

IF YOUR BABY IS BREATHING, hold her in the recovery position (above). Make sure you hold her securely, with her head tilted slightly downward to keep the airway open, while you wait for medical help to arrive.

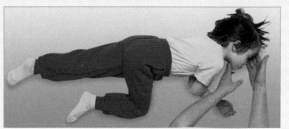

THEN BEND HER TOP LEG TO form a right angle and afterward move her bottom arm into a position that will prevent her from rolling forward. Tilt her head backward slightly in order to keep her airway open.

ABC FOR INFANTS LESS THAN 1 YEAR OF AGE

If your baby seems to be unconscious, try to get some kind of response: call his name and gently tap or flick the sole of one of his feet. Never shake a baby. If possible, ask a helper to dial 911 or call EMS after you have checked the breathing. If you are alone, give breaths or CPR for one minute before dialing 911 or calling EMS.

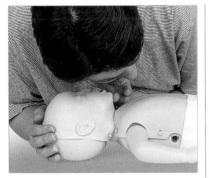

1 OPEN AIRWAY, CHECK BREATHING

Lay your baby down on a flat surface. Tilt the head back slightly with one hand. Remove any visible objects from the mouth. With one finger of the other hand, lift the chin. Check for signs of breathing: look along the chest for movement; listen for sounds of breathing; lean over and feel for any breath on your cheek.

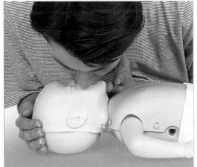

2 GIVE TWO RESCUE BREATHS

If there is no breathing, give rescue breaths immediately. Take a deep breath, seal your lips over the mouth and nose and blow steadily into the mouth. Watch the chest rise. Remove your mouth and let the chest fall. Give 2 of these "effective" breaths, taking a fresh breath yourself after each one. If no air enters, readjust the head using the chin lift technique and try again.

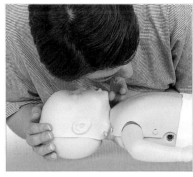

3 CHECK FOR SIGNS OF CIRCULATION

Check for a pulse and other signs of circulation, such as breathing, coughing, or movement. If there are signs but no breathing, continue to give rescue breaths and assess response every minute. If there are no signs, begin CPR (steps 4, 5). If you cannot get your breaths into your baby, or you know she has choked, go to p.329.

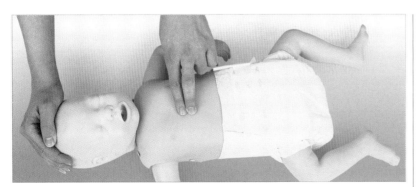

4 GIVE FIVE CHEST COMPRESSIONS

Place two fingers of one hand on the breastbone, one finger's width below a line joining the nipples. Avoid the bottom tip of the breastbone. Press down sharply with your fingertips to one third of the depth of the chest and release the pressure but do not remove your fingers. Do this five times in about three seconds.

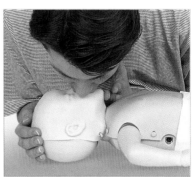

5 GIVE ONE RESCUE BREATH

Give one rescue breath, then repeat step 4. Repeat this cycle of 5 compressions to each breath until help arrives, your baby moves or breathes, or you are too exhausted to continue.

ABC FOR CHILDREN 1–8 YEARS OF AGE

If your child seems unconscious, try to get a response: call his name and gently tap his shoulder. If possible, ask a helper to dial 911 or call EMS after you have checked the breathing. If you are on your own, carry out rescue breaths and/or CPR for a minute before calling 911 or EMS.

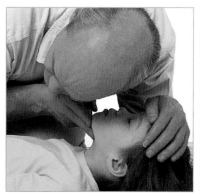

1 CHECK AIRWAY AND BREATHING
Tilt the head back with a hand on the forehead. Then lift the chin. Look, listen, and feel for breathing. If there is breathing, place your child in the recovery position.

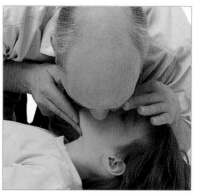

2 GIVE RESCUE BREATHS
If there's no breath, pinch the nose, and blow steadily into the mouth until the chest rises. Remove mouth and let chest fall. If no air enters, readjust the airway and retry. If this fails, treat for choking (*see p.329*).

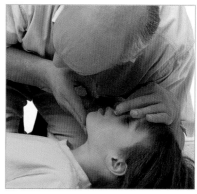

3 SIGNS OF CIRCULATION
Check the pulse and look for other signs of circulation, such as breathing, coughing, or movement. If there is no pulse, begin CPR (steps 4, 5, and 6).

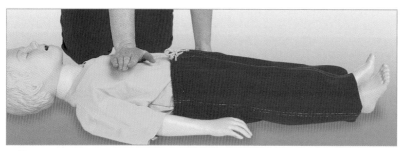

4 FIND POSITION ON BREASTBONE AND GIVE COMPRESSIONS
Place the heel of one hand over the lower half of the breastbone. Lift your fingers to avoid pressing on the ribs. Do not press near the bottom tip of the breastbone. Depress to one-third of the depth of the chest. Do this five times at a rate of 100 times per minute. Then proceed to step 5.

COMPRESSIONS FOR CHILDREN OVER 8
Position the heel of one hand as in step 4 and the heel of the other on top, and interlock your fingers. Lean over and depress the chest about 4 cm (2 in). Do this 15 times at a rate of 100 compressions per minute. Proceed to step 5.

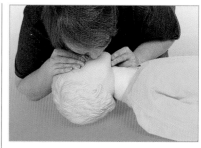

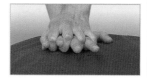

5 GIVE RESCUE BREATHS
Pinch the nose, lift the chin, seal your lips over the mouth, and give one rescue breath. Repeat steps 4 and 5 for a minute in a cycle of 5 compressions to one rescue breath (or 15 compressions to 2 rescue breaths for children over 8 years) until help arrives, the child takes a spontaneous breath, or you are too exhausted to continue.

CHOKING

A choking child may cough and gasp or make high-pitched squeaks because he is unable to speak or breathe. His face may turn red, and then blue. Encourage him to cough. Call 911 or EMS. Start treatment only if he shows signs of distress or loses consciousness.

TREATING A CHOKING INFANT (LESS THAN 1 YEAR)

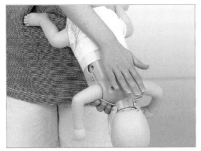

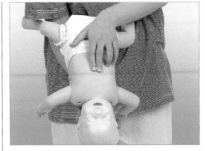

1 GIVE 5 BACK SLAPS
Lay your baby face down along one of your arms, with the head lower than the body. Support the chin between your fingers. Carefully but firmly, give 5 sharp slaps on the middle of his back with the heel of your hand. Pick out any objects you can see from your baby's mouth.

2 GIVE 5 CHEST THRUSTS
If back slaps do not work, turn him over and put two fingers on the breastbone, below the nipple line. Carefully give five inward and forward thrusts. Repeat this sequence until the object is removed. If your baby loses consciousness, begin CPR (*see sidebar*).

☐ **WARNING**

Choking emergency

Call 911 or EMS immediately if a baby or child loses consciousness while choking. As you wait, follow the ABC sequence (*see p.327 for babies and p.328 for children*).

- **First, open the airway**. If you see an object, carefully try to remove it.
- **Then check for breathing**. If there is no breathing, give 2 rescue breaths.
- **If your breaths fail to go in, start chest compressions** – alternate 5 of these with one rescue breath (*see ABC for infants, step 5 & ABC for children, step 5*).
- **After every set of compressions**, check the mouth for obstructions. Continue until help arrives.

TREATING YOUR CHOKING CHILD

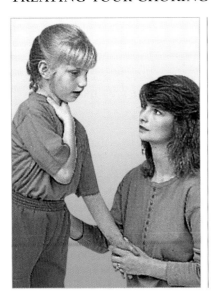

1 DETERMINE WHETHER YOUR CHILD IS CHOKING
If you suspect that your child is choking, ask her "Are you choking?" If she can speak or cough, do not interfere. If she is having severe distress, proceed to Step 2.

2 GIVE 5 ABDOMINAL THRUSTS
Stand behind her and position your fist over her upper abdomen. Place your other hand over your fist and thrust sharply inward and upward 5 times. Repeat this sequence until the object is removed. If she becomes unconscious, start CPR (*see p.328*) and call 911 or EMS.

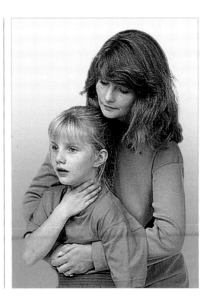

NEAR DROWNING

When a child inhales water, breathing is prevented and drowning may result. This may happen if your baby or child falls into a pool, pond, or bath. Even 2.5cm (1in) of water is enough to cover the nose and mouth. You should always be within arm's reach of young children whenever they are near water, no matter how shallow. Children should never swim alone.

1 REMOVE CHILD FROM WATER
Carry her with her head lower than her chest to reduce the risk of inhaling water. If water gushes from her mouth, let it drain of its own accord. Don't try to force water from her stomach because the child may vomit and then inhale it.

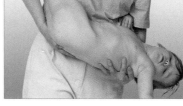
Keep her head lower than her chest.

2 GET HER DRY
Make sure you get her dry and warm as quickly as possible. You may have to treat her for hypothermia (*see p.333*).

3 SEEK MEDICAL CARE
Get medical attention even if she seems to have recovered. The inhaled water can irritate her lungs and may cause them to swell later.

COPING WITH AN UNCONSCIOUS CHILD
You should always consider the possibility of neck or spinal injuries with near drowning and keep the head, neck, and back aligned. Check both her airway and breathing and look for signs of circulation (*see pp.326–329*). Be ready to resuscitate with rescue breaths (*see p.327 for a baby and p.328 for older children*). You may find that getting air into her lungs may be harder than you expected because of the water she has inhaled and the coldness of her body.

Your child may vomit swallowed water during CPR. If so, turn your child to the recovery position until vomiting has stopped. Then reassess the need for CPR.

If an unconscious child is still breathing, put her into the recovery position (*see p.326*) and dial 911 or call EMS immediately.

SWALLOWED OBJECTS

Young children commonly swallow objects such as coins, small toys, or buttons. These usually present no danger and emerge in the stools. However, without prompt attention, swallowed miniature "button" batteries can cause severe damage. If the object is large or sharp, it may damage the digestive tract.

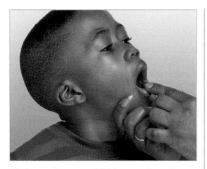
Find out what your child has swallowed.

1 SPEAK TO HIM
Reassure your child so that he does not panic, and then try to find out exactly what object he has swallowed.

2 SEEK MEDICAL ADVICE
If the swallowed object was small and smooth, you should consult your doctor. Depending on the answer, go to step 3 or 4.

3 SEEK MEDICAL CARE
If you know or suspect your child has swallowed a button battery, seek urgent medical care.

4 SUMMON HELP
If the object is large or sharp, or if he finds it hard to breathe or swallow, call 911 or EMS. Do not let him eat or drink in case he needs a general anesthetic at the hospital.

INHALING OBJECTS
A child may choke when a small object, such as a peanut, goes into the lungs. A violent cough may expel it. If your child has a persistent dry cough, difficulty breathing, or continues to choke, take emergency steps (*see* Choking, *p.329*).

INHALING TOXIC FUMES

If your child inhales toxic fumes and gases she can suffer breathing difficulties, confusion, and a shortage of oxygen. Her skin may turn blue-gray. The fumes may come from glue, cleaning solvents, vehicle exhaust, smoke, or emissions from defective heaters. If there is a fire, smoke, or fumes, do not put yourself at risk, and call the fire department.

1 SIT HER UPRIGHT
Help her into a position where she finds it easiest to breathe. Support her in an upright position. Make sure there is plenty of fresh air, and encourage her to keep breathing as normally as possible.

2 DIAL 911 OR CALL EMS
Call for urgent medical assistance as soon as you can.

3 MONITOR HER CONDITION
As you wait, monitor her breathing, pulse, and consciousness. Be prepared to perform rescue breaths.

UNCONSCIOUSNESS

If she becomes unconscious, check her airway, breathing, and signs of circulation (*see ABC, pp.326–328*). If she is breathing, place her in the recovery position (*see p.326*).

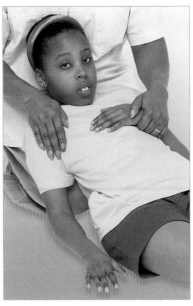
Support your child in an upright position.

ANIMAL BITES

Bites from animals, such as dogs and rodents, often puncture the skin and can expose your child to infections, such as tetanus. The most serious infection is rabies. Seek advice immediately regarding the possible need for antirabies injections.

SUPERFICIAL BITES

Bites that don't break the skin may be treated at home.

1 WASH THE WOUND
Thoroughly wash the wound with warm, soapy water.

2 DRY AND COVER THE WOUND
Gently pat the wound dry and cover with a bandage or sterile dressing.

3 SEEK MEDICAL HELP
Consult your doctor if there is bleeding or signs of infection.

DEEP BITES

Bites that penetrate deep into the tissues beneath the skin need to be checked by a physician.

1 DRESS THE WOUND
Put a clean pad over the wound and press down on it to control the bleeding. (*See p.338* if the bleeding is severe.)

2 RAISE THE LIMB
Raise the injured part of the body above the level of the child's heart to reduce blood flow to the wound.

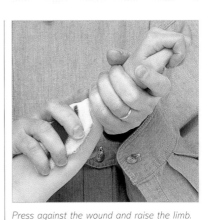
Press against the wound and raise the limb.

3 COVER THE BITE
Use either a clean pad or a sterile dressing. Bandage it firmly.

4 SEEK MEDICAL HELP
Take your child to the emergency department or to your doctor's office or clinic immediately.

SHOCK

The body enters a state of shock when circulation fails and organs are deprived of oxygen. Severe infection, severe bleeding (internal or external), or a burn or scald are the most likely causes. A loss of body fluids ("hypovolemia") from diarrhea or vomiting can also be a cause. The skin turns pale, cold, and sweaty. A rapid pulse grows weaker; breathing is fast and shallow. After these symptoms come restlessness, extreme thirst, and, eventually, unconsciousness.

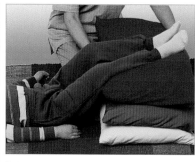

Raise your child's legs above the heart.

1 LAY YOUR CHILD DOWN
Lay your child down on his back, with his head low to improve the blood supply to the brain. Stay calm yourself and reassure and comfort your child. Call 911 or EMS and ask for medical assistance.

2 RAISE HIS LEGS
Gently raise your child's legs above the level of his heart. Prop them up on a chair, several pillows, or a stack of cushions. Make sure that his head is kept lower than his chest.

3 LOOSEN HIS CLOTHES
Loosen any tight or constricting clothes around his neck, chest, and waist. If he is thirsty, do not give him anything to drink – instead, moisten his lips with water.

4 KEEP HIM WARM
Wrap your child in a blanket or a coat, but do not give him a direct source of heat such as a hot water bottle.

5 STAY WITH HIM
Do not leave your child unattended. If possible, ask someone else to dial 911 or call EMS.

6 COMFORT HIM
Continue to reassure and comfort your child. If possible, encourage him to talk with you. Monitor his breathing, pulse, skin color, and level of consciousness.

7 USE THE ABC SEQUENCE
If he becomes unconscious, open his airway, check his breathing, and look for signs of circulation (*see* ABC, *pp.326–328*). Be prepared to resuscitate him with rescue breaths. If he is breathing, place him in the recovery position (*see p.326*).

ELECTROCUTION

Children who play with electrical sockets or wires, or who splash water onto an electrical appliance, are in danger of electrocution. The electrical current may stop your child's breathing or even the heart, and may burn the skin where it enters and leaves the body.

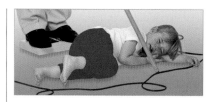

Push the cable away from the child.

1 TURN OFF ELECTRICITY
Switch off the main electricity supply if you can. If you are unable to do this, then stand on dry insulating material such as a thick telephone book and use a wooden broom handle or chair to push the limbs of your child apart from the source of electricity.

2 REMOVE HER FROM SOURCE
Do not touch your child and only pull at her clothes as a last resort. Wrap a dry towel around her feet and pull her away from the source of the electricity. If she appears to be unharmed, then encourage her to relax and rest. Seek medical help immediately.

3 USE THE ABC SEQUENCE
If she becomes unconscious, check her airway, breathing, and signs of circulation (*see* ABC, *pp.326–328*). Be ready to give her rescue breaths. If she is breathing, put her into the recovery position (*see p.326*).

HYPOTHERMIA

When the body's temperature falls below 95°F (35°C), moderate hypothermia sets in. If the temperature falls still further to below 86°F (30°C), the hypothermia can be fatal. The symptoms and treatment are different for babies and older children.

BABIES

A baby is unable to regulate her own temperature properly and may develop hypothermia even in a cold room. Her skin may look pink and healthy but feels cold. She seems limp, quiet, and disinterested in feeding.

1 SEEK MEDICAL HELP
Call your doctor immediately. You should warm your baby gradually. Carry her into a warm room and wrap her in blankets. Cover your baby's head with a hat and cuddle her.

CHILDREN

Prolonged exposure to cold outdoors, either in water or in air when the wind-chill factor is high, is the most likely cause of hypothermia in children. Their skin becomes pale, cold, and dry. Shivering is accompanied by listlessness or confusion. Breathing is slow and shallow while the pulse weakens.

1 SEEK MEDICAL HELP
Call your doctor. Do not try to warm your child too quickly by using a hot water bottle or other source of direct heat.

2 BATHE HER
Give your child a warm bath. When the color of her skin returns to normal, dry her and wrap her in warm blankets.

3 DRESS HER
Put clothes on your child, including socks and gloves. Add extra layers to her head, neck, and trunk. Put her to bed. Warm the room and give her a warm drink.

4 USE THE ABC SEQUENCE
If your child becomes unconscious, check her airway, breathing, and signs of circulation (see ABC, p.328). You should be prepared to resuscitate your child with rescue breaths. Call 911 or EMS.

HEAD INJURIES

A head injury may involve a temporary loss of consciousness or a severe delayed reaction. If a reaction occurs hours, or even days, later when confusion and a headache set in, or your child's breathing, pulse, and pupils are abnormal, you should seek immediate medical attention.

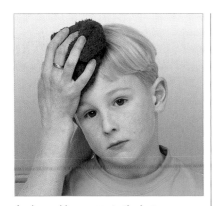

Apply a cold compress to the bump.

1 APPLY A COMPRESS
If your child gets a bump on his head, sit him down and apply a cold compress. If he does not recover fully within a few minutes, call your doctor.

2 SUMMON HELP
If your child briefly loses consciousness and then recovers fully, he may have a concussion. Ensure he rests. Call your doctor immediately.

UNCONSCIOUSNESS

If a child loses consciousness due to the head injury, check his airway using the following jaw thrust method because there may also be a spinal injury. Kneel behind your child's head and place your hands on each side of his face, over the ears and with your fingertips at the angles of the jaw. Gently lift the jaw to open the airway but be careful to avoid tilting his neck. Check his breathing and look for signs of circulation (see p.328). Be ready to give rescue breaths to resuscitate him. If he is breathing, continue to support his head. Call 911 or EMS.

3 SEEK TREATMENT
If he does not recover fully in a few minutes, seek immediate medical treatment.

BROKEN BONES

Children's bones are still growing and may split, bend, or crack as well as break completely. If you suspect that your child has a broken bone (fracture), try not to move the affected area.

CLOSED FRACTURES

If the skin has not been punctured, the fracture is said to be closed.

1 SUPPORT THE INJURY
Ask your child to lie still and support the injured part with your hands. To immobilize it, you should try to bandage it to an uninjured part – bandage a fractured arm against the body. You should always secure the bandage on the uninjured side of the limb.

2 TREAT FOR SHOCK
If there are any signs of shock (see p.332), lay your child down and raise his legs – unless it causes him some pain.

3 SEEK MEDICAL HELP
Get immediate medical attention. You should not let your child eat or drink without first consulting the doctor.

OPEN FRACTURES

If the skin has been pierced by the bone, or there is a wound near the fracture, the fracture is said to be open.

1 COVER THE WOUND
Use a large pad or sterile dressing and press to control bleeding. If the bone protrudes, do not press it. Drape a piece of gauze over the top and press either side.

2 COVER THE DRESSING
Place a clean pad over the dressing and cover it with a bandage. If the bone is protruding, build up pads of clean, nonfluffy material around it so that you can bandage over and protect the bone from pressure.

3 TREAT FOR SHOCK
Immobilize the injured part (see step 1, left) as soon as you can. If there are signs of shock (see p.332), lay your child down and raise his legs.

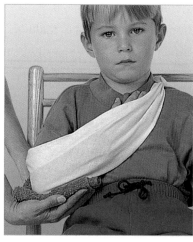

An elevation sling should be used for broken hands and collarbones

4 SEEK MEDICAL HELP
Dial 911 or call EMS or, if the injury is not too serious, contact your doctor first. Do not let your child eat or drink because he may need a general anesthetic.

5 CHECK HIS CIRCULATION
Periodically check the circulation in the limb beyond the bandage. If circulation seems impaired, then reapply the bandage more loosely.

BROKEN COLLARBONE

Broken collarbones often occur during an athletic activity. You can immobilize a broken collarbone by making a triangular bandage into a sling on the arm of the affected side.

1 APPLY A SLING
Put the fingers of the hand on the injured side on the other shoulder. Hold one end of the bandage here, and drape the long edge down the body. The point should be below the elbow on the injured side.

2 SECURE THE SLING
Tuck the bandage under his forearm and elbow, supporting the arm on the injured side, and bring it up across the back. Secure it over the shoulder on the uninjured side. Make sure a few fingers are visible.

3 CHECK THE CIRCULATION
Tuck in excess fabric at the elbow behind the sling or pin it to the front of the sling. Keep checking the circulation in the fingers; if they become pale, cold, or numb, reapply the sling more loosely.

4 SEEK MEDICAL HELP
Take your child to the doctor's office, the emergency department, or an urgent-care center.

BROKEN LEG

If your child breaks a bone in a leg, either the thighbone or a bone in the lower leg, make sure you support it to prevent further injury. Do not try to straighten the leg. If the knee is injured, try to put some padding underneath it for support.

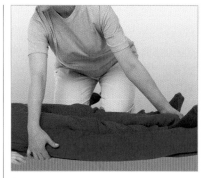

Place padding on either side of the leg.

1 SUPPORT THE LEG
Place plenty of padding, such as rolled-up towels or blankets, or folded newspaper, on both sides of the injured leg and then dial 911 or call EMS immediately.

2 PREVENT MOVEMENT
Support the injured leg above and below the location of the fracture to prevent movement, which could cause further injury and internal bleeding, until help arrives.

DISLOCATED JOINTS

A strong force or blow to a joint can move a bone out of position and tear ligaments. More seriously, nerves can be damaged and bones broken. Do not try to put the bone back into place yourself or move your child until you have immobilized the affected joint.

1 SUPPORT THE JOINT
Have your child keep as still as possible. Support the dislocated joint in a position that is most comfortable for him.

2 IMMOBILIZE THE JOINT
Use padding and bandages. If an arm is affected try to use a sling. Treat your child for shock if you need to (*see p.332*).

3 SEEK MEDICAL HELP
Take your child to the nearest emergency department, where a medical expert will put the dislocated bone back into place. Do not allow your child eat or drink anything because he may need a general anesthetic. Check the circulation near the bandage regularly – if it is impaired, loosen the bandage.

STRAINS & SPRAINS

A strain occurs when a muscle or tendon attached to a joint is overstretched or torn. A sprain occurs when a violent or sudden movement overstretches or tears a ligament in a joint. In either case, follow the RICE sequence – Rest, Ice, Compression, and Elevation. You can also use this treatment for deep bruising.

1 SUPPORT THE INJURY
Rest – your child must rest the affected part of the body. Make sure he sits or lies down. Support the injured part in a comfortable position.

2 COOL THE INJURY
Ice – apply a cold compress, such as ice or a bag of frozen peas wrapped in a cloth, to the affected part for 10–15 minutes. This helps reduce pain, swelling, and bruising.

3 COMPRESS THE INJURY
Compression – bandage a thick layer of cotton padding firmly around the injured area. Regularly check the circulation – if it is impaired, reapply the bandage.

4 RAISE THE INJURY
Elevation – raise and support the affected part to reduce the flow of blood and minimize further swelling. If he is in severe pain, or if he cannot use the injured part at all, seek medical attention.

BURNS & SCALDS

Burns are commonly caused by flames, hot objects, or electricity. Scalds are burns involving steam or hot liquids. Potent chemicals, such as household detergents or cleaners, can cause chemical burns. If your child suffers a burn, seek medical help.

MINOR BURNS

Small burns and scalds that damage only the superficial layers of skin will heal naturally. Consult your doctor to make sure. Do not apply ointments, grease, butter, or lotions to the burn.

1 COOL THE BURN
Pour cold water on the burn for about 10 minutes. Remove anything that might constrict the injured area. Cover the burn with a sterile dressing or a nonfluffy pad to keep infection out. Bandage loosely.

2 LEAVE A BLISTER
If a blister forms, leave it alone – bursting it may introduce infection. If it breaks, cover it with a large, nonadhesive bandage until it heals.

SEVERE BURNS

Your main priorities are to stop the burning, dial 911 or call EMS, and relieve your child's pain. Treat any associated injuries if you can and minimize the risk of infection.

1 COOL THE BURN
Pour copious amounts of cold water on to the burn for 10 minutes or more to cool the burn and help to relieve the pain. Do not overcool since it can cause hypothermia. Dial 911 or call EMS as soon as you can.

2 SEEK MEDICAL HELP
Help your child lie down and prevent the burned area from touching the floor.

3 CUT AWAY CLOTHES
Gently remove such items as shoes, belt, or watch, before tissues start to swell. Use blunt-tipped scissors to cut away burned clothing, except where it sticks to the skin.

4 APPLY A DRESSING
Protect the injury from infection with a sterile dressing – but do not apply lotion or adhesive tape to the burn. If you do not have a dressing, use a folded triangular bandage, a clean piece of cloth, or a strip of plastic wrap. The dressing must not stick to the burn. Cover a hand or foot with a clean plastic bag, secured to itself, not to the skin. Do not cover a facial burn since you may cause distress and make breathing difficult.

5 CHECK FOR OTHER INJURIES
Assess any other injuries. Do not let him eat or drink and treat him for shock (*see p.332*). Reassure the child until medical help arrives.

SUNBURN

Sunburned skin is itchy, red, and tender to the touch. Babies and young children are especially prone to sunburn, so make sure they are protected with sunscreen, a hat, and clothing.

1 TAKE INTO THE SHADE
Bring a sunburned child into the shade or into a cool room. Give him a cool drink and encourage him to take frequent sips rather than swallowing the drink quickly.

2 COOL THE BURN
Apply cool compresses to the burn or give him a cool bath. If you see blistering, contact your doctor.

3 TREAT HEAT EXHAUSTION
If your child is restless, dizzy, or flushed, or complains of a headache, he may be suffering from heat exhaustion. Try to bring his temperature back to normal. You should sponge his body down repeatedly with cold or tepid water. If your child's condition deteriorates, you should dial 911 or call EMS.

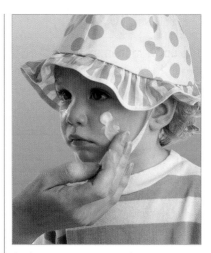
Apply sunscreen to prevent burns.

FOREIGN OBJECTS IN THE EAR OR NOSE

If a child pushes an object into one of her ears, it could get stuck, causing pain, inflammation, and temporarily decreased hearing. If pushed in too far, it may damage the eardrum. Children also often put objects in their nostrils, where they can become lodged.

1 SPEAK TO YOUR CHILD
Reassure your child and ask her what, if anything, she has put into her ear or nose. Button batteries, such as those in hearing aids and watches, are particularly dangerous as they may release a strong alkali that can damage tissue. If you suspect this is the foreign body involved, go immediately to the nearest emergency department. If your child cannot tell you what the object is, look closely and try to find out what is trapped in the ear canal or nostril. Do not try to extract it even if you can see it.

2 OBJECT IN THE EAR
Do not put liquid or anything else into the ear. Call your doctor or take your child to the nearest emergency department.

3 OBJECT IN THE NOSE
Ask your child to sit down, lean her head forward, and blow her nose. This may dislodge the object. If it remains stuck, do not try to remove it yourself, as you might push it further back. Call a doctor or go to the nearest emergency department.

FOREIGN OBJECTS IN THE EYE

Working together, the eyelids and tears are remarkably good at protecting the cornea and membranes of the eyes, but sometimes a speck of dust or some other foreign object gets past the defenses and is not removed. You may be able to remove these tiny objects yourself, but consult your pediatrician if you have any concerns.

1 LET THE EYE WATER
Sit your child down and get her to face the light. Tell her not to rub the eye but to blink frequently and let it water with tears.

2 LOOK AT THE EYE
If this doesn't work, stand behind your child and ask her to tilt her head back. Lean over and carefully separate the eyelids with your finger and thumb. Ask her to look right, left, up, and down as you examine her eye for the object.

3 RINSE THE EYE
If the object is on the white of the eye, rinse it away by pouring clean water into the inner corner of the eye.

4 REMOVE THE OBJECT
If the object remains lodged in your child's eye, you should moisten the corner of a tissue or handkerchief. Carefully dab the object on the surface of her eye – it should stick to the tissue or handkerchief – and then lift it clear of the eye.

5 SEEK MEDICAL HELP
If the object is under the upper lid, pull this eyelid over the lower lid. Or ask her to blink under gently running water. If you are still unsuccessful, seek medical help. Do not try to remove an object that sticks to the eye, is embedded in the eyeball, or rests over the iris or pupil. Get medical attention urgently.

CHEMICAL IN THE EYE
If a chemical enters your child's eye, flush it out under gently running cold water for about 10 minutes. Try to prevent the water from splashing on to her face or from entering the unaffected eye. Bandage the injured eye, then get medical help.

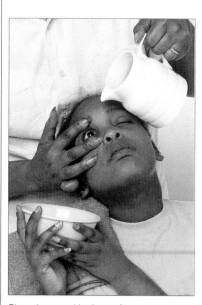

Rinse the eye with plenty of water.

BRUISES

Children often come home with bruises caused by a fall or bumping into a hard object. Bruises that develop rapidly respond well to first aid. If the bruise is on your child's arm, the swelling may be relieved by putting the arm in a sling.

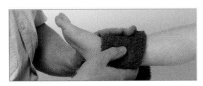

Put a cold compress on the bruise.

1 RAISE THE INJURED PART
Lift up the affected part of the body to a comfortable position and allow it to rest. At the same time, this decreases the circulation and helps minimize the swelling.

2 USE A COLD COMPRESS
Apply firm pressure with your hand on a cold compress for as long as 30 minutes. This will minimize the swelling by reducing the flow of blood to the bruise. You can use a cold pad made from cloth dampened with cold water, or an ice pack made from ice or a bag of frozen vegetables wrapped in a dry cloth. When the compress warms up you will need to replace it.

CUTS & ABRASIONS

Small cuts and abrasions are treatable at home. Control bleeding using pressure and elevation, and then cover the wound with a bandage. The most important thing is to prevent infections, such as tetanus, so be sure the child is up to date with immunizations.

1 STOP THE BLEEDING
Press a pad against the wound with your hand until the bleeding stops, and then raise the affected part of the body.

2 CLEAN AND COVER WOUND
Clean the wound with plain water. Gently pat it dry with clean gauze and then cover it with a sterile dressing.

3 USE A BANDAGE
Remove the dressing and replace it with a bandage that has a pad larger than the wound.

4 SEEK MEDICAL HELP
Get medical attention if the bleeding doesn't stop, if an object is embedded in the wound, or if the wound was caused by a bite or a dirty object.

SEVERE BLEEDING

Bleeding usually stops quickly. However, if it is profuse, you may need to control it to prevent shock (*see p.332*). To reduce the risk of wound infection, wash your own hands before and after treatment and wear gloves if possible.

1 STOP THE BLEEDING
Press a pad against the wound with your hand until the bleeding stops.

2 RAISE THE INJURED PART
You should lift the affected part of the body until it is higher than the heart.

3 SECURE THE PAD
Fasten the pad firmly in place and cover with a sterile dressing. If the blood soaks through the dressing, apply a new one to the wound. If the blood continues to come through, remove the dressing and start again since the pressure is not sufficient.

4 SUPPORT THE INJURY
Lay your child down and support the injury in a raised position. Seek immediate medical care.

EMBEDDED OBJECT

If an object is embedded in the wound, do not remove it since you may cause more damage. Cover the wound lightly with gauze and surround it with bandage rolls built up to the same height as the object. Secure them in place by bandaging on either side of the wound. Seek medical attention immediately.

NOSEBLEEDS

Tiny blood vessels in the membranes that line the nostrils may rupture when treated roughly. This can happen during a sneeze or a bang on the nose, or if your child picks or blows her nose too vigorously. A nosebleed is only dangerous if a child loses a lot of blood or if the blood is thin and watery following a head injury.

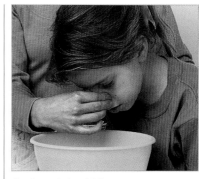

Gently pinch the child's nose.

1 POSITION YOUR CHILD
Sit your child down. Ask her to lean forward over a bowl or sink to allow the blood to flow freely from her nose. Do not let her lean back, because blood may trickle down her throat and cause her to vomit.

2 PINCH THE NOSTRILS
Encourage her to breathe through her mouth while you pinch the soft part of her nostrils with your thumb and forefinger. If she is old enough she may be able to pinch her own nose. Ask her to spit any blood into the bowl.

3 TALK TO HER
Reassure her and encourage her not to sniff, swallow, cough, or even speak. This will allow time for clots to form. Her nostrils will need to be pinched for about 10 minutes.

4 STOP THE BLEEDING
Release the nostrils to see if the nosebleed has stopped. If it has not, her nostrils will have to be pinched again for two more periods of about 10 minutes. If the nosebleed lasts for longer than 30 minutes, consult your doctor or take her to the nearest emergency department.

5 CLEAN THE BLOOD
If the nosebleed has stopped, ask her to remain leaning forward. Clean the blood from around her nose with a washcloth and tepid water.

6 ENSURE SHE RESTS
Your child now needs to rest for a while. Most importantly, she should avoid blowing her nose or doing anything that will disrupt the clotting process.

SPLINTERS

Your child's hands, knees, and feet are all prone to getting splinters, usually of wood but occasionally of glass or even metal. If the splinter is in the top layer of skin, you can remove it with clean tweezers. But if it proves difficult to extract or if it is more deeply embedded in the skin or over a joint, then consult your doctor. In the case of a large splinter, make sure your child is up to date on his tetanus vaccination.

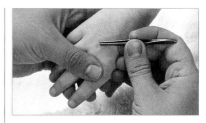

Grip the splinter with the tweezers.

1 CLEAN THE SKIN
You should carefully clean around the area where the splinter entered your child's skin. Use soap and warm water. Take care not to embed the splinter further into the skin.

2 USE TWEEZERS
Look closely to see at what angle the splinter entered the skin. Grip the splinter with clean tweezers as close to the skin as you can. Make sure you pull the splinter out at the same angle as it entered.

3 LET IT BLEED
Squeeze the wound gently so that it may bleed a little in order to bring out any dirt.

4 COVER THE WOUND
Clean and dry the puncture wound and then cover it with a bandage.

MAKING SENSE OF HEALTH CARE INFORMATION

WITH THE ADVENT OF MODERN-DAY COMMUNICATIONS, there is a wealth of information as close as your telephone, computer, or library. It is important to sort through this material to get accurate and up-to-date information.

About Web site addresses

The last three letters in a Web site address can tell you what type of organization or company has set up the site.

.gov Government-information Web sites that often provide large amounts of information for the general public.

.org Nonprofit organization Web sites may contain useful information. However, not all organizations publish reliable materials. Search for information on nonprofit organization Web sites that you have heard of before and have good reputations.

.edu Academic or education-based Web sites may have educational materials for parents.

.com Commercial Web site addresses are often designed to sell you something. They are not necessarily a source of reliable information.

SEEKING INFORMATION

When you're trying to help your child stay healthy or recover from an illness, it may be challenging to decide what medicines to give or what treatments to try. You and your doctor are partners in keeping your child healthy so it is important to have as many facts as possible when making health care choices. You may need to determine which sources, in addition to your doctor, you can trust. Commercials and magazine ads for products often claim to help and heal. TV and newspapers report on the "latest" studies showing which treatments work and don't work. Web sites claim to have "cutting-edge" health information.

One challenge of parenting is sorting through all of the available information about children's health. Some sources can be trusted while others should be questioned. Read more to learn how to understand these many sources of health-care information.

UNDERSTANDING THE LANGUAGE OF ADVERTISERS

Advertisers try many ways to get you to buy the products they are selling. They may use certain words or phrases to interest you.

"#1 Pediatrician Recommended" or "Doctor Recommended" are marketing terms that try to get you to buy a product. Although the product may be recommended by a group of doctors, what the advertisers don't tell you are how many doctors or how long ago the recommendation was made.

"Patented Design" means that the maker and/or inventor of a product have proven to the government that they were the first to create the product. In return, the government gives a patent, and says that only the patent-holder can make or sell the product for a certain period. A patent doesn't necessarily mean that the product is the best, is safe, or will work.

"The Canadian Paediatric Society Web site, www.cps.ca, is a good starting point."

"Clinically Shown" is a phrase that means the product was tested on patients as part of a study to see if the product worked. There are many ways to conduct studies. However, if the people doing the study don't follow strict scientific rules for doing research, the study results may have little meaning.

CONSIDER THE SOURCE

It's important to ask the following questions when evaluating a source. In general, sources you can trust include accredited medical schools, government agencies, professional medical associations, and recognized national disorder/disease-specific organizations. Don't rely mainly on the name of the organization, though – do your own research.

The doctors or researchers being interviewed may sound like experts, but they may not be experts on the particular issue being discussed. Also, if they are being paid for their support of a product, this could influence their recommendations.

Preliminary vs. confirmed findings – a "breakthrough" finding may seem promising but still has to be replicated and reviewed over time. Don't let a headline make you think that "new study" is the same as "proven." Another word of caution: "new" doesn't mean improved. Sometimes newer medicines are not an improvement over older medicines and may cost much more.

GOOD SCIENCE

Scientific studies require careful planning. Researchers need to follow specific procedures and processes. Studies must follow certain rules to be considered scientifically credible.

First, the testing must take place in carefully controlled conditions. Researchers have to make sure to

control factors that could affect the results. For example, if researchers want to know how a medicine affects a child, they have to make sure the child isn't taking any other medicines at the same time.

Researchers also need to determine how many people should be included in the study. Study size varies according to the kind of study and the number of people needed to demonstrate an effect.

The group of people receiving treatment should be compared to a control group to truly test if the treatment has any effect. A control doesn't receive the new treatment but they may be given either a placebo (sugar pill) or an alternative treatment.

Good clinical studies should be replicated. That means other researchers should be able to do the same study again using different subjects and get similar results. We know we can trust the findings when different studies come to the same conclusions.

Well-done, scientifically sound studies should go through peer review. This means other experts on the topic being studied should review each study and make sure that all the proper scientific standards were met.

EVALUATING NEW TREATMENTS OR MEDICINES

When you come across a new treatment or medicine, consider the following examples as warnings that the treatment may not be effective or safe. You should be suspicious if advertising for the product claims it will work for everyone, cites only one study or uses a story about one person's experience or testimonials as proof that it works, claims it is a

"cure," or if the product is available from only one source.

Do not use a product if it comes without directions for proper use, does not list contents or ingredients, or has no information or warnings about side effects. Use caution if a product isn't approved by Health Canada or if a treatment is described as "harmless" or "natural." Remember that most medications are made from natural sources. A "natural" treatment doesn't necessarily work and may actually be harmful to your child or may interact with other medication.

USING THE INTERNET

The Internet can be a valuable source of medical information and advice, but you can't trust everything you read. The Internet also is the source of a lot of health-related theories and opinions that haven't been proven. Begin your search for information with the most reliable, general-information web sites and expand from there. The Canadian Paediatric Society (CPS) Web site, **www.cps.ca**, is a good starting point. Some useful addresses are included in the resource section of this book.

RESOURCES

To make informed decisions about your child's health, it is important to have accurate information (*see* Making Sense of Health-Care Information, *pp.340–341.*) A wealth of information can be found from the sources listed below under general resources. Also listed are resources for individual topics. Keep in mind these resources should not be used as a substitute for the medical care and advice of your doctor.

GENERAL RESOURCES

Canadian Health Network
Web site: www.canadian-health-network.ca

Canadian Medical Association
Web site: www.cma.ca
1867 Alta Vista Drive
Ottawa, ON K1G 3Y6
Tel: (800) 457-4205
Tel: (613) 731-9331

Canadian Paediatric Society
Web site: www.cps.ca
100-2204 Walkley Rd.
Ottawa, ON K1G 4G8
Tel.: (613) 526-9397

Centers for Disease Control and Prevention
Web site: www.cdc.gov
1600 Clifton Road
Atlanta, GA 30333
Tel: (888) 232-3228
Tel: (800) 311-3435

Health Canada
Web site: www.hc-sc.gc.ca
Tunney's Pasture
A.L. 0900C2
Ottawa, ON K1A 0K9
Tel: (613) 957-2991
TTY: 1-800-267-1245

Health Canada – Division of Childhood and Adolescence
Web site: www.hc-sc.gc.ca/dca-dea
Tunney's Pasture
A.L. 1909C2
Ottawa, ON K1A 1B4
Tel: (613) 952-1220

Healthfinder®
www.healthfinder.gov

KidsHealth.org
www.kidshealth.org

Medbroadcast.com
Web site: www.medbroadcast.com

MEDLINEplus
Web site: www.medlineplus.gov
Consumer health site; a service of the US National Library of Medicine and the National Institutes of Health.

National Library of Medicine
Web site: www.nlm.nih.gov
8600 Rockville Pike
Bethesda, MD 20894
Tel: (888) FIND-NLM
Tel: (301) 594-5983
The world's largest medical library, located on the campus of the National Institutes of Health.

US Food and Drug Administration
Web site: www.fda.gov
5600 Fishers Lane
Rockville, MD 20857
Tel: (888) INFO-FDA

ALLERGY & ASTHMA
Asthma Society of Canada
Web site: www.asthma.ca
130 Bridgeland Avenue, Suite 425
Toronto, ON M6A 1Z4
Tel: 1-866-787-4050 / (416) 787-4050

Canadian Society of Allergy and Clinical Immunology
Web site: www.csaci.medical.org/
774 Echo Drive
Ottawa, ON K1S 5N8
Tel: (613) 730-6272

ARTHRITIS
The Arthritis Society
Web site: www.arthritis.ca
393 University Avenue, Suite 1700
Toronto, ON M5G 1E6
Tel: (416) 979-7228

See also MUSCULOSKELETAL SYSTEM

ATTENTION DEFICIT HYPERACTIVITY DISORDER
Centers for Disease Control and Prevention
National Center on Birth Defects and Developmental Disabilities
Web site: www.cdc.gov/ncbddd/adhd

Children and Adults with Attention Deficit Disorders
CH.A.D.D. Canada Inc.
Web site: www.chaddcanada.org
1376 Bank Street
Ottawa, ON K1H 1B3
Tel: (613) 731-1209

AUTISM
Autism Society Canada
Web site: www.autismsocietycanada.ca/
P.O. Box 65, Orangeville, ON, L9W 2Z5
Tel: (866) 874-3334
Tel: (519) 942-8720

Centers for Disease Control and Prevention
National Center on Birth Defects and Developmental Disabilities
Autism Information Center
Web site:
www.cdc.gov/ncbddd/dd/ddautism.htm

BIRTH DEFECTS

Canadian Organization for Rare
Disorders
Web site: www.cord.ca
P.O. Box 814
Coaldale, AB T1M 1M7
Tel: (877) 302-7273
Tel: (403) 345-4544

Centers for Disease Control
and Prevention
National Center on Birth Defects
and Developmental Disabilities
Web site: www.cdc.gov/ncbdd

See also GENETICS

BLOOD

Canadian Hemophilia Society
Web site: www.hemophilia.ca
625 President Kennedy Avenue,
Suite 505
Montreal, QC H3A 1K2
Tel: (800) 668-2686
Tel: (514) 848-0503

See also CANCER, GENETICS

BREASTFEEDING

La Leche League Canada
Web site: www.lalecheleaguecanada.ca
18C Industrial Drive
P.O. Box 29
Chesterville, ON K0C 1H0
Tel: (800) 665-4324
Tel: (613) 448-1842

CANCER

Canadian Cancer Society
Web site: www.cancer.ca
10 Alcorn Avenue, Suite 200
Toronto, ON M4V 3B1
Tel: (416) 961-7223

National Cancer Institute of Canada
Web site: www.ncic.cancer.ca
10 Alcorn Avenue, Suite 200
Toronto, ON M4V 3B1
Tel: (416) 961-7223

CHILD CARE

American Academy of Pediatrics
Healthy Child Care America
Web site: www.healthychildcare.org

Canadian Child Care Federation
Web site: www.cccf-fcsge.ca
201-383 Parkdale Avenue
Ottawa, ON K1Y 4R4
Tel: (800) 858-1412
Tel: (613) 729-5289

Caring for Kids
Web site: www.caringforkids.cps.ca
Canadian Paediatric Society
100-2204 Walkley Rd.
Ottawa ON K1G 4G8
Tel.: (613) 526-9397

COMPLEMENTARY & ALTERNATIVE THERAPIES

National Center for Complementary
and Alternative Medicine
Web site: www.nccam.nih.gov
NCCAM Clearinghouse, PO Box 7923
Gaithersburg, MD 20898
Tel: (888) 644-6226

DENTISTRY

American Dental Association
Web site: www.ada.org
211 East Chicago Avenue
Chicago, IL 60611
Tel: (312) 440-2500

Canadian Dental Association
Web site: www.cda-adc.ca
1815 Alta Vista Drive
Ottawa, ON K1G 3Y6
Tel: (613) 523-1770

DIABETES

Canadian Diabetes Association
Web site: www.diabetes.ca
National Life Building
1400-522 University Avenue
Toronto ON M5G 2R5
Tel: (800) 226-8464
Tel: (416) 363-0177

Juvenile Diabetes Research
Foundation Canada
Web site: www.jdfc.ca
7100 Woodbine Avenue, Suite 311
Markham, ON L3R 5J2
Tel: (877) 287-3533
Tel: (905) 944-8700

DIGESTIVE SYSTEM

Canadian Digestive Health
Foundation
Web site: www.cdhf.ca
2902 South Sheridan Way
Oakville, ON L6J 7L6
Tel: 905 829-3949
Tel: 1 866 819-2333

DISABILITY

Canadian Association for Community
Living
Web site: www.cacl.ca
Kinsmen Building, York University
4700 Keele Street
Toronto, ON M3J 1P3
Tel: (416) 661-9611
TTY: (416) 661-2023

Council of Canadians with
Disabilities
Web site: www.ccdonline.ca
926-294 Portage Avenue
Winnipeg, MB R3C 0B9
Voice/TTY: (204) 947-0303

DRUG & ALCOHOL ABUSE

Canadian Centre on Substance Abuse
Web site: www.ccsa.ca
Canadian Centre on Substance Abuse
75 Albert Street, Suite 300
Ottawa, ON K1P 5E7
Tel: (613) 235-4048

Centre for Addiction and Mental
Health
Web site: www.camh.net
33 Russell Street
Toronto, ON M5S 2S1
Tel: (800) 463-6273
Tel: (416) 595-6111

EAR, NOSE, & THROAT

Canadian Academy of Audiology – Consumer Information
Web site: www.canadianaudiology.ca/
consumer-information.html
250 Consumers Road, Suite 301
Toronto, ON M2J 4V6
Tel: (800) 264-5106
Tel: (416) 494-6672

Canadian Association of Speech-Language Pathologists and Audiologists
Web site: www.caslpa.ca
401- 200 Elgin Street
Ottawa, ON K2P 1L5
Tel: (800) 259-8519
Tel: (613) 567-9968

EYES & VISION

Canadian National Institute for the Blind
Web site: www.cnib.ca
1929 Bayview Avenue
Toronto, ON M4G 3E8
Tel: (416) 486-2500

Canadian Ophthalmological Society
Web site: www.eyesite.ca
610-1525 Carling Avenue
Ottawa, ON K1Z 8R9
Email: cos@eyesite.ca

FIRST AID

Canadian Poison Control Centres
Web site: www.napra.org/docs/0/95/157/
164/349.asp

Canadian Red Cross Society
Web Site: www.redcross.ca
170 Metcalfe Street, Suite 300
Ottawa, ON K2P 2P2
Tel: (613) 740-1900

FITNESS

Canada's Physical Activity Guide for Children and Youth
Web site: www.hc-sc.gc.ca/hppb/paguide/
child_youth/partners/boiler3.html
Health Canada - Physical Activity Unit
Tunney's Pasture
Jeanne Mance Building, 7th Floor
A.L. 1907C1
Ottawa, ON K1A 0K9
Tel: (613) 941-3109

FOOD & DRUG INFORMATION

Health Canada – Health Products and Food Branch
Web site: www.hc-sc.gc.ca/hpfb-
dgpsa/index_e.html
Health Canada
A.L. 0900C2
Ottawa, ON K1A 0K9
Tel: (613) 957-2991
TTY: 1-800-267-1245

GENETICS

Canadian Organization for Rare Disorders
Web site: www.cord.ca
P.O. Box 814
Coaldale, AB T1M 1M7
Tel: (877) 302-7273
Tel: (403) 345-4544

See also BIRTH DEFECTS

HEALTH CARE CHOICES & ACCESS

Kirby Study on the State of the Health Care System in Canada
Web site:
www.parl.gc.ca/common/Committee_Sen
Home.asp?Language=E&Parl=37&Ses=1
&comm_id=47

Romanow Commission on the Future of Health Care in Canada
Web site: www.hc-sc.gc.ca/english/care/
romanow/index1.html

HEART & CIRCULATION

Heart and Stroke Foundation of Canada
Web site: www.heartandstroke.ca
222 Queen Street, Suite 1402
Ottawa, ON K1P 5V9
Tel: (613) 569-4361

National Heart, Lungs, and Blood Institute
Web site: www.nhlbi.nih.gov
PO Box 30105
Bethesda, MD 20824
Tel: (800) 575-WELL
Tel: (301) 592-8573

INFECTIOUS DISEASES

Health Canada - Bureau of Infectious Diseases
Web site: www.hc-sc.gc.ca/pphb-
dgspsp/bid-bmi/index.html
Health Canada
A.L. 0900C2
Ottawa, ON K1A 0K9
Tel: (613) 957-2991
TTY: 1-800-267-1245

LEARNING DISABILITIES

Learning Disabilities Association of Canada
Web site: www.ldac-taac.ca
323 Chapel Street
Ottawa, ON K1N 7Z2
Tel: (613) 238-5721

LUNG PROBLEMS

Canadian Lung Association
Web site: www.lung.ca
3 Raymond Street, Suite 300
Ottawa, ON K1R 1A3
Tel: (613) 569-6411

National Heart, Lung, and Blood Institute
Web site: www.nhlbi.nih.gov
PO Box 30105
Bethesda, MD 20824
Tel: (800) 575-WELL
Tel: (301) 592-8573

MENTAL HEALTH
American Academy of Child and Adolescent Psychiatry
Web site: www.aacap.org
3615 Wisconsin Ave., N.W.,
Washington, D.C. 20016
Tel: (202) 966-7300

Canadian Mental Health Association
Web site: www.cmha.ca
8 King Street East, Suite 810
Toronto, ON M5C 1B5
Tel: (416) 484-7750

Health Canada – Mental Health Promotion Unit
Web site: www.hc-sc.gc.ca/hppb/
mentalhealth
Mental Health Promotion Unit
Health Canada
Tunney's Pasture, 1907-C1
Ottawa, Ontario K1A 1B4

MUSCULOSKELETAL SYSTEM
Canadian Orthopaedic Association
Web site: www.coa-aco.org
1440 St. Catherine Street West,
Suite 718
Montreal, QC H3G 1R8
Tel: (514) 874-9003

The Arthritis Society
Web site: www.arthritis.ca
393 University Avenue
Suite 1700
Toronto, ON M5G 1E6
Tel: (416) 979-7228

NEUROLOGICAL DISORDERS
National Institute of Neurological Disorders
Web site: www.ninds.nih.gov
PO Box 5801
Bethesda, MD 20824
Tel: (800) 352-9424

NUTRITION
Dietitians of Canada
Web site: www.dietitians.ca
480 University Avenue, Suite 604
Toronto, ON M5G 1V2
Tel: (416) 596-0857

Food and Nutrition – Health Canada
Web site: www.hc-
sc.gc.ca/english/lifestyles/food_nutr.html
Health Canada
A.L. 0900C2
Ottawa, ON K1A 0K9
Tel: (613) 957-2991
TTY: 1-800-267-1245

National Institute of Nutrition
Web site: www.nin.ca
408 Queen Street, 3rd Floor
Ottawa, ON K1R 5A7
Tel: (613) 235-3355

SAFETY & HEALTH
Health Canada – Product Safety Program
Web site: www.hc-sc.gc.ca/hecs-
sesc/psp/index.htm
5th floor MacDonald Building,
123 Slater Street,
Ottawa, ON K1A 0K9
AL: 3505D1
Tel: (613) 946-6465

Transport Canada – Road Safety
Web site: www.tc.gc.ca/roadsafety/site/
menu.htm
330 Sparks Street
Ottawa, ON K1A 0N5
Tel: (613) 990-2309
TTY: 1-888-675-6863

SCHOOL HEALTH
Health Canada – School Health
Web site: www.hc-sc.gc.ca/dca-dea/7-
18yrs-ans/index_e.html
Tunney's Pasture, 1909C2
Ottawa, ON K1A 1B4
Tel: (613)-952-1220

SKIN CARE
Canadian Dermatology Association
Web site: www.dermatology.ca
1385 Bank Street, Suite 425
Ottawa ON K1H 8N4
Tel: (800) 267-3376
Tel: (613) 738-1748

TRAVEL HEALTH
Population and Public Health Branch – Health Canada
Information for Travellers
Web site: www.hc-sc.gc.ca/pphb-
dgspsp/tmp-pmv/pub_e.html

World Health Organization – International Travel and Health
Web site: www.who.int/ith/

URINARY SYSTEM
Kidney Foundation of Canada
Web site: www.kidney.ca
300-5165 Sherbrooke Street West
Montréal, QC H4A 1T6
Tel: (800) 361-7494
Tel.: (514) 369-4806

National Kidney and Urologic Diseases Information Clearinghouse
Web site: http://kidney.niddk.nih.gov
3 Information Way, Bethesda, MD 20892
Tel: (800) 891-5390
Tel: (301) 654-4415

Please note: Inclusion on this list does not imply an endorsement by the Canadian Medical Association. The CMA is not responsible for the content unless specifically indicated. Addresses, phone numbers, and Web site addresses are as current as possible, but may change at any time.

INDEX

ACKNOWLEDGMENTS

CANADIAN MEDICAL ASSOCIATION
President Albert J. Schumacher, MD
Secretary General and CEO William G. Tholl
Acting Director, Publications Lorne Ross
Editor-in-chief, Publications John Hoey, MD
Program Manager, Book Publishing Christine A. Pollock
Assistant Nunzia Parent
Information Services Elizabeth Czanyo

Consultants
Maurice Bouchard, MD, FRCPC
Barbara A. Bulleid, MD, FRCPC
Michael Burger, MDCM, FRCPC
Marvin Gans, MD, FRCPC
Norman Goldberg, MD, FRCPC
Alan P. Hudak, MD, FRCPC
Aline Levi, MDCM
Tilak Raj Malhotra, MB, FRCPC
Geneviève Moineau, MD, FRCPC
John M. Stoffman, MD, FRCPC
Peter Strachan, MD, FRCPC
Lionel J. Weinstein, MD, FRCPC

The CMA acknowledges the valuable contributions of
Denise Beatty, RD, Health Canada, and Human Resources
and Skill Development Canada.

DK Publishing would like to thank:
Anna Barlow, Debbie Beckerman, Tanya Carr, Tracey Godridge, Harriet
Griffey, Professor James Law, Dr. Sarah Temple, Dr. Bernard Valman;
Caroline Buckingham, Jemima Dunne, Jane Perlmutter, and Sue
Bosanko for the index.

Illustrator Debbie Maizels
Picture researcher Anna Bedewell
Picture librarians Romaine Werblow and Hayley Smith

Models Sharon, Cleveland, Leanne, Alexander and Dominic Williams;
Sam and Bradley Jones; Rachel Ann Hawkins; Jessica Casey; Niel,
Kirsty and Grace Stannard; Nathan, Martha and Luke Jenkinson; Noa,
Ella and Gil Krikler; Sally, Louis, Cicely, Harvey and Sydney Barron; the
Jeffrey family; Shelley and Jake Goswell; Derek, Lisa and Alexander
Butterworth; Jasper Cumiskey; Robin and Thomas Engelhard; Joshua and
Charlie Ojeda-Siena; Max and Evie Register; Chris and Kiara Lambrias;
Jake, Rosie and Lauren Couch; Laura Davenport, David Ainsworth and
Luke Ainsworth; Katy Wilson; Helen Drake with Grace; Julia Major and
Charlie Coulthard; Leo, Noah and JJ Stiles; Holden and Hope Jones; Lucy
Butterworth with Isabelle and Chloe; Kate Limm; pupils of Weston Park
Primary School, London, and Muswell Hill Primary School, London.

Picture credits The publisher would like to thank the following for
their kind permission to reproduce their photographs:
(Abbreviations key: t=top, b=bottom, r=right, l=left, c=center, a=above)
47: Getty Images: Rosanne Olson (tr); 51: Corbis: Norbert Schaefer (b);
55: Getty Images: Christopher Bissell (t); 161: Science Photo Library:
Jim Varney (tr); 163: Getty Images: Bruce Ayres (tl); 168-9: Corbis:
Philip James Corwin; 183: alamy.com: Stock Connection, Inc (bc); 187:
Bubbles (br), Imagingbody.com (c), Meningitis Research Foundation
(cca), Science Photo Library: Dr. P. Marazzi (cra), The Wellcome
Institute Library, London (cr), (bcr); 193: Mike Wyndham (tl), (bc);
216-217: Getty Images: James Darell; 218: Getty Images: Richard Price
(br); 219: Getty Images: Charles Thatcher; 223: Science Photo Library
(cr); 225: Science Photo Library: Damien Lovegrove; 226: Science Photo
Library: BSIP Chassenet (bl): Mark Thomas (bc); 227: The Wellcome
Institute Library, London; 230: Science Photo Library: Dr. P. Marazzi
(cl), (bl); 231: Science Photo Library: St Bartholomew's Hospital (ca),
The Wellcome Institute Library, London (bl); 232: The Wellcome
Institute Library, London; 233: Science Photo Library: Dr. P. Marazzi
(br), The Wellcome Institute Library, London (cla); 234: Science Photo
Library: Dr. P. Marazzi; 235: Science Photo Library: Hattie Young (cla);
The Wellcome Institute Library, London (br); 236: C. James Webb (c),
The Wellcome Institute Library, London (br), (cl); 237: The Wellcome
Institute Library, London (cr), (bl); 238: The Wellcome Institute
Library, London (cla), (br); 240: Medical Slide Library; 243: Science
Photo Library (br); The Wellcome Institute Library, London (cr); 244:
Science Photo Library: Dr. P. Marazzi; 245: Science Photo Library: Dr. P.
Marazzi; 247: Science Photo Library: Dr. P. Marazzi; 248: Science Photo
Library: Dr. P. Marazzi (tr); 256: Science Photo Library: Professors P.M
Motta & F.M Magliocca (cl); 259: The Wellcome Institute Library,
London (tc); 260: Science Photo Library (bl); 261: Mike Wyndham (c);
262: Medical Slide Library (bc), Science Photo Library: Professors P.M
Motta & F.M Magliocca (tl); 264: Science Photo Library: Lowell
Georgia (tl); 265: The Wellcome Institute Library, London (tr); 266:
The Wellcome Institute Library, London (cl), (bl); 267: The Wellcome
Institute Library, London (cl); 268: Dr. Jean Watkins (cr); 272: Science
Photo Library: CNRI (tr); 284: Science Photo Library: Dr. P. Marazzi
(bl), Princess Margaret Rose Orthopaedic Hospital (bc); 287: The
Wellcome Institute Library, London (br); 288: The Wellcome Institute
Library, London (cr); 291: Mediscan (cl); 295: Science Photo Library:
Will and Deni McIntyre (br); 297: Mediscan (cr); 300: Science Photo
Library: James King-Holmes (tr); 305: Science Photo Library: Tek
Image (tr); 306: Science Photo Library: Andrew Syred (bl); 307: The
Wellcome Institute Library, London (cr); 313: Science Photo Library:
Dr. Gopal Murti (br); 316: Science Photo Library: Simon Fraser (tr);
319: Corbis: Rob Lewine (tl), Science Photo Library: Mark Clarke/Bath
Chinese Medical Centre (tr); 320: Science Photo Library: Sheila
Terry (tl); 321: Science Photo Library: Cordelia Molloy (tr): Gaillard,
Jerrican (b); 322: alamy.com: Frank Krahmer (tl), Science Photo
Library: Georgette Douwma (bl); 323: Getty Images: Mary Kate Denny
(tr); 324: Science Photo Library: Antonia Reeve; 326: Getty Images:
Arthur Tilley; 328: Corbis: LWA-Stephen Welstead (br).

All other images © Dorling Kindersley Limited.
For further information see: www.dkimages.com